VOLUME

# 3

# Dementia

## Second Edition

*Edited by*

## Mario Maj
*University of Naples, Italy*

## Norman Sartorius
*University of Geneva, Switzerland*

*WPA Series*
Evidence and Experience in Psychiatry

**WILEY**

*Other Wiley Editorial Offices*

John Wiley & Sons Inc., 111 River Street, Hoboken, NJ 07030, USA

Jossey-Bass, 989 Market Street, San Francisco, CA 94103-1741, USA

Wiley-VCH Verlag GmbH, Boschstr. 12, D-69469 Weinheim, Germany

John Wiley & Sons Australia Ltd, 33 Park Road, Milton, Queensland 4064, Australia

John Wiley & Sons (Asia) Pte Ltd, 2 Clementi Loop #02-01, Jin Xing Distripark, Singapore
129809

John Wiley & Sons Canada Ltd, 22 Worcester Road, Etobicoke, Ontario, Canada M9W
1L1

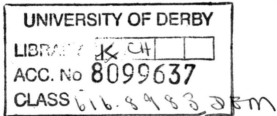

*British Library Cataloguing in Publication Data*

A catalogue record for this book is available from the British Library

ISBN 0-470-84963-0

Typeset in 10/12pt Times by Kolam Information Services Pvt. Ltd, Pondicherry, India
Printed and bound in Great Britain by TJ International, Padstow, Cornwall.
This book is printed on acid-free paper responsibly manufactured from sustainable forestry
in which at least two trees are planted for each one used for paper production.

# Contents

# Review Contributors

**Dr Ove Almkvist** *Division of Geriatric Medicine B84, Huddinge Hospital, 14186 Huddinge, Sweden*

**Professor Franz Baro** *Catholic University of Leuven, Psychiatric Centre Sint-Kamillus, Broeders van Liefde, Krijkelberg 1, B-3360 Bierbeck, Belgium*

**Dr Maciej Bobinski** *Institute for Basic Research in Developmental Disabilities, 1050 Forest Hill Road, Staten Island, NY 10314, USA*

**Professor Kenneth L. Davis** *Department of Psychiatry, Mount Sinai School of Medicine, Box 1230, One Gustave L. Levy Place, New York, NY 10029-6574, USA*

**Dr Emile Franssen** *Aging and Dementia Research and Treatment Center, New York University School of Medicine, New York, NY 10016, USA*

**Professor A. Scott Henderson** *National Health and Medical Research Council, Centre for Mental Health Research, The Australian National University, Canberra, ACT 0200, Australia*

**Dr Bengt Jönsson** *Stockholm School of Economics, Box 6501, S-113 83 Stockholm, Sweden*

**Dr Linus Jönsson** *Division of Geriatric Medicine, Neurotec, Karolinska Institute, S-171 76 Stockholm, Sweden*

**Dr Anthony F. Jorm** *National Health and Medical Research Council, Psychiatric Epidemiology Research Centre, The Australian National University, Canberra, ACT 0200, Australia*

**Professor Barry Reisberg** *Aging and Dementia Research and Treatment Center, New York University School of Medicine, New York, NY 10016, USA*

**Dr Steven C. Samuels** *Department of Psychiatry, Mount Sinai School of Medicine, Box 1230, One Gustave L. Levy Place, New York, NY 10029-6574, USA*

**Dr Muhammad A. Shah** *Aging and Dementia Research and Treatment Center, New York University School of Medicine, New York, NY 10016, USA*

**Dr Jerzy Weigel** *Institute for Basic Research in Developmental Disabilities, 1050 Forest Hill Road, Staten Island, NY 10314, USA*

**Dr Anders Wimo**   *Division of Geriatric Medicine, Neurotec, Karolinska Institute, S-171 76 Stockholm, Sweden*

**Dr Henryk M. Wisniewski**   *Institute for Basic Research in Developmental Disabilities, 1050 Forest Hill Road, Staten Island, NY 10314, USA*

# Preface

The increase in the absolute and relative number of elderly people will be accompanied by a significant rise of the number of people with dementia. Since life expectancy at all ages is increasing faster in developing countries, the number of people with dementia will grow faster there.

The spreading of HIV infection and the prolonged survival of patients with AIDS and with other chronic diseases will further increase the number of cases of dementia. It has been estimated, for example, that—unless new and effective treatments are applied on a large scale—the number of people with dementia in Africa will, in a few years, exceed the total number of hospital beds on the continent.

Due to its progressive and disabling course, dementia also places an enormous burden on families and other carers, so that the losses in social and economic productivity due to dementia far exceed the estimates based on the epidemiological investigations of the disorder.

On the other hand, our knowledge of dementia has significantly increased. The diagnosis of the dementia syndromes has been considerably refined. New types of the disorder, such as the Lewy body dementia, have been described. Our understanding of the risk factors and the pathogenesis of Alzheimer's disease has considerably improved. Clinical and neuropsychological tools for the early diagnosis and the staging of dementia have been developed, and their usefulness in ordinary practice has been demonstrated. Promising leads for pharmacological treatment have been developed, and much has been done to facilitate the life and work of carers, by increasing training and support programmes in numbers and quality in many countries. Psychosocial interventions have also been developed and seen to be helpful in maintaining a person with dementia at a particular level of functioning without further loss and in improving the quality of life of the patients and their caregivers.

The application of new knowledge in clinical practice, however, remains inadequate almost everywhere in the world. In many countries, the vast majority of people with dementia derive no benefits from the above-mentioned advances and their living conditions are often extremely poor. Many live with their families without any kind of support from the health care system.

Psychiatrists are, on the whole, much less skilled in the early diagnosis and proper management of dementia than in the diagnosis and treatment of other disorders, such as depression or schizophrenia. The awareness of available psychosocial interventions is scarce and the pharmacological treatment is often inappropriate.

The WPA series *Evidence and Experience in Psychiatry* has been initiated as part of the effort of the World Psychiatric Association to bridge the gap between research evidence and clinical practice concerning the most prevalent mental disorders. Because of its increasing frequency, severity and ubiquity, and because the application of knowledge is so limited, dementia should be a priority for research, teaching and care. We hope that this volume will contribute to making it such.

**Mario Maj**
**Norman Sartorius**

# Definition and Epidemiology of Dementia: A Review

## A. Scott Henderson and Anthony F. Jorm

*National Health and Medical Research Council, Centre for Mental Health Research, The Australian National University, Canberra, Australia*

## INTRODUCTION

Dementia is a disorder of the brain. This is an important assertion to make from the outset, because many members of the general public and even some health professionals still believe something else. Some attribute the cognitive and behavioural changes to senility. Others believe that the impaired memory is due to past psychic traumas which, if talked through, will bring cure. But the behavioural changes in dementia are not under conscious control, nor are they due to laziness or "letting go". In this review, an account is given of what dementia is, its course and how it is distributed in the population. Dementia must have been affecting people ever since humans began to survive in appreciable numbers into old age. But it is a condition that has come into prominence only during the late twentieth century, because of the unprecedented increase in the numbers of people all over the world who survive to become very elderly.

"Dementia" originally meant "out of one's mind", from the Latin *de* (out of) and *mens* (the mind). Early in the nineteenth century, Esquirol [1] gave a succinct definition of dementia as "a cerebral affection...characterised by a weakening of the sensibility, understanding, and will" (cited by Caine *et al* [2]). In describing with such words how the condition can be recognized, Esquirol drew attention not only to the cognitive features of the disorder, with impairment of memory and thinking in day-to-day life, but also to its other manifestations, such as apathy, deterioration in social behaviour, occasional aggressiveness, delusional ideas and hallucinations. These show how widespread the changes are in the brain. The impact of

*Dementia, Second Edition.* Edited by Mario Maj and Norman Sartorius.
© 2002 John Wiley & Sons Ltd.

dementia on individuals, families and communities has been profound, and this will continue until dementia can not only be effectively treated, but prevented.

## DEFINITION OF DEMENTIA

Following extensive consultations with experts in some 40 countries, the World Health Organization (WHO) published the *Clinical Descriptions and Diagnostic Guidelines for Mental and Behavioural Disorders*, as part of the *International Classification of Diseases* (10th Revision) (ICD-10) [3]. This was followed by the more compact *Diagnostic Criteria for Research* [4]. A summary of the ICD-10 *Diagnostic Guidelines* for dementia [3] is that each of the following should be present:

1. A decline in memory to an extent that it interferes with everyday activities, or makes independent living either difficult or impossible.
2. A decline in thinking, planning and organizing day-to-day things, again to the above extent.
3. Initially, preserved awareness of the environment, including orientation in space and time.
4. A decline in emotional control or motivation, or a change in social behaviour, as shown in one or more of the following: emotional lability, irritability, apathy or coarsening of social behaviour, as in eating, dressing and interacting with others.

The diagnostic criteria for dementia are essentially similar in the *Diagnostic and Statistical Manual* (4th edition) of the American Psychiatric Association (DSM-IV) [5], although the two systems may give somewhat different prevalence estimates, even when they are applied to the same data from the same population. The evidence so far is that the ICD-10 criteria are more strict and therefore identify fewer cases [6,7].

## Differential Diagnosis

There are several disorders that may present with clinical features similar to dementia. Some of them may even co-occur with dementia. Because they call for different treatment and have a very different course, it is of the greatest importance that clinicians be able to identify these alternative diagnoses and distinguish them from dementia. The WHO Guidelines [3] recommend that the following alternative diagnoses be considered:

1. A depressive disorder, which may exhibit many of the features of an early dementia, especially memory impairment, slowed thinking, apathy and lack of spontaneity.
2. Delirium, which typically is acute in onset with clouding of consciousness, fluctuating in degree.
3. Mild or moderate mental retardation.
4. States of subnormal cognitive functioning attributable to a severely impoverished social environment and limited education.
5. Iatrogenic mental disorders due to medication.

## The Continuum of Normal Ageing, Cognitive Impairment and Dementia

Although persons with a dementia are often spoken of as though they were a qualitatively different group from the normal elderly, there is no evidence for a discrete break between the two. Yet it is often implied in clinical and administrative circles that elderly persons fall into two neat groups: those with and those without dementia. In some ways, dementia in the elderly represents an exaggeration of certain cognitive and behavioural changes that commonly occur with ageing. There is a continuum from normal functioning through to severe dementia. A useful scheme for describing the stages of dementia is that proposed by Berg [8]. This can be applied cross-sectionally to all the elderly in a community, or those in some form of care. But it can also be applied to determine the progression of cognitive and behavioural changes in a cohort of the elderly followed over time. Berg's table summarizing the clinical and social features is shown in Table 1.1.

The majority of elderly persons come under the first column in Table 1.1 and have no dementia. They are by far the largest group. There are then those who have some changes in memory and thinking, sometimes with very mild changes in behaviour and personality as well. There is no doubt that nearly all people undergo a deterioration in memory and a slowing of mental processes in very late life, and some experience these changes earlier than others for reasons that are not yet well-understood. Various terms have emerged to describe such states. The term ''benign senescent forgetfulness'' was introduced by Kral [9] to describe one group of such states. Although it was not well defined by him, the term has persisted because it fulfils a need and has no sinister connotations. Other concepts have since been introduced. ''Age-associated memory impairment'' [10] has been shown to be an unsatisfactory construct. Christensen *et al* [11,12] showed that the ICD-10 experimental entity called ''mild cognitive disorder'' is not really a syndrome in its own right,

**TABLE 1.1** Clinical Dementia Rating (CDR) of Berg [8]

| | No dementia CDR 0 | Questionable dementia CDR 0.5 | Mild dementia CDR 1 | Moderate dementia CDR 2 | Severe dementia CDR 3 |
|---|---|---|---|---|---|
| Memory | No memory loss or slight inconstant forgetfulness | Consistent slight forgetfulness; partial recollection of events; "benign" forgetfulness | Moderate memory loss, more marked for recent events; defect interferes with everyday activities | Severe memory loss; only highly learned material retained; new material rapidly lost | Severe memory loss; only fragments remain |
| Orientation | Fully oriented | Fully oriented except for slight difficulty with time relationships | Moderate difficulty with time relationships; oriented for place at examinations; may have geographical disorientation elsewhere | Severe difficulty with time relationships; usually disoriented in time, often to place | Oriented to person only |
| Judgement and problem solving | Solves everyday problems well; judgement good in relation to past performance | Slight impairment in solving problems, similarities, differences | Moderate difficulty in handling problems, similarities, differences; social judgement usually maintained | Severely impaired in handling problems, similarities, differences; social judgement usually impaired | Unable to make judgements or solve problems |
| Community affairs | Independent function at usual level in job, shopping, business and financial affairs, volunteer and social groups | Slight impairment in these activities | Unable to function independently at these activities though may still be engaged in some; appears normal to casual inspection | No pretence of independent function outside home. Appears well enough to be taken to functions outside a family home | Appears too ill to be taken to functions outside a family home. No significant function in home |
| Home and hobbies | Life at home, hobbies, intellectual interests well maintained | Life at home, hobbies, intellectual interests slightly impaired | Mild but definite impairment of function at home; more difficult chores abandoned; more complicated hobbies and interests abandoned | Only simple chores preserved; very restricted interests, poorly sustained | No significant function in home |
| Personal care | Fully capable of self-care | | Needs prompting | Requires assistance in dressing, hygiene, keeping of personal effects | Requires much help with personal care; frequent incontinence |

Score only as decline from previous usual level due to cognitive loss, not impairment due to other factors.

but correlates with affective and other non-cognitive factors. But there is surely some face validity in the proposition that there is a state of progressive cognitive decline which people traverse on their way to eventually fulfilling the diagnostic criteria for a dementia. For this reason, it will be important to assess the validity and natural history of the entities called "mild neurocognitive disorder" and "age-related cognitive decline" proposed in the DSM-IV. A useful review of this important issue has been provided by Ritchie *et al* [13].

There is then the older person who goes to a doctor or clinic *complaining of a failing memory*. With the greater public awareness of dementia that has emerged in recent years, such complaints have become more frequent, particularly where the individual has some personal experience of others with a dementia. The crucial question is whether there is objective evidence of decline in memory and/or other cognitive processes. If there is, then the complaint indicates that the individual has been aware of the deterioration. While this is recognized as happening in the earlier stage of Alzheimer's disease, there is now abundant evidence from surveys of the elderly in the general population that memory complaints are more often a symptom of *being depressed in mood* than a pointer to an incipient dementia [14–18]. By contrast, among persons going to doctors, it seems that the complaint can sometimes be a predictor of further decline in memory and thinking [19,20]. The conclusion from this research is that people who complain of a failing memory deserve to be assessed further, to see if they are also depressed in mood, or if there is objective evidence of cognitive decline.

For dementia itself, there are three levels in Berg's Clinical Dementia Rating (CDR) (Table 1.1): mild, moderate and severe. This description is in step with the levels specified in the ICD-10 *Diagnostic Criteria for Research* [4]. Unfortunately, the three adjectives—mild, moderate and severe—are not always used consistently within one country, let alone between countries. As a result, what one clinician may say is mild dementia, another may call moderate. It is very important that clinicians and administrators use the same words consistently. The most appropriate standards are those in the ICD-10, because they are truly international in the way they have been agreed upon.

## DEMENTIA SYNDROMES

Numerous dementia syndromes can occur in the elderly. The most common is Alzheimer's disease (AD), followed by vascular dementia, mixed dementia, Lewy body dementia and then the fronto-temporal dementias.

## Dementia in Alzheimer's Disease (AD)

Until around 1970, AD was thought to be a rare dementia affecting people under 65. At that time, the common senile dementia of the elderly was believed to be due to arteriosclerosis causing a slow strangulation of the brain's blood supply. However, following the important neuropathological study of Tomlinson *et al* [21], it was established that persons with senile dementia had the same brain changes as in AD. Following this work, the term "senile dementia of the Alzheimer type" (SDAT) was often used to describe elderly cases with Alzheimer brain changes. However, in recent years the term "Alzheimer's disease" has come to be used to refer to all cases, irrespective of age. The account which follows is based on the *Clinical Descriptions and Diagnostic Guidelines* of the ICD-10 [3].

AD has characteristic neuropathological and neurochemical features. It is usually insidious in onset and develops slowly but steadily over a period of years. The onset can be in middle adult life or even earlier (AD with early onset), but the incidence is higher in later life (AD with late onset). In cases with onset before the age of 65–70, there is the likelihood of a family history of a similar dementia, a more rapid course, and prominence of features of temporal and parietal lobe damage, including dysphasia or dyspraxia. In cases with a later onset, the course tends to be slower and to be character-ized by more general impairment of higher cortical functions. McKhann *et al* [22] have also provided guidelines to the clinical diagnosis of AD. Dementia in AD is at present irreversible.

The changes in the brain revealed by magnetic resonance imaging (MRI) are shown in Figure 1.1. This shows $T_1$-weighed MRI coronal sections of the brains of two persons: on the left a normal; on the right, a 75-year-old man with moderately severe AD. Features to note in the latter are the generalized widening of the sulci, marked 1; the considerable enlargement of the lateral ventricles, marked 2; and, most notable of all, the pronounced bilateral atrophy of the hippocampus, marked 3. The hippocampal atrophy is an early and sensitive feature of AD, the hippocampus being important for memory function.

## Vascular Dementia

This group of dementias result from strokes destroying areas of the brain that subserve memory and intelligence. These events can be acute, or can take place more gradually and cumulatively. Dementia may follow several small strokes (multi-infarct dementia), or a single infarct or inadequate blood flow (ischaemia) to a critical brain area. In subcortical vascular dementia, ischaemic changes take place in the deep white matter of the

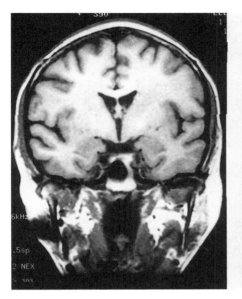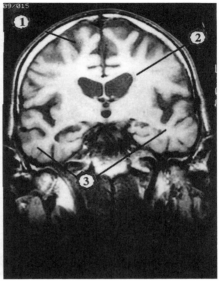

FIGURE 1.1   $T_1$ weighed magnetic resonance imaging coronal sections of a normal brain (on the left) and of the brain of a 75-year-old man with Alzheimer's disease (on the right)

cerebral hemispheres. Where diffuse demyelination of the white matter occurs, it is termed Binswanger's encephalopathy.

Vascular dementia is distinguished from dementia in AD by its history of onset, clinical features and subsequent course. Typically, there is a history of transient ischaemic attacks with brief impairment of consciousness, fleeting pareses, or visual loss. The dementia may also follow a succession of acute cerebro-vascular accidents, or, less commonly, a single major stroke. Some impairment of memory and thinking then becomes apparent. Onset, which is usually in later life, can be abrupt, following one particular ischaemic episode, or there may be more gradual emergence. The dementia is usually the result of infarction of the brain due to vascular disease, including hypertensive cerebrovascular disease. The infarcts are usually small but cumulative in their effect.

Vascular dementia is diagnosed when a person shows evidence of dementia, together with the following features [4]:

1.   Deficits in higher cognitive functions are unevenly distributed, with some functions affected and others relatively spared. Thus, memory may be quite markedly affected, while thinking, reasoning and information processing may show only mild decline.

2. There is clinical evidence of focal brain damage, manifest as at least one of the following: unilateral spastic weakness of the limbs; unilaterally increased tendon reflexes; an extensor plantar response; or pseudobulbar palsy.
3. There is evidence from the history, examination or tests of significant cerebrovascular disease, which may reasonably be judged to be aetiologically related to the dementia (e.g. a history of stroke or evidence of cerebral infarction).

## Mixed Dementia

It is quite common for features of both AD and vascular dementia to be present in the same person at the same time, and it may be difficult to determine which came first. Hofman *et al* [23] have shown that vascular factors play a significant role in the development of AD.

## Dementia with Lewy Bodies

Lewy body dementia is a relatively recent addition to the types of dementia, but may be more common than first thought, possibly accounting for 10–15% of all dementias. It is characterized by a progressive course. In addition, there is variability in attention and alertness, visual hallucinations and parkinsonism. The diagnostic criteria were first proposed by McKeith *et al* [24,25]. There may be falls or transient loss of consciousness, delusions and a sensitivity to neuroleptic drugs. The latter include the newer atypical antipsychotics. Subsequent work has shown that the diagnostic criteria needed better sensitivity [26]. McKeith *et al* [27] have now brought out improved criteria, reached by international consensus. A concise overview of the latest information on Lewy body dementia by McKeith *et al* [28] lays emphasis on the clinical importance of making the diagnosis correctly. This is because it allows identification of patients who are at risk of severe adverse reactions to neuroleptics, but who may benefit considerably from drugs that enhance cholinergic neurotransmission.

## Other Causes of Dementia

Less common causes of dementia include Parkinson's disease, severe alcohol abuse, Creutzfeldt–Jakob disease, Huntington's disease, Pick's disease and the increasingly recognized frontal or fronto-temporal lobe dementias. In the frontal lobe group, the typical picture is of a slowly progressive dementia dominated at first by personality and behavioural changes with disinhibition, apathy, stereotypy and lack of insight [29]. Memory and spatial function are relatively spared.

## Dementia Due to AIDS

A dementia syndrome can develop in persons suffering from AIDS [30]. This usually begins in the later stages of the disease, progressing quickly over a few weeks or months to death. Dementia from AIDS is found almost exclusively in younger adults rather than the elderly.

## WHAT HAPPENS OVER TIME? THE COURSE OF DEMENTIA

All of the dementias are progressive disorders, but there can be great variability in the course, as Hope *et al* [31] have emphasized on the basis of their longitudinal study of 100 cases. From a social and public health perspective, the most significant fact is that people with dementia are surviving longer than earlier in the twentieth century [32]. In vascular dementia, a person may show some impairment in memory and behaviour, but get no worse unless another episode occurs, when the blood supply is further reduced. Likewise, in AD, some may become worse quite rapidly— over 2–3 years—while others may have a much slower course over a decade or more. In general, dementia takes about 7 years from being first recognized to the advanced stages. At present, clinicians are not able to predict the prognosis with any accuracy in AD. The 5-year prospective study by Becker *et al* [33] of 204 patients, initially diagnosed as having AD, found that the accuracy of these baseline diagnoses was 86%, rising to 91% with follow-up information. The criterion was neuropathology post-mortem.

For cognitive decline not amounting to dementia, a better understanding of the ageing process is being acquired. In one community-based survey, studying changes in cognitive function in some 730 older persons over a period of 3–4 years, cognitive performance deteriorated steadily with age, but there was marked variability between individuals. Decline did not differ in men and women, but was almost universal in persons over 85 years [34]. There are some promising developments in finding drugs that may slow the progress in AD and in vascular dementia. It may even be possible soon to identify who is most likely to respond to particular medications. A possibility with particular public health appeal is to immunize people as younger adults to block the deposition of $\beta$-amyloid protein in the brain [35].

## THE PREVALENCE AND INCIDENCE OF DEMENTIA

Prevalence and incidence may be understood using the analogy of a granary. The amount of cereal in the granary at a particular time corresponds to the prevalence, while the rate of intake to the granary is analogous to the incidence, and survival is the length of time a grain of cereal remains in the granary.

### Estimating Prevalence Rates

To determine how many persons there are in a particular community who have a dementia is a disarmingly simple ambition. But it requires the following: a research team, including some clinicians; the capacity to identify the true denominator, which is all persons aged, say, 70 years and over, in a defined geographic area, including their year of birth, so that age-specific estimates can be made; a method for sampling these elderly persons, so that each has an equal probability of being assessed; and an instrument for accurately ascertaining who has the features for dementia specified in ICD-10 or DSM-IV. It is not possible to determine the presence of dementia by interviewing only the elderly person: to establish decline in cognitive performance or change in behaviour, collateral information is necessary, usually obtained from a relative. Then, if the study seeks to estimate the prevalence of specific dementias such as AD, further clinical information is needed, ideally obtained by a standardized examination by a clinician. Few groups have such resources. In short, any survey of dementia and cognitive decline in the community elderly is extremely demanding on resources, infrastructure and experience in methodology.

Despite these awesome requirements, over 100 studies have been reported from throughout the world estimating the prevalence of dementia in general population samples. Because the number of studies is so large, researchers have carried out meta-analyses in which the data from a group of studies are pooled to arrive at better estimates of prevalence. There have now been three such meta-analyses. These have focused on those studies which report prevalence rates for specific age groups (e.g. 65–69, 70–74, etc.), rather than for the elderly as a total group. Studies of the elderly as a total group hide the fact that prevalence is much higher in the "old-old" than in the "young-old". They are therefore of much less value.

TABLE 1.2  Prevalence rates (%) for dementia estimated from three different meta-analyses

| Age group (years) | Jorm et al [36] | Hofman et al [37] | Ritchie et al [38] | Ritchie and Kildea [39] |
|---|---|---|---|---|
| 60–64 | 0.7 | 1.0 | 0.9 | – |
| 65–69 | 1.4 | 1.4 | 1.6 | 1.5 |
| 70–74 | 2.8 | 4.1 | 2.8 | 3.5 |
| 75–79 | 5.6 | 5.7 | 4.9 | 6.8 |
| 80–84 | 11.1 | 13.0 | 8.7 | 13.6 |
| 85–89 | 23.6* | 24.5* | 16.4* | 22.3 |
| 90–94 | | | | 33.0 |
| 95–99 | | | | 44.8 |

* Rates for ages 85+.

In the first meta-analysis, Jorm et al [36] used data from 22 studies from throughout the world. They found that the actual prevalence rates differed greatly from study to study, but underlying all studies was a consistent trend for prevalence to increase exponentially with age. The prevalence rate for dementia was found to double with every 5.1 years of age. The exponential rise was somewhat steeper for AD (doubling every 4.5 years of age) than for vascular dementia (doubling every 5.3 years of age). The implication of these findings was that there is no single set of "true" prevalence rates. The prevalence rates found in a particular study will be affected by the methodology used, in particular where the boundary between dementia and normal ageing is placed. However, it is possible to give a summary of age-specific prevalence rates which reflects the average across the studies. These average prevalence rates are shown in Table 1.2.

The second meta-analysis, by Hofman et al [37], pooled data from 12 European studies carried out between 1980 and 1990. This meta-analysis differed from the first one in that it excluded non-European and older studies. Nevertheless, as shown in Table 1.2, the estimated prevalence rates were strikingly similar to the ones derived from the earlier meta-analysis.

The third meta-analysis, by Ritchie et al [38], used data from three studies which had been carried out since 1980 and which used the DSM-III diagnostic criteria for dementia. By restricting the studies to those which used the same diagnostic criteria, the authors found much less variability in prevalence rates than had Jorm et al [36]. Surprisingly, they also found lower prevalence rates in the upper age ranges than had the other two meta-analyses. However, the number of studies included was small. The estimated prevalence rates from Ritchie et al [38] are also shown in Table 1.2.

Later, Ritchie and Kildea [39] carried out a meta-analysis of nine studies that used DSM-III criteria and included samples of people aged over 80. Their aim was to more precisely estimate prevalence rates at extreme ages. The rates from these studies are also shown in Table 1.2. Ritchie and Kildea fitted various curves to the data and found that the rise in prevalence was not exponential over age 95, but showed some levelling off. They found that a modified logistic curve provided the best fit to the data. However, as can be seen in Table 1.2, the rates up to age 85+ are very close to those of Jorm et al [36] and Hofman et al [37], but higher than those of Ritchie et al [38].

## Prevalence Rates of Alzheimer's Disease (AD)

There have also been several meta-analyses focusing specifically on AD. In the first of these, Rocca et al [40] pooled data from six European studies. The rates were 0.3% at 60–69 years, 3.2% at 70–79 years and 10.8% at 80–89 years.

The second meta-analysis, by Corrada et al [41], analysed 15 studies using a logistic model. They found considerable variability between studies, depending on the methodology used. However, the odds of having AD increased by 18% for every year of age. Actual rates for each age group were not reported.

The most recent meta-analysis, by the US General Accounting Office [42], involved fitting a logistic model to data from 18 studies. They found that the rates doubled with every 5 years of age up to age 85 and were higher in women than men. Table 1.3 shows the rates for all levels of severity and for moderate–severe cases for specific age groups.

TABLE 1.3   Prevalence rates (%) for Alzheimer's disease estimated from a meta-analysis by the US General Accounting Office [42]

| Age (years) | All severity levels | | Moderate-severe cases | |
|---|---|---|---|---|
| | Males | Females | Males | Females |
| 65 | 0.6 | 0.8 | 0.3 | 0.6 |
| 70 | 1.3 | 1.7 | 0.6 | 1.1 |
| 75 | 2.7 | 3.5 | 1.1 | 2.3 |
| 80 | 5.6 | 7.1 | 2.3 | 4.4 |
| 85 | 11.1 | 13.8 | 4.4 | 8.6 |
| 90 | 20.8 | 25.2 | 8.5 | 15.8 |
| 95 | 35.6 | 41.5 | 15.8 | 27.4 |

## Prevalence of Dementia in Younger Persons

It can be inferred from Table 1.2 that dementia is rare below the age of 60. Nevertheless, this younger group is an important one to consider, because they have somewhat different service needs. While the prevalence of dementia in older people is best estimated by community surveys, this method is not suitable for rare disorders, because of the very large sample that would be required. For younger people, we must rely on counting cases that have come to medical attention. Since these younger individuals will in most industrialized countries receive thorough medical investigation, this approach to estimating prevalence is quite reasonable. Table 1.4 shows data on dementia below age 60 from a medical case register in Rochester in the United States [43].

## Projected Increases in Prevalence

Because the world's population is progressively ageing, more people are falling into the age groups where dementia prevalence is highest. Thus, the ageing of the population will in itself produce a large increase in the number of dementia cases, even without any change in the age-specific prevalence rates. Jorm and Korten [44] have used their meta-analysis of prevalence to project future increases in dementia cases by applying it to suitable age-specific population projections. The method they used does not need to assume particular age-specific prevalence rates (like those in Table 1.2), but only that the increase in prevalence rate with age is exponential in form, with a doubling every 5.1 years of age. This method can be applied to various countries even if their absolute prevalence rates are very different.The method gives the percentage increase in dementia cases over a base year. It is instructive to compare the projected increase in dementia cases for more developed and less developed countries. This can be done by applying

TABLE 1.4  Prevalence rates for dementia below age 60 in Rochester, USA (according to Kokmen *et al* [43])

| Age group (years) | Prevalence of dementia (per 100 000 population) |
| --- | --- |
| 0–44 | 0 |
| 45–49 | 77 |
| 50–54 | 40 |
| 55–59 | 86 |

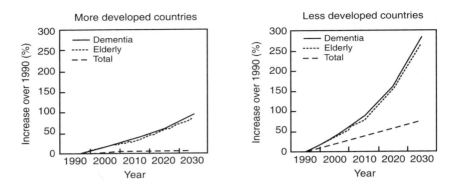

**FIGURE 1.2** Projected increases in dementia cases, elderly population and total population for the more developed countries and less developed countries, 1990–2030

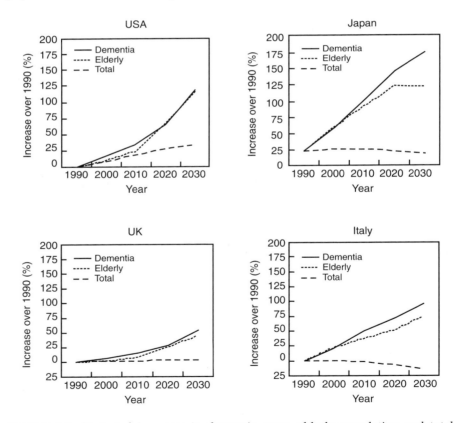

**FIGURE 1.3** Projected increases in dementia cases, elderly population and total population for four more developed countries, 1990–2030

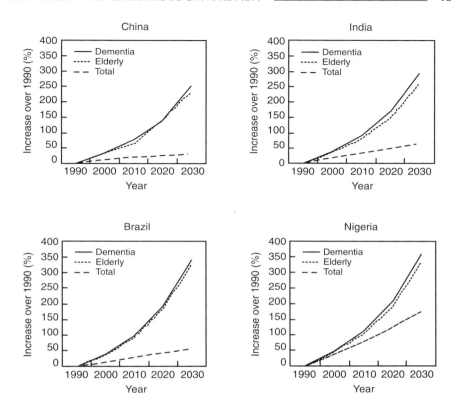

FIGURE 1.4 Projected increases in dementia cases, elderly population and total population for four less developed countries, 1990–2030

the prevalence rates from the Jorm *et al* [36] meta-analysis to the latest United Nations' population projections for various countries [45]. Figure 1.2 shows the results. It can be seen that the more developed countries are projected to have low total population growth, but a sharp rise in the number of elderly and even greater rise in people with dementia. This is because the old-old, who are most likely to suffer from dementia, are expected to increase at a faster rate than either the total population or the young-old. The less developed countries will experience much greater growth in total population, but an even steeper growth in the elderly and people with dementia. Figures 1.3 and 1.4 show the projections for some specific countries. These projections make clear that the biggest growth in dementia for the twenty-first century will be in the less developed countries which currently have predominantly young populations.

## Is Prevalence or Incidence Changing?

All these projections assume, of course, that the age-specific prevalence rates for dementia do not change in the future. If either the incidence rate or the survival duration of dementia were to change, then so would the prevalence rate. Whether there will be future changes in incidence or survival is unknowable, although there is the hope that prevention programs will eventually reduce incidence. However, we can look back for any trends of this sort in the recent past. Studies from Sweden [46] and the USA [47] have failed to find any changes in incidence over recent decades, although one American study showed a slight increase in the prevalence of cases coming to medical attention during the 1980s [48]. The authors of this study concluded that the increase in prevalence could be due to better recognition of dementia by physicians and families rather than any true increase.

## Incidence of Dementia

Incidence studies are much scarcer than prevalence studies, undoubtedly because such studies are costly and take many years to complete. However, the number of studies has now cumulated to the point where meta-analyses are possible. The first of these was carried out by Jorm and Jolley [49] and involved 23 studies. Data were pooled separately for different regions of the world and for males and females. Incidence was found to rise exponentially with age up to 90 years, after which there were insufficient data to draw any firm conclusions. Table 1.5 shows the results for dementia and Table 1.6 for AD.

TABLE 1.5   Incidence rates (%) for dementia from two meta-analyses

| Age group (years) | Europe mild +* | Europe moderate +* | USA moderate +* | East Asia mild +* | All cases ** |
|---|---|---|---|---|---|
| 55–59 | – | – | – | – | 0.03 |
| 60–64 | – | – | – | – | 0.11 |
| 65–69 | 0.91 | 0.36 | 0.24 | 0.35 | 0.33 |
| 70–74 | 1.76 | 0.64 | 0.50 | 0.71 | 0.84 |
| 75–79 | 3.33 | 1.17 | 1.05 | 1.47 | 1.82 |
| 80–84 | 5.99 | 2.15 | 1.77 | 3.26 | 3.36 |
| 85–89 | 10.41 | 3.77 | 2.75 | 7.21 | 5.33 |
| 90–94 | 17.98 | 6.61 | – | – | 7.29 |
| 95+ | – | – | – | – | 8.68 |

 * According to Jorm and Jolley [9].
** According to Gao et al [50].

TABLE 1.6    Incidence rates (%) for Alzheimer's disease from two meta-analyses

| Age group (years) | Europe mild +* | Europe moderate +* | USA mild +* | USA moderate +* | East Asia mild +* | All cases ** |
|---|---|---|---|---|---|---|
| 60–64 | – | – | – | – | – | 0.06 |
| 65–69 | 0.25 | 0.10 | 0.61 | 0.16 | 0.07 | 0.19 |
| 70–74 | 0.52 | 0.22 | 1.11 | 0.35 | 0.21 | 0.51 |
| 75–79 | 1.07 | 0.48 | 2.01 | 0.78 | 0.58 | 1.17 |
| 80–84 | 2.21 | 1.06 | 3.84 | 1.48 | 1.49 | 2.31 |
| 85–89 | 4.61 | 2.26 | 7.45 | 2.60 | 3.97 | 3.86 |
| 90–94 | 9.66 | 4.77 | – | – | – | 5.49 |
| 95+ | – | – | – | – | – | 6.68 |

  * According to Jorm and Jolley [9].
 ** According to Gao et al [50].

The second meta-analysis, by Gao et al [50], was carried out at the same time as the first, but involved only the 12 studies that used the DSM-III or DSM-III-R criteria for dementia and the National Institute of Neurological and Communicative Disorders—Alzheimer's Disease and Related Disorders Association (NINCDS-ADRDA) criteria for AD. The rise in incidence with age was not found to be exponential, with some slowing of the rate of increase at older ages. Table 1.5 shows the estimated rates for dementia and Table 1.6 for AD. The differences between the two meta-analyses result because Gao et al pooled data for different levels of severity and different regions of the world, while Jorm and Jolley separated them. It can be seen from the tables that the rates of Gao et al fall in between the mild+ and the moderate+ rates of Jorm and Jolley.

## Survival with Dementia

Although dementing diseases are often not listed on death certificates as causes of death, they clearly reduce a person's life expectancy. Published studies consistently show a reduction in survival. Tabl
shows the results of an American study of survival base
case register for the city of Rochester. It can be see
dementia had poorer survival than others of the same
studies comparing survival in AD and vascular de
survival is poorer for the latter group [51]. In people
shorter for older cases than for younger ones, as m
the reduction in life expectancy is proportionately grea
cases.

TABLE 1.7   Survival in dementia cases from the point of medical detection (adapted from Schoenberg *et al* [52])

|  | 1 year (%) | 5 years (%) | 10 years (%) |
|---|---|---|---|
| Survival of people with dementia | 93 | 49 | 16 |
| Expected survival in population | 92 | 64 | 37 |

# RISK AND PROTECTION FACTORS FOR DEMENTIA

One way of stemming the rising tide of dementia cases would be to find effective methods of preventing the diseases that result in dementia. A reduction in the prevalence rate for dementia would help to counteract the increase due to an ageing population. We must therefore ask whether prevention of dementia is a possibility.

If the causes of dementia in the elderly were understood, it would be possible to use this knowledge to develop preventive strategies. However, even in the absence of a full understanding of its causes, it is possible to base prevention around factors known to increase or decrease the risk of developing dementia. Some risk and protection factors cannot be easily modified and so provide no basis for preventive action. For example, we might know that a family history of dementia increases risk for AD, but there is nothing we can do to modify this risk, at least so far. Gene therapy for dementia remains a distant prospect. Some other factors are modifiable and it is these that are important for prevention. This strategy is already used to prevent other common health problems such as cancer and heart disease.

## Risk Factors for Alzheimer's Disease (AD)

In recent years, a number of studies have been carried out to investigate risk factors for AD. An international collaborative project has pooled the data from many of these studies in order to allow a more powerful evaluation of potential risk factors [53]. At this stage, we can say that there are only four "confirmed" risk factors, where the evidence is beyond reasonable doubt. However, there are several other "possible" risk factors where evidence is less certain. There are also some factors that possibly provide protection. Identifying these is particularly important for future preventive efforts.

*Confirmed Risk Factors*

*Old age.* This is by far the most important risk factor for AD. As discussed earlier, the incidence of the disease rises sharply with age, at least up to age 90. There is controversy about what happens in extreme old age. Some authorities believe everyone would develop AD if they lived long enough, whereas others believe that the incidence rate eventually levels out and that some individuals will never develop the disease over a feasible life-span.

*Family history of AD.* A family history of AD is probably the most import-ant risk factor apart from old age. First-degree relatives (siblings and children) of people with AD have around 3.5 times the risk of developing the disorder themselves [54]. However, the actual percentage risk depends on how long a relative lives. Someone with a family history of AD who lives only to age 50 may have a lower risk than someone with no family history who lives to 100. Table 1.8 shows the risk of first-degree relatives develop-ing AD according to what age they live to.

There is also evidence that the risk to relatives varies depending on the age at which the index case developed AD. Relatives of people developing AD in their 40s or 50s have a greater risk than relatives of cases developing the disease in their 80s. In rare families, AD shows an autosomal dominant pattern of inheritance, meaning that a first-degree relative of someone affected will have a 50% chance of developing the disease. These families usually show onset of the disease in middle age. A number of genes have now been identified which are responsible for the disease in these families (see below).

TABLE 1.8   Risk that a first-degree relative of a patient with Alzheimer's disease develops the disease (adapted from Lautenschlager *et al* [55])

| Age relative lives to (years) | Risk to relative (%) |
| --- | --- |
| 60 | 1 |
| 65 | 2 |
| 70 | 5 |
| 75 | 9 |
| 80 | 16 |
| 85 | 24 |
| 90 | 33 |
| 95 | 38 |

*Down's syndrome.* Chromosome 21 contains the β-amyloid precursor gene which plays an important role in the amyloid plaques that appear in the brain in AD. Because people with Down's syndrome have trisomy of chromosome 21, they invariably develop the brain changes of AD by age 40. However, the prevalence of AD is much less than 100% even by age 50 [56].

*Apolipoprotein E (ApoE) and other genes.* It is now known that some early-onset cases of AD are caused by single genes [57]. The genes identified at this stage are mutations of the β-amyloid precursor gene on chromosome 21 and of the presenilin genes on chromosomes 1 and 14. However, these genes account for only a small percentage of AD cases. The vast majority, which have onset after age 65, probably have complex causes involving both genetic and environmental influences. It is now known that the apolipoprotein E gene (ApoE for short) on chromosome 19 is involved in these complex cases. This gene has three different alleles, labelled ε2, ε3 and ε4, with the ε3 allele being the most common. Each person has two alleles, one of which is inherited from the mother and one from the father. Thus, individuals may have any of the following combinations of ApoE alleles: ε2/ε2, ε2/ε3, ε2/ε4, ε3/ε3, ε3/ε4 and ε4/ε4. People with one ε4 allele have an increased risk of developing AD, while those with two ε4 alleles have an even greater risk. There is some evidence that the ε2 allele is associated with a decreased risk. A meta-analysis found that, in Caucasians, the ε4/ε4 genotype was associated with 15 times the risk compared to the common ε3/ε3 genotype, while the ε3/ε4 genotype was associated with three times the risk [58]. Having an ε2/ε2 or ε2/ε3 genotype reduced the risk by 40%. However, it must be emphasized that the ε4 allele is only a risk factor for AD, not in itself a sufficient cause. Although individuals carrying two ε4 alleles are at increased risk, some do not develop the disease. Conversely, individuals with no ε4 alleles may still develop the disease. Because the relationship between ApoE and AD is imperfect, determining a person's ApoE genotype is not recommended for predicting the future likelihood of developing the disease [59]. There is debate about whether ApoE testing might be useful as an adjunct in the diagnosis of AD in people already presenting with the symptoms of dementia, particularly when current methods of diagnosis can already be better than 85% accurate [60].

## Other Possible Risk Factors

There are a large number of other possible risk factors for which the evidence is still uncertain. These include national and ethnic background, head trauma, aluminium in the water supply, occupational exposure to electromagnetic fields [61], history of depression [62,63], family history of

Down's syndrome [53], herpes simplex infection [64], advanced maternal age [65], fingerprint patterns [66] and hypothyroidism [67]. It is beyond the scope of this report to examine all of these; only the first four are discussed here because of the current scientific interest in them.

*National and ethnic differences.* Most of the research that has been carried out on AD has been in countries with predominantly Caucasian populations. However, the incidence of AD could be different in other countries or in other ethnic groups. This could be because of different environmental exposures throughout life, including dietary patterns, or because of different gene frequencies in the contrasted populations. A meta-analysis of incidence studies found that East Asian countries had a lower incidence of dementia, and a lower incidence of AD at younger ages, than countries with predominantly Caucasian populations [49]. Japanese studies have often found that vascular dementia is more prominent than AD [68]. However, Japanese-Americans, who have oriental ancestry but have adopted American culture, are more like Caucasians in having a preponderance of AD [69]. Recent studies in Japan indicate that the Japanese may have gradually moved to the Caucasian pattern of dementia [70], although Hatada *et al* [71] attribute the change largely to different ascertainment practices in recent years. Overall, the findings suggest that there may be some important genetic or environmental factors which produce a different pattern of dementing diseases. Possible factors are the higher intake of salt in the Japanese diet (predisposing them to high blood pressure and vascular dementia) and the lower frequency of the ApoE $\varepsilon$4 allele in the Japanese (lowering their risk of AD).

Another interesting study has compared the prevalence and incidence of dementia in Black Americans and Nigerians [72,73]. Both groups are of West African ancestry, but they have very different lifestyles. The Nigerians have been found to have a lower prevalence and incidence of AD and of dementia generally.

The Cree Indians in Canada have also been found to have a lower prevalence of AD than White Canadians, but they did not differ in the prevalence of all dementias because they had more alcoholic dementia [74]. It is important to note, however, that the Cree study has reported a lower *prevalence* of AD, not a lower *incidence*. The difference in prevalence could be due to a lower incidence in the Cree or to shorter survival after developing AD.

Ganguli *et al* [75] and Chandra *et al* [76] undertook a methodologically sophisticated survey of 5126 individuals aged 55 years and over in Ballabgarh, Northern India. By DSM-IV and NINCDS–ADRDA criteria, they found a prevalence of only 1.07% (CI 0.72–1.53) for AD in persons aged 65 and over. Neither gender nor literacy were associated with prevalence, but this rose with age for both AD and all dementias. Their conclusion was that the low prevalence compared to Western estimates could be due to shorter survival of cases, but it is also possible that the incidence is lower, speculatively attributable to differences in the underlying distribution of risk and protective factors.

*Head trauma.* A few studies have found that AD cases are more likely than normal people to have previously experienced a head injury with loss of consciousness. It has also been found that $\beta$-amyloid can be deposited extensively in the brain following severe head injury, supporting a role for head trauma as a risk factor [77]. However, many other studies have failed to support this link, although the trend of the data has been in the same direction. Pooling of data from seven studies found that a history of head trauma was 80% more common in AD cases than in normal controls [78]. Head trauma in the 10 years before onset of dementia was found to be more important as a risk factor than head trauma earlier in life. Although the pooled data support head trauma as a risk factor, it cannot be regarded as a definite risk factor, because history of head trauma was ascertained by reports of relatives rather than from medical records. It is possible that relatives of demented people are more likely to remember incidents of head trauma because it provides a plausible explanation for the dementia. Two studies have looked at head trauma using medical records and have found no link to AD [79,80]. However, a recent study suggested that head trauma may be a risk factor only in individuals who carry the ApoE $\varepsilon$4 allele; in other individuals head trauma did not increase risk [81]. It has also been found that $\beta$-amyloid was more likely to be deposited in the brain after injury in persons who carried the $\varepsilon$4 allele [82]. Such an effect might explain the inconsistency in earlier research.

*Aluminium.* There is considerable controversy about the role of aluminium in AD [83]. There is no doubt that accumulation of aluminium in the brain due to environmental exposure has toxic effects, but the brain changes involved are different from those found in AD. Aluminium is one of the most abundant elements in the earth's crust, so some degree of exposure is inevitable. Average daily intake of aluminium has been estimated at 20.5 mg, with 20 mg coming from food, 0.5 mg from fluid intake and 0.01 mg from inhalation [84]. There are rare instances where individuals have been exposed to very high levels of aluminium in their occupations. For example, gold miners in Canada were required to inhale aluminium powder in an attempt to prevent the lung disease silicosis [85]. These miners were found to have a greater incidence of cognitive impairment than miners who had not used the powder. However, there was no evidence of a specific link to AD. Much of the research on aluminium and AD has centred on aluminium in the water supply. Aluminium is naturally present in the water supply, but is also often added during water treatment as a flocculant to improve the clarity of the water. Several studies have reported a higher incidence of AD in regions with more aluminium in the water, particularly if the water is also acidic. However, the methodology of these studies has been criticized. One problem with the idea that aluminium in water could be a risk factor is that water provides only a tiny percentage of the aluminium in the diet. However, the aluminium added during water treatment is soluble, unlike the aluminium which naturally occurs in water. In this soluble form it may be more readily absorbed by the body. In some countries, the water supply authorities have closely monitored the evidence that the aluminium added during treatment might conceivably contribute to AD. Despite the weakness of the evidence, it might be prudent to keep the aluminium content of drinking water as low as practicable [86]. Even though the evidence is weak, we need to be cautious because of the widespread public health risk if there is a link.

*Electromagnetic fields.* There is evidence from several studies that AD cases were more likely to have worked in occupations where exposure to electromagnetic fields was high [87]. These occupations involve working with electric motors very close to the body, and include carpenter, electrician, machinist and seamstress. It has been hypothesized that electromagnetic fields may upset intracellular calcium ion homeostasis, which may promote the cleavage of amyloid precursor protein into $\beta$-amyloid [61]. However, other studies have not consistently supported an association [88,89]. What is needed are studies that directly examine exposure to electromagnetic fields rather than inferring exposure from the type of occupation.

## Possible Protection Factors for Alzheimer's Disease (AD)

Protection factors are those that are associated with a reduced risk of developing a disease. At present, there are no factors which are definitely known to provide protection against AD. However, there is suggestive evidence about several, including use of anti-inflammatory drugs, use of estrogen replacement therapy and a high level of education or intelligence.

### Anti-inflammatory Drugs

These drugs include the non-steroidal anti-inflammatory drugs (NSAIDs) and the steroids, commonly used to treat inflammatory diseases such as arthritis. Several studies have been carried out looking at the association between these drugs and AD. Pooling the data across the studies has indicated that individuals who take anti-inflammatory drugs over a long period, or suffer from arthritis, may have nearly 50% lower risk of AD [90,91]. However, because the studies have not consistently shown a protective effect, this association must still be regarded as uncertain. Randomized controlled trials are needed to establish whether there is protective effect, but the side effects of anti-inflammatory drugs make such trials difficult.

## Estrogen Replacement Therapy

Animal studies have shown that estrogen has several protective effects on the brain, including increased cerebral blood flow, stimulation of the cholinergic neurotransmitter system, acting as a co-factor with nerve growth factors, prevention of neural atrophy, and reversal of damage caused by glucocorticoids [92]. There is also some epidemiological evidence suggesting that estrogen replacement therapy in post-menopausal women may have a protective effect. A meta-analysis of such studies found that estrogen reduced the risk of AD by around 30% [93]. However, women who take estrogen tend to be better educated and may differ in other ways. As discussed below, education may itself be protective. Randomized trials are needed to establish whether there is an effect. Currently in the United States, the Women's Health Initiative Memory Study is looking at the effects of estrogen replacement therapy on the incidence of dementia in over 8000 women [94].

## High Education or Intelligence

Better educated people are well known to perform better on dementia screening tests like the Mini-Mental State Examination. However, there is controversy about whether these people are protected against AD and other dementing diseases or whether they are simply better at doing cognitive tests. Several studies have found that better educated people have a lower incidence of AD or cognitive decline, but this is not a universal finding [95–97]. One hypothesis is that education does not protect against Alzheimer brain changes, but rather allows the individual to compensate better for the effects of these changes [98]. In other words, better educated persons can tolerate greater loss of brain cells before they begin to show the effects of dementia in their everyday behaviour. There is some evidence to support this hypothesis [99]. Because education is correlated with intelligence, it could be pre-morbid intelligence rather than education that is protective. For example, one longitudinal study has found that pre-morbid intelligence is a better predictor of dementia than education [100]. While the evidence on

education and pre-morbid intelligence is generally interpreted i
compensation for brain pathology, a recent study of AD in Ame
went further to suggest that higher verbal ability in early adulthood actuany
protects against AD processes in old age [101]. Verbal ability was assessed
from samples of writing that the nuns had made as young adults. Among
the nuns who died and came to autopsy, all of those with confirmed AD had
low verbal ability, compared to none of those without the disease. Any
protective effects of education or intelligence could be mediated by brain
reserve [102]. Intelligence is known to be correlated with brain size, and
individuals who have a larger brain or head size appear to have reduced
risk of dementia.

## Risk Factors for Vascular Dementia

There has been much less investigation of risk factors for vascular dementia
than for AD. The study of risk factors is complicated because there are
several different types of vascular dementia, each of which is difficult to
diagnose. The clear distinction between vascular and Alzheimer's dementia
also appears shaky in the light of evidence that AD involves atherosclerotic
changes [23]. The most common form of vascular dementia is multi-infarct
dementia which is due to strokes. Therefore the risk factors for stroke might
also be presumed to apply to this type of vascular dementia. The limited
evidence available on risk factors for vascular dementia is consistent with
this. According to a review of the evidence by Gorelick [103], the only
confirmed risk factor is old age. However, there is evidence for several
other putative risk factors: race/ethnic group (orientals, African-Americans), low education, hypertension, cigarette smoking, myocardial infarction, diabetes mellitus, hypercholesterolaemia, and various factors related to
the nature and extent of cerebrovascular disease.

In another recent review of the evidence, Skoog [104] has concluded that
probable risk factors for the multi-infarct form of vascular dementia are
hypertension, diabetes mellitus, advanced age, male sex, smoking and
cardiac diseases. In addition, hypertension is a risk factor for the type of
vascular dementia associated with changes to the white matter of the brain.

More recently, it has been found that the $\varepsilon4$ allele of the ApoE gene is a
possible risk factor for vascular dementia as well as for AD [105].

## PROSPECTS FOR PREVENTION OF DEMENTIA

In considering the prevention of diseases common in old age, it is useful
to make a distinction between "age-dependent" and "age-related" diseases

[106]. Age-dependent diseases are those in which the disease process is an intrinsic part of ageing. Everyone would develop these diseases if they lived long enough. Age-related diseases, on the other hand, may become more common with age, but are not necessarily related to the ageing process. Age-related diseases can be prevented if an individual is not exposed to the causative agent. By contrast, age-dependent diseases cannot be completely prevented. They can be postponed by slowing down the disease process or avoiding environmental risk factors, but their eventual occurrence is inevitable. With age-dependent diseases the aim of prevention is to extend the period of life free of disablement by delaying disease onset. Whether the major dementing diseases are age-related or age-dependent is still a matter of debate. However, if the age-dependent view is correct, preventive efforts will not reduce the demand for health and welfare programmes to deal with dementia, but might progressively advance the age group at which these become necessary.

Whether the goal of prevention is elimination of disease or postponement of onset, this is most likely to be achieved by reducing exposure to risk factors or promoting exposure to protection factors. This strategy has been successful in other areas, such as the prevention of lung and skin cancer. Prevention can be aimed at changing exposure in the whole population (such as education campaigns on sun exposure as a risk factor for skin cancer) or targeted specifically at high-risk groups (for example, use of low-dose aspirin to prevent heart attacks and stroke) [107].

With AD, genetic factors are clearly of great importance, but environmental factors also play some role. Reducing exposure to possible environmental factors like head trauma is an obvious approach, although this is already a public health goal in its own right, quite apart from any possible association with AD. The greatest interest currently is in the possible protection factors like anti-inflammatory drugs, estrogen replacement therapy and education. Controlled trials will be necessary to confirm whether anti-inflammatory drugs and estrogen replacement therapy have a protective effect. Any preventive effect on AD will have to be balanced against the side effects of these drugs. If education and intelligence are confirmed to be protection factors, this will have important implications for the future incidence of dementia, because levels of education and IQ test scores are rising over successive generations. The possibility of immunization against AD has now emerged [35]. This is highly attractive but as yet entirely unevaluated.

Vascular dementia presents the greatest scope for prevention, because there are a number of risk factors which are modifiable. Control of hypertension and smoking are the interventions most likely to be successful. There is evidence that stroke mortality in Australia is declining at around

5% a year [108]. If so, this decline should also be reducing mortality from vascular dementia.

## SUMMARY

### Consistent Evidence

- It is methodologically possible to estimate the prevalence of dementia, and specifically of AD and vascular dementia, in general population samples. Estimates of incidence are much more taxing.
- There is an unprecedented growth in the world's elderly.
- The dementias are progressive disorders.
- There are four known risk factors for AD: age, family history of dementia, Down's syndrome, and apoE $\varepsilon$4 genotype.

### Incomplete Evidence

- There are probably different prevalence rates of dementia in different populations, but it is not known if this is due to different incidence rates, different survival times of established cases, or both.
- There are a number of possible risk factors for AD: region or ethnicity, head injury, aluminium, and electromagnetic fields.
- There are a number of possible protective factors for AD: anti-inflammatory drugs, estrogen, and high intelligence or education.

### Areas Still Open to Research

- If there are different incidence rates of dementia between populations, this may be due to differences in the underlying distribution of protective and risk factors. These call for a concerted research effort.
- Methods for preventing the dementias must be found, but none have yet been established.

## ACKNOWLEDGEMENTS

The authors express their appreciation to Dr L. Berg for permission to reproduce Table 1.1 and to Professor Perminder S. Sachdev, University of New South Wales, Sydney, Australia, for Figure 1.1.

# REFERENCES

1. Esquirol J.E. (1845) A treatise on insanity. In *Documentary History of Psychiatry. A Source Book on Historical Principles* (Ed. C.E. Goshen), pp. 314–369, Lea and Blanchard, New York.

2. Caine E.D., Grossman H., Lyness J.M. (1995) Delirium, dementia, and amnestic and other cognitive disorders and mental disorders due to a general medical condition. In *Comprehensive Textbook of Psychiatry* (Eds H.I. Kaplan, B.J. Sadock), pp. 705–754, Williams and Wilkins, Baltimore.

3. World Health Organization (1992) *The ICD-10 Classification of Mental and Behavioural Disorders. Clinical Descriptions and Diagnostic Guidelines*, World Health Organization, Geneva.

4. World Health Organization (1993) *The ICD-10 Classification of Mental and Behavioural Disorders. Diagnostic Criteria for Research*, World Health Organization, Geneva.

5. American Psychiatric Association (1994) *Diagnostic and Statistical Manual of Mental Disorders*, 4th edn, American Psychiatric Association, Washington, DC.

6. Henderson A.S., Easteal S., Jorm A.F., Mackinnon A.J., Korten A.E., Christensen H., Croft L., Jacomb P.A. (1995) Apolipoprotein E allele e4, dementia and cognitive decline in a population sample. *Lancet*, **346**: 1387–1390.

7. Erkinjuntti T., Ostbye T., Steenhuis R., Hachinski V. (1997) The effect of different diagnostic criteria on the prevalence of dementia. *N. Engl. J. Med.*, **337**: 1667–1674.

8. Berg L. (1988) Mild senile dementia of the Alzheimer type: diagnostic criteria and natural history. *Mt. Sinai J. Med.*, **55**: 87–96.

9. Kral V.A. (1962) Senescent forgetfulness, benign and malignant. *Can. Med. Assoc. J.*, **86**: 257–260.

10. Crook T., Bartus R.T., Ferris S.H., Whitehouse P., Cohen G.D., Gershon S. (1986) Age-associated memory impairment: proposed diagnostic criteria and measures of clinical change—Report of a National Institute of Mental Health Work Group. *Develop. Neuropsychol.*, **2**: 261–276.

11. Christensen H., Henderson A.S., Jorm A.F., Mackinnon A.J., Scott R., Korten A.E. (1995) ICD-10 mild cognitive disorder: epidemiological evidence of its validity. *Psychol. Med.*, **25**: 105–120.

12. Christensen H., Henderson A.S., Korten A.E., Jorm A.F., Jacomb P.A., Mackinnon A.J. (1997) ICD-10 mild cognitive disorder: its outcome three years later. *Int. J. Geriatr. Psychiatry*, **12**: 581–586.

13. Ritchie K., Touchon J. (2000) Mild cognitive impairment: conceptual basis and current nosological status. *Lancet*, **355**: 225–228.

14. Bolla K.I., Lindgren K.N., Bonaccorsy C., Bleecker M.L. (1991) Memory complaints in older adults. *Arch. Neurol.*, **48**: 61–64.

15. Christensen H. (1991) The validity of memory complaints by elderly persons. *Int. J. Geriatr. Psychiatry*, **6**: 307–312.

16. Hanninen T., Reinikainen K.J., Helkala E.-L., Koivisto K., Mykkanen L., Laakso M., Pyrorala K., Riekkinen P.J. (1994) Subjective memory complaints and personality traits in normal elderly subjects. *J. Am. Geriatr. Soc.*, **42**: 1–4.

17. Jorm A.F., Christensen H., Henderson A.S., Korten A.E., Mackinnon A.J., Scott R. (1994) Complaints of cognitive decline in the elderly: a comparison of reports by subjects and informants in a community sample. *Psychol. Med.*, **24**: 365–374.

18. Jorm A.F., Christensen H., Korten A.E., Henderson A.S., Jacomb P.A., Mackinnon A. (1997) Do cognitive complaints either predict future cognitive decline or reflect past cognitive decline? A longitudinal study of an elderly community sample. *Psychol. Med.*, **27**: 91–98.
19. Schmand B., Jonker C., Hooijer C., Lindeboom J. (1996) Subjective memory complaints may announce dementia. *Neurology*, **46**: 121–125.
20. Schofield P., Marder K., Dooneief G., Bell K., Chun M., Ramachandran G., Jacobs D.M., Sano M., Stern Y. (1996) Subjective memory complaints predict decline in memory and cognition at 1-year follow-up in individuals with cognitive impairment. *Neurology*, **46**: A434.
21. Tomlinson B., Blessed G., Roth M. (1970) Observations on the brains of demented old people. *J. Neurol. Sci.*, **11**: 205–242.
22. McKhann G., Drachman D., Folstein M., Katzman R., Price D., Stadlan E.M. (1984) Clinical diagnosis of Alzheimer's disease: Report of the NINCDS–ADRDA work group under the auspices of Department of Health and Human Services Task Force on Alzheimer's Disease. *Neurology*, **34**: 939–944.
23. Hofman A., Ott A., Breteler M.M.B., Bots M.L., Slooter A.J.C., van Harskamp F., van Duijn C., Van Broeckhoven C., Grobbee D.E. (1997) Atherosclerosis, apolipoprotein E, and prevalence of dementia and Alzheimer's disease in the Rotterdam study. *Lancet*, **349**: 151–154.
24. McKeith I.G., Perry R.H., Fairbairn A.F., Jabeen S., Perry E.K. (1993) Operational criteria for senile dementia of Lewy body type (SDLT). *Psychol. Med.*, **22**: 911–922.
25. McKeith I.G., Galasko D., Kosaka K., Perry E.K., Dickson D.W., Hansen L.A., Salmon D.P., Lowe J., Mirra S.S., Byrne E.J. *et al* (1996) Consensus guidelines for the clinical and pathologic diagnosis of dementia with Lewy bodies (DLB): report of the Consortium on DLB international workshop. *Neurology*, **47**: 1113–1124.
26. Luis C.A., Barker W.W., Gajaraj K., Hardwood D., Petersen R., Kashuba A., Waters C., Jimison P., Pearl G., Petito C. *et al.* (1999) Sensitivity and specificity of three clinical criteria for dementia with Lewy bodies in an autopsy-verified sample. *Int. J. Geriatr. Psychiatry*, **14**: 526–533.
27. McKeith I.G., Perry E.K., Perry R.H. (1999) Report of the second dementia with Lewy body international workshop: diagnosis and treatment. Consortium on Dementia with Lewy Bodies. *Neurology*, **53**: 902–905.
28. McKeith I.G., O'Brien J.T., Ballard C. (1999) Diagnosing dementia with Lewy bodies. *Lancet*, **354**: 1227–1228.
29. Gustafson L. (1987) Frontal lobe degeneration of non-Alzheimer type. II. Clinical picture and differential diagnosis. *Arch. Gerontol. Geriatr.*, **6**: 209–223.
30. Maj M. (1990) Organic mental disorders in HIV-1 infection. *AIDS*, **4**: 831–840.
31. Hope T., Keene J., Fairburn C.G., Jacoby R., McShane R. (1999) Natural history of behavioural changes and psychiatric symptoms in Alzheimer's disease. A longitudinal study. *Br. J. Psychiatry*, **174**: 39–44.
32. Blessed G., Wilson D. (1982) The contemporary natural history of mental disorder in old age. *Br. J. Psychiatry*, **141**: 59–67.
33. Becker J.T., Boller F., Lopez O.L., Saxton J., McGonigle K.L. (1994) The natural history of Alzheimer's disease: description of study cohort and accuracy of diagnosis. *Arch. Neurol.*, **51**: 585–594.
34. Korten A.E., Henderson A.S., Christensen H., Jorm A.F., Rodgers B., Jacomb P., Mackinnon A.J. (1997) A prospective study of cognitive function in the elderly. *Psychol. Med.*, **27**: 919–930.
35. St George-Hyslop P.H., Westaway D.A. (1999) Antibody clears senile plaques. *Nature*, **400**: 116–117.

36. Jorm A.F., Korten A., Henderson A.S. (1987) The prevalence of dementia: a quantitative integration of the literature. *Acta Psychiatr. Scand.*, **76**: 465–479.
37. Hofman A., Rocca W.A., Brayne C., Breteler M.M.B., Clarke M., Cooper B., Copeland J.R.M., Dartigues J.F., da Silva Droux A., Hagnell O. *et al* (1991) The prevalence of dementia in Europe: a collaborative study of 1980–1990 findings. *Int. J. Epidemiol.*, **20**: 736–748.
38. Ritchie K., Kildea D., Robine J.-M. (1992) The relationship between age and the prevalence of senile dementia: a meta-analysis of recent data. *Int. J. Epidemiol.*, **21**: 763–769.
39. Ritchie K., Kildea D. (1995) Is senile dementia "age-related" or "ageing-related"?—evidence from meta-analysis of dementia prevalence in the oldest old. *Lancet*, **346**: 931–934.
40. Rocca W.A., Hofman A., Brayne C., Breteler M.M., Clarke M., Copeland J.R.M., Dartigues J.-F., Engedal K., Hagnell O., Heeren T.J. *et al* (1991) Frequency and distribution of Alzheimer's disease in Europe: a collaborative study of 1980–1990 prevalence findings. *Ann. Neurol.*, **30**: 381–390.
41. Corrada M., Brookmeyer R., Kawas C. (1995) Sources of variability in prevalence rates of Alzheimer's disease. *Int. J. Epidemiol.*, **24**: 1000–1005.
42. United States General Accounting Office (1998) *Alzheimer's Disease: Estimates of Prevalence in the United States*. US General Accounting Office, Washington, DC.
43. Kokmen E., Beard C.M., Chandra V., Offord K.P., Schoenberg B.S. (1989) Case-control study of Alzheimer's disease in Rochester, Minnesota (1960–1974). *Neurology*, **39**: 179.
44. Jorm A.F., Korten A.E. (1988) A method for calculating projected increases in the number of dementia sufferers. *Aust. N. Zeal. J. Psychiatry*, **22**: 183–189.
45. United Nations Department of Economic and Social Affairs (1997) *The Sex and Age Distribution of the World Population: The 1996 Revision*. United Nations, New York.
46. Rorsman B., Hagnell O., Lanke J. (1986) Prevalence and incidence of senile and multi-infarct dementia in the Lundby Study: a comparison between the time periods 1947–1957 and 1957–1972. *Neuropsychobiology*, **15**: 122–129.
47. Kokmen E., Chandra V., Schoenberg B.S. (1988) Trends in incidence of dementing illness in Rochester, Minnesota, in three quinquennial periods, 1960–1974. *Neurology*, **38**: 975–980.
48. Beard C.M., Kokmen E., O'Brien P.C., Kurland L.T. (1995) The prevalence of dementia is changing over time in Rochester, Minnesota. *Neurology*, **45**: 75–79.
49. Jorm A.F., Jolley D. (1998) The incidence of dementia: a meta-analysis. *Neurology*, **51**: 728–733.
50. Gao S., Hendrie H.C., Hall K.S., Hui S. (1998) The relationships between age, sex, and the incidence of dementia and Alzheimer disease: a meta-analysis. *Arch. Gen. Psychiatry*, **55**: 809–815.
51. Jorm A.F. (1990) *The Epidemiology of Alzheimer's Disease and Related Disorders*, Chapman and Hall, London.
52. Schoenberg B.S., Okazaki H., Kokmen E. (1981) Reduced survival in patients with dementia: a population study. *Trans. Am. Neurol. Assoc.*, **106**: 306–308.
53. van Duijn C.M., Hofman A. (1991) Risk factors for Alzheimer's disease: a collaborative re-analysis of case-control studies. *Int. J. Epidemiol.*, **20** (Suppl. 2).
54. van Duijn C.M., Clayton D., Chandra V., Fratiglioni L., Graves A.B., Heyman A., Jorm A.F., Kokmen E., Kondo K., Mortimer J.A. *et al* (1991) Familial aggregation of Alzheimer's disease and related disorders: a collaborative re-analysis of case-control studies. *Int. J. Epidemiol.*, **20**: S13–S20.

55. Lautenschlager N.T., Cupples L.A., Rao V.S., Auerbach S.A., Becker R., Burke J., Chui H., Duara R., Foley E.J., Glatt S.L. *et al* (1996) Risk of dementia among relatives of Alzheimer's disease patients in the MIRAGE study: what is in store for the oldest old? *Neurology*, **46**: 641–650.
56. Zigman W.B., Schupf N., Sersen E., Silverman W. (1996) Prevalence of dementia in adults with and without Down syndrome. *Am. J. Ment. Retard.*, **100**: 403–412.
57. Plassman B.L., Breitner J.C.S. (1996) Recent advances in the genetics of Alzheimer's disease and vascular dementia with an emphasis on gene–environmental interactions. *J. Am. Geriatr. Soc.*, **44**: 1242–1250.
58. Farrer L.A., Cupples L.A., Haines J.L., Hyman B., Kukull W.A., Mayeux R., Myers R.H., Pericak-Vance M.A., Risch N., van Duijn C.M. (1997) Effects of age, sex, and ethnicity on the association between apolipoprotein E genotype and Alzheimer disease. *JAMA*, **278**: 1349–1356.
59. American College of Medical Genetics/American Society of Human Genetics Working Group on ApoE and Alzheimer Disease (1995) Statement on use of apolipoprotein E testing for Alzheimer disease. *JAMA*, **274**: 1627–1629.
60. Post S.G., Whitehouse P.J., Binstock R.H. (1997) The clinical introduction of genetic testing for Alzheimer's disease: an ethical perspective. *JAMA*, **277**: 832–836.
61. Sobel E., Davanipour Z. (1996) Electromagnetic field exposure may cause increased production of amyloid beta and eventually lead to Alzheimer's disease. *Neurology*, **47**: 1594–1600.
62. Jorm A.F., van Duijn C.M., Chandra V., Fratiglioni L., Graves A., Heyman A., Kokmen E., Kondo K., Mortimer J.A., Rocca W.A. *et al* (1991) Psychiatric history and related exposures as risk factors for Alzheimer's disease: a collaborative re-analysis of case-control studies. *Int. J. Epidemiol.*, **20**: S43–S47.
63. Kessing L. V., Olsen E.W., Mortensen P.B., Andersen P.K. (1999) Dementia in affective disorder: a case-register study. *Acta Psychiatr. Scand.*, **100**: 176–185.
64. Itzhaki R.F., Lin W.-R., Shang D., Wilcock G.K., Faragher B., Jamieson G.A. (1997) Herpes simplex virus type 1 in brain and risk of Alzheimer's disease. *Lancet*, **349**: 241–244.
65. Rocca W.A., van Duijn C.M., Clayton D., Chandra V., Fratiglioni L., Graves A.B., Heyman A., Jorm A.F., Kokmen E., Kondo K. *et al* (1991) Maternal age and Alzheimer's disease: a collaborative re-analysis of case-control studies. *Int. J. Epidemiol.*, **20**: S21–S27.
66. Weinreb H.J. (1986) Dermatoglyphic patterns in Alzheimer's disease. *J. Neurogenetics*, **3**: 233–246.
67. Breteler M.M.B., van Duijn C.M., Chandra V., Fratiglioni L., Graves A.B., Heyman A., Jorm A.F., Kokmen E., Kondo K., Mortimer J.A. *et al* (1991) Medical history and the risk of Alzheimer's disease: a collaborative re-analysis of case-control studies. *Int. J. Epidemiol.*, **20**: S36–S42.
68. Jorm A.F. (1991) Cross-national comparisons of the occurrence of Alzheimer's and vascular dementias. *Eur. Arch. Psychiatry Neurol. Sci.*, **240**: 218–222.
69. White L., Petrovich H., Ross W., Masaki K.H., Abbott R.D., Teng E.L., Rodriguez B.L., Blanchette P.L., Havlik R.J., Wergowske G. *et al* (1996) Prevalence of dementia in older Japanese-American men in Hawaii. *JAMA*, **276**: 955–960.
70. Homma A., Hasegawa K. (2000) Epidemiology of vascular dementia in Japan. In *Cerebral Vascular Disease and Dementia: Pathology, Neuropsychiatry and Management* (Eds E. Chiu, L. Gustafson, D. Ames, M. Folstein), pp. 33–46, Dunitz, London.
71. Hatada K., Okazaki Y., Yoshitake K., Takada K., Nakane Y. (1999) Dementia: further evidence of westernization of dementia prevalence in Nagasaki, Japan, and family recognition. *Int. Psychogeriatrics*, **11**: 123–138.

72. Hendrie H.C., Osuntokun B.O., Hall K.S., Ogunniyi A.O., Hui S.L., Unverzagt F.W., Gureje O., Rodenberg C.A., Baiyewu O., Musick B.S. *et al* (1995) Prevalence of Alzheimer's disease and dementia in two communities: Nigerian Africans and African Americans. *Am. J. Psychiatry*, **152**: 1485–1492.

73. Hendrie H.C. (1998) Indianapolis–Ibadan dementia project. *Neurobiol. Aging*, **19**: S65.

74. Hendrie H.C., Hall K.S., Pillay N., Rodgers D., Prince C., Norton J., Brittain H., Nath A., Blue A., Kaufert J. *et al* (1993) Alzheimer's disease is rare in Cree Indians. *Int. Psychogeriatrics*, **5**: 5–14.

75. Ganguli M., Chandra V., Gilby J.E., Ratcliff G., Sharma S.D., Pandav R., Seaberg E.C., Belle S. (1996) Cognitive test performance in a community-based non-demented elderly sample in rural India: the Indo–US Cross-National Dementia Epidemiology Study. *Int. Psychogeriatrics*, **8**: 507–524.

76. Chandra V., Ganguli M., Pandav R., Johnston M.S., Belle S., De Kosky S.T. (1998) Prevalence of Alzheimer's and other dementias in rural India: the Indo–US study. *Neurology*, **51**: 1000–1008.

77. Roberts G.W., Gentlemen S.M., Lynch A., Graham D.I. (1991) $\beta$A4 amyloid protein deposition in brain after head trauma. *Lancet*, **338**: 1422–1423.

78. Mortimer J.A., Van Duijn C.M., Chandra V., Fratiglioni L., Graves A.B., Heyman A., Jorm A.F., Kokmen E., Kondo K., Rocca W.A. *et al* (1991) Head trauma as a risk factor for Alzheimer's disease: a collaborative re-analysis of case-control studies. *Int. J. Epidemiol.*, **20**: S28–S35.

79. Breteler M.M.B., de Groot R.R.M., van Romunde L.K.J., Hofman A. (1995) Risk of dementia in patients with Parkinson's disease, epilepsy, and severe head trauma: a register-based follow-up study. *Am. J. Epidemiol.*, **142**: 1300–1305.

80. Williams D.B., Annegers J.F., Kokmen E.O., Brien P.C., Kurland L.T. (1991) Brain injury and neurologic sequelae: a cohort study of dementia, parkinsonism, and amyotrophic lateral sclerosis. *Neurology*, **41**: 1554–1557.

81. Mayeux R., Ottman R., Maestre G., Ngai C., Tang M.X., Ginsberg H., Chun M., Tycko B., Shelanski M. (1995) Synergistic effects of traumatic head injury and apolipoprotein-E4 in patients with Alzheimer's disease. *Neurology*, **45**: 555–557.

82. Nicoll J.A., Roberts G.W., Graham D.I. (1995) Apolipoprotein E epsilon 4 allele is associated with deposition of amyloid beta-protein following head injury. *Nature Med.*, **1**: 135–137.

83. Doll R. (1993) Review: Alzheimer's disease and environmental aluminium. *Age Ageing*, **22**: 138–153.

84. Anonymous (1992) Is aluminium a dementing ion? *Lancet*, **339**: 713–714.

85. Rifat S.L., Eastwood M.R., McLachlan D.R.C., Corey P.N. (1990) Effect of exposure of miners to aluminium powder. *Lancet*, **336**: 1162–1165.

86. Douglas R. (1998) Alzheimer's disease, drinking water and aluminium content. *Australasian J. Ageing*, **17**: 2–3.

87. Sobel E., Dunn M., Davanipour D.V.M., Qian Z., Chiu H.C. (1996) Elevated risk of Alzheimer's disease among workers with likely electromagnetic field exposure. *Neurology*, **47**: 1477–1481.

88. Feychting M., Pedersen N.L., Svedberg P., Floderus B., Gatz M. (1998) Dementia and occupational exposure to magnetic fields. *Scand. J. Work Environ. Health*, **24**: 46–53.

89. Savitz D.A., Checkoway H., Loomis D.P. (1998) Magnetic field exposure and neurodegenerative disease mortality among electric utility workers. *Epidemiology*, **9**: 398–404.

90. Breitner J.C.S. (1996)  Inflammatory processes and anti-inflammatory drugs in Alzheimer's disease: a current appraisal. *Neurobiol. Aging*, **17**: 789–794.

91. McGeer P.L., Schulzer M., McGeer E.G. (1996)  Arthritis and anti-inflammatory agents as possible protective factors for Alzheimer's disease: a review of 17 epidemiologic studies. *Neurology*, **47**: 425–432.

92. Burns A., Murphy D. (1996)  Protection against Alzheimer's disease? *Lancet*, **348**: 420–421.

93. Yaffe K., Sawaya G., Lieberburg I., Grady D. (1998)  Estrogen therapy in postmenopausal women: effects on cognitive function and dementia. *JAMA*, **279**: 688–695.

94. Shumaker S.A., Reboussin B.A., Espeland M.A., Rapp S.R., McBee W.L., Dailey M., Bowen D., Terrell T., Jones B.N. (1998)  The Women's Health Initiative Memory Study (WHIMS): a trial of the effect of estrogen therapy in preventing and slowing the progression of dementia. *Contr. Clin. Trials*, **19**: 604–621.

95. Farmer M.E., Kittner S.J., Rae D.S., Bartko J.J., Regier D.A. (1995)  Education and change in cognitive function. The epidemiologic catchment area study. *Ann. Epidemiol.*, **5**: 1–7.

96. Stern Y., Gurland B., Tatemichi T.K., Tang M.X., Wilder D., Mayeux R. (1994)  Influence of education and occupation on the incidence of Alzheimer's disease. *JAMA*, **271**: 1004–1010.

97. White L., Katzman R., Losonczy K., Salive M., Wallace R., Berkman L., Taylor J., Fillenbaum G., Havlik R. (1994)  Association of education with incidence of cognitive impairment in three established populations for epidemiological studies of the elderly. *J. Clin. Epidemiol.*, **47**: 363–374.

98. Mortimer J.A. (1988)  Do psychosocial risk factors contribute to Alzheimer's disease? In *Etiology of Dementia of Alzheimer's Type* (Eds A.S. Henderson, J.H. Henderson), pp. 39–52, Wiley, Chichester.

99. Stern Y., Alexander G.E., Prohovnik I., Mayeux R. (1992)  Inverse relationship between education and parietotemporal perfusion deficit in Alzheimer's disease. *Ann. Neurol.*, **32**: 371–375.

100. Schmand B., Smit J.H., Geerlings M.I., Lindeboom J. (1997)  The effects of intelligence and education on the development of dementia. A test of the brain reserve hypothesis. *Psychol. Med.*, **27**: 1337–1344.

101. Snowdon D.A., Kemper S.J., Mortimer J.A., Greiner L.H., Wekstein D.R., Markesbery W.R. (1996)  Linguistic ability in early life and cognitive function and Alzheimer's disease in late life. *JAMA*, **275**: 528–532.

102. Schofield P. (1999)  Alzheimer's disease and brain reserve. *Australasian J. Ageing*, **18**: 10–14.

103. Gorelick P.B. (1997)  Status of risk factors for dementia associated with stroke. *Stroke*, **28**: 459–463.

104. Skoog I. (1994)  Risk factors for vascular dementia: a review. *Dementia*, **5**: 137–144.

105. Slooter A.J.C., Tang M.-X., van Duijn C.M., Stern Y., Ott A., Bell K., Breteler M.M.B., Van Breckhoven C., Tatemichi T.K., Tycko B. *et al* (1997)  Apolipoprotein E ε4 and the risk of dementia with stroke. *JAMA*, **277**: 818–821.

106. Brody J.A., Schneider E.L. (1986)  Disease and disorders of aging: an hypothesis. *J. Chron. Dis.*, **39**: 871–876.

107. Rose G. (1992)  *The Strategy of Preventive Medicine*, Oxford University Press, Oxford.

108. Australian Institute of Health and Welfare (1996)  *Australia's Health 1996*, Australian Government Publishing Service, Canberra.

# Commentaries

## 1.1
## The Continuing Evolution of Dementia Epidemiology
Mary Ganguli[1]

Henderson and Jorm have raised several provocative issues, all of which cry out for well-designed, adequately powered, longitudinal studies in representative populations. For example, they offer a model of normal aging and dementia at either end of a continuum of cognitive function, with quantitative rather than qualitative differences between them. Undoubtedly, it is hard to distinguish between the cognitive impairments associated with normal aging and early or incipient dementia, and certainly, both conditions involve quantitatively different progressive memory loss and plaque and tangle counts in the brain. However, to conclude that dementia represents accelerated aging is also to suggest, without proof, that dementia is an inevitable consequence of aging. Within the average life span, there is in fact evidence of qualitative differences between normal aging and dementia. Functionally, for example, memory loss in normal elderly appears to be largely a retrieval deficit which can be overcome by cuing, while in Alzheimer's disease (AD) there is an encoding deficit which makes retrieval virtually impossible. Further, AD patients have deficits in both semantic and episodic memory, while normal elderly lose primarily episodic memory [1]. Structurally, for example, there are qualitative differences between AD and normal aging brains in the patterns of neuron loss within different regions of the hippocampus [2].

Twenty years ago, depression and dementia were regarded as almost mutually exclusive; clinicians were urged to diagnose and treat "depressive pseudodementia" and be reassured by the resolution of the cognitive impairment along with the depressive symptoms. Unfortunately, over time the majority of these patients went on to develop dementia. Today, a body of case-control research clearly shows depression and dementia to be independently associated with each other, while a few longitudinal studies suggest that depression precedes dementia more often than would be expected by chance. Perhaps depression is an independent risk factor for dementia, e.g. through prolonged hypercortisolemia, which can damage the hippocampus. Alternatively, it may be a prodrome of dementia, either

[1] *Department of Psychiatry, University of Pittsburgh School of Medicine, Pittsburgh, PA 15213, USA*

through disruption of serotonergic circuits by the general neurodegenerative process or through psychological mechanisms related to the patient's growing struggle to cope with failing cognitive abilities [3].

Alzheimer's and vascular dementias co-occur frequently and appear to share risk factors; it is often hard to distinguish between them [4]. Definitions of vascular dementia are still evolving. In a group of nuns with AD pathology at autopsy, clinical manifestations were observed during life primarily among those who also had subcortical infarcts [5]. It is easy to assume that risk factors for vascular dementia are the same as risk factors for stroke; the more intriguing question is why some individuals develop dementia after stroke while others do not. As advances occur in the treatment of acute stroke and subsequent survival, it becomes increasingly important to identify risk and protective factors for dementia after stroke.

Studies from developing countries suggest that the prevalence of dementia is lower in populations with shorter life-expectancy. This finding may reflect the smaller proportion of individuals who live into the age of risk for dementia, and, further, may be the ones with fewer risk factors. It may also be related to shorter survival once the disease has manifested itself. There is clearly potential for discovering new risk and protective factors in these populations. There is also a chilling possibility that an increasing burden of chronic disease, including dementia, is the price we pay for improving standards of living and life expectancy across the planet.

Henderson and Jorm demonstrate the dramatic evolution of epidemiology beyond the simple counting of cases it is too often believed to be. Dementia is a classic example of Morris's [6] "uses of epidemiology". Alzheimer's original single case report [7] shows his belief that the disease subsequently named for him was a rare condition of middle-aged people. The landmark epidemiological studies of the Newcastle group [8], half a century later, completed the clinical picture of the disease by demonstrating it to be a relatively common condition of older people. At the end of the twentieth century, research into disease mechanisms, risk and protective factors, prevention and treatment is on an exponential course. Epidemiology is gaining momentum in its vital role of examining the real-world implications of clinical and laboratory discoveries, and of identifying patterns and associations in the population at large for further exploration in the clinic and laboratory.

## REFERENCES

1. Craik F.I.M., Anderson N.D., Kerr S.A., Li K.Z.H. (1995) Memory changes in normal ageing. In *Handbook of Memory Disorders* (Eds A.D. Baddeley, B.A. Wilson, F.A. Watts), pp. 211–241, Wiley, Chichester.

2.  West M.J., Coleman P.D., Flood D.G., Troncoso J.C. (1997)   Is Alzheimer's disease accelerated aging? Patterns of age and Alzheimer's disease related neuronal losses in the hippocampus. In *Connections, Cognition, and Alzheimer's Disease* (Eds B.T. Hyman, C. Duyckaerts, Y. Christen), pp. 141–147, Springer, Berlin.
3.  Chen P. Ganguli M., Mulsant B.H., DeKosky S.T. (1999)   The temporal relationship between depressive symptoms and dementia: a community-based prospective study. *Arch. Gen. Psychiatry*, **56**: 261–266.
4.  Skoog I. (1998)   Status of risk factors for vascular dementia. *Neuroepidemiology*, **17**: 2–9.
5.  Snowdon D.A., Greiner L.H., Mortimer J.A., Riley K.P., Greiner P.A., Markesbery W.R. (1997)   Brain infarction and the clinical expression of Alzheimer disease. The Nun Study. *JAMA*, **277**: 813–817.
6.  Morris J.N. (1975)   *Uses of Epidemiology*, Livingstone, Edinburgh.
7.  Alzheimer A. (1907)   Uber eine eigenartige Erkrankung de Hirnrinde. *Allgemeine Zeitschrift fur Psychiatrie und Psychisch-Gerichtliche Medizin*, **64**: 146–148.
8.  Kay D.W.K., Beamish P., Roth M. (1964)   Old age mental disorders in Newcastle Upon Tyne. Part I: A study of prevalence. *Br. J. Psychiatry*, **110**: 146–158.

1.2
# Dementia: Hope for the Future

Simon Lovestone[1]

In their review Henderson and Jorm note that dementia has only come to prominence in the late twentieth century. This is something of an understatement; my impression is that the increase in public awareness has really only come in the last 10 years; and there is still some way to go. Why is this? Surely part of the reason is, as Henderson and Jorm suggest, the unprecedented increase in the elderly. However, two other factors must be mentioned: the Alzheimer Societies and science. Both provide hope, and perhaps hope is necessary for the public to confront the devastation of Alzheimer's disease (AD), for the media to engage with the subject, and for professionals to spend entire life-times working in the area. The lay societies have contributed immensely by providing tangible and emotional support for carers and relatives, and by engaging with health care organizations and governments to provide ever better care. Science provides hope of a different kind—hope for understanding that might lead to prevention or cure.

Perhaps the first indication that such optimism is justified comes from the acetylcholinesterase inhibitors. These compounds, directly resulting from the discovery that it is the cholinergic system that is lost first and most in AD, modify the symptoms of AD, but were not expected to alter

[1] *Institute of Psychiatry, De Crespigny Park, London SE5 8AF, UK*

the disease pathogenesis itself. The effect is almost certainly time-limited, but in those individuals responding to the drug there is a small improvement or temporary stabilization in both cognition and function. These modest effects are hugely important. For the first time AD can now be considered a treatable disorder. The compounds are relatively expensive and, although widely licensed for use, are only patchily available. Doubts remain regarding cost–benefit and effects on the quality of life for patients and carers. However, one almost inevitable result, wherever the compounds are in use, is that the profile of AD will be raised further, that primary care health-teams will recognize more dementia, and that the possibility of early intervention with appropriate services and carer supports will increase. These developments should not be underestimated.

However, it is approaches that will modify the disorder itself that are needed. Henderson and Jorm note that autosomal dominant AD is very rare. However, genetic discoveries from these occasional families have contributed to the huge advances in understanding, which suggest that disease-modification therapies will become available sooner rather than later. The discovery that mutations in the amyloid precursor protein (APP) and pre-senilin genes both give rise to dementia and both alter the processing of the APP, resulting in more Ab peptide, are good evidence that this is a critical step in the process [1]. Henderson and Jorm are right to point to the potential for vaccines as hugely exciting, but other, more conventional pharmacological approaches, reducing the fibrillization of the Ab peptide or modifying the metabolism of the APP molecule, are already well advanced [2].

In the review, a categorical approach is adopted, splitting the dementias into their separate diseases, although the case of mixed AD and vascular dementia is noted. In fact, increasing evidence suggests that isolated vascular pathology causing dementia is considerably less common than mixed pathology. Understanding the relationship between the different pathologies is important, as illustrated by the case of the frontotemporal degenerations, some of which have neurofibrillary pathology similar to AD but without amyloid deposits. These disorders have been called the tauopathies, as the neurofibrillary tangles are composed of the protein tau. Confirmation of the amyloid cascade hypothesis was provided by the discovery that mutations in tau cause some variants of these disorders [3]. Thus we now know that changes in APP precede changes in tau in AD, but that the changes in tau are a sufficient cause of dementia. Just what these changes are is being actively researched but might include the phosphorylation of tau or altered aggregation. In both cases the normal function of tau in the brain is altered. Preventing these changes is another route towards disease modification, and at least in the case of tau phosphorylation we already have compounds that reduce phosphorylation and restore function in cells [4]. Understanding other complex interrelationships between the dementias will, I suspect, result in more insights to common pathogenic pathways.

Epidemiological science also provides hope, as Henderson and Jorm outline, by identifying risk factors that might be modified. One factor not mentioned is diabetes, which in multiple studies, including longitudinal, does seem to significantly increase risk [5]. The observation that insulin resistance also increases risk [6] suggests that it is not the long-term sequelae of diabetes, such as vascular damage, but something to do with the disorder itself that affects the pathogenesis of AD. Here molecular and epidemiological sciences may merge, as considerable knowledge already exists regarding the insulin signalling events and, importantly, insulin has been shown to alter the properties of tau, reducing phosphorylation through inhibition of glycogen synthase kinase-3.

Epidemiology and molecular science are also coming together through genetics and there is considerable hope that this will yield important insights into personal vulnerability to the environmental risk and protective factors highlighted by Henderson and Jorm. Certainly there are more genetic factors to be identified. Apolipoprotein E contributes only half of the genetic variance of AD, and the next few years will see more genes identified by association studies and by genome scanning approaches. As the human genome mapping project matures and maps of single nucleotide polymorphisms (the subtle differences in genes that accounts for all inherited variation) are produced, this work will accelerate. We can expect many false positives and will have to ensure that repeated replication within studies in different populations and between studies is achieved. Such appears to be the case for the angiotensin converting enzyme (ACE) gene that we identified as a risk factor for AD [7], again bringing together genetics and epidemiology, as ACE plays a critical role in the vasopressor response, and hypertension and related factors appear to be risk factors for AD.

Clearly dementia is a prevalent disorder and with the projected rise in the elderly is set to increase substantially. However, there are considerable grounds for optimism. The advocates for those with dementia are growing stronger and the ears of governments and others are increasingly attuned to the need for better care and more research. The research is accelerating at a dizzying pace and the first fruits of this research have reached the clinic already. A significant step forward would come from the first drug shown to alter the pathogenesis of AD and many potential such compounds are already well-developed. There is one important catch, however. Any such drug will inevitably carry the huge costs of research and development and be correspondingly expensive. As Henderson and Jorm point out, the very countries least able to afford such costs will be the ones experiencing the largest growth in dementia. Hope, as always, is tempered by politics and economics.

# REFERENCES

1. Storey E., Cappai R. (1999) The amyloid precursor protein of Alzheimer's disease and the Ab peptide. *Neuropathol. Appl. Neurobiol.*, **25**: 81–97.
2. Mills J., Reiner P.B. (1999) Regulation of amyloid precursor protein cleavage. *J. Neurochem.*, **72**: 443–460.
3. Goedert M., Crowther R.A., Spillantini M. (1998) Tau mutations cause fronto-temporal dementias. *Neuron*, **21**: 955–958.
4. Lovestone S., Davis D.R., Webster M.-T., Kaech S., Brion J.-P., Matus A., Anderton B.H. (1999) Lithium reduces tau phosphorylation—effects in living cells and in neurons at therapeutic concentrations. *Biol. Psychiatry*, **45**: 995–1003.
5. Stewart R., Liolitsa D. (1999) Type 2 diabetes mellitus, cognitive impairment and dementia. *Diabet. Med.*, **16**: 93–112.
6. Kuusisto J., Koivisto K., Mykkänen L., Helkala E.L., Vanhanen M., Hänninen T., Kervinen K., Kesäniemi Y.A., Riekkinen P.J., Laakso M. (1997) Association between features of the insulin resistance syndrome and Alzheimer's disease independently of apolipoprotein E4 phenotype: cross sectional population based study. *Br. Med. J.*, **315**: 1045–1049.
7. Kehoe P.G., Russ C., McIlroy S., Williams H., Holmans P., Holmes C., Liolitsa D., Vahidassr D., Powell J., McGleenon B. *et al* (1999) Variation in *DCP1*, encoding ACE, is associated with susceptibility to Alzheimer disease. *Nature Genet.*, **21**: 71–72.

1.3
## Dementia: Much Information, Many Unanswered Questions

Lissy F. Jarvik[1]

With the aging of the population worldwide, the dementias are assuming ever greater importance, and the costs of treating them are about to have a major impact on national budgets. Dementia is not only the most frequent psychiatric diagnosis among the old, but the only psychiatric disorder more prevalent in geriatric than in younger age groups. Henderson and Jorm discuss the complex issues of prevalence, incidence and the distinction between them, as well as their antecedents and consequences, in a manner which is bound to leave even the uninitiated reader well informed. Their expertise is clearly apparent. Overall, their chapter represents the state of

[1] *Department of Biobehavioral Sciences, Neuropsychiatric Institute and Hospital, University of California, Los Angeles, CA, USA*

the art, provides much information and raises many questions, as illustrated by a small sampling below:

1. Is dementia the inevitable consequence of the natural aging process? The authors leave the question open. Yet, the impressive data they assembled show that even though the prevalence of dementia increases with advancing age, it never comes close to 100% (e.g., 45% at ages 95–99). And we know that Jeanne Calment, who died when 122 years old—with widely publicized fully documented age and mental status—was not demented according to repeated neuropsychologic examinations.

2. What are the prospects for preventing dementia? There are promising leads, but no method has as yet been established. This data-based conclusion is vitally important at a time when there is great temptation to recommend remedies with as yet unproven side effects and unknown long-term consequences; for example, the vaccination of individuals at risk for the development of Alzheimer's disease (AD).

3. Does education protect against dementia? What is the relationship between education, premorbid intelligence, and neuronal endowment? Henderson and Jorm introduce us to the current controversies assigning pre-eminence to one or another of these factors. It is possible also that we are dealing with complex interactions of several factors. Not only do the more intelligent tend to get better educated but, judging by animal data [1], intellectual activity may enhance synaptic connections at any time throughout life. The high correlation between linguistic ability in the third decade of life and the autopsy diagnosis of AD in the seventh decade and beyond is intriguing. As described in the review, this observation, stemming from a study of nuns, has been taken to suggest that high verbal ability protects against AD. However, it is conceivable also that low verbal ability may be a very early result of an otherwise asymptomatic AD process, or the operation of pleiotropic genes. In an old prospective study [2] with a group far less educated than the college-trained nuns, and first examined neuropsychologically at age 60 or older (then functioning within the normal range), verbal ability also distinguished between those with and without a subsequent (20 years later) diagnosis of dementia (based on clinical, not autopsy findings). Exploring very early as well as later differences in verbal abilities as predictors of cognitive decline, especially when combined with neuroimaging (e.g. [3]), may provide new clues. Expanding the search into adjacent areas, e.g. dyslexia [4], may also prove highly profitable.

4. What is the relation of depression to dementia? Is it a risk factor? An early symptom of dementia, both Alzheimer and vascular types? A reaction of the dementing individual to the perceived mental decline?

The coexistence of two independent, possibly interacting processes? These questions are currently without answers.

5. The distinction between cognitive decline which does and does not progress to dementia remains elusive. Identifying valid differences will relieve much fear and apprehension among the older population and is likely to enhance understanding of both.

6. Henderson and Jorm make an important contribution in pointing to the evidence for multiple risk factors in the development of dementia. Even though the complex interplay of endogenous and exogenous risk factors was noted by dementia researchers decades ago (e.g. [5]), current treatment approaches still continue to focus on monotherapy. That is surprising since the idea is not a new one (e.g. [6]) and, since the adoption of multipronged approaches has proved to be so successful in cancer therapy, I do not see how we can justify continuing to pursue the same old paths tried so often and found wanting. Finally, there is another venue to be added. Since neuroimaging has demonstrated that behavioural changes (e.g. behavioural therapy of obsessive-compulsive disorder [7]) can lead to brain changes as well as the reverse, it behooves us to explore the combination of psychologic interventions with other techniques.

In conclusion, the fact that Henderson and Jorm have raised so many questions which are still without answers should spur us on to creative innovations which will yield successful treatments for many victims of dementia before the twenty-first century has a chance to achieve maturity.

## REFERENCES

1. Bennett E.L., Diamond M.C., Krech D., Rosenzweig M.R. (1996) Chemical and anatomical plasticity of brain. *J. Neuropsychiat. Clin. Neurosci.*, **8**: 459–470.
2. La Rue A., Jarvik L.F. (1987) Cognitive function and prediction of dementia in old age. *Int. J. Aging Hum. Develop.*, **25**: 79–89.
3. Small G.W., La Rue A., Komo S., Kaplan A., Mandelkern M.A. (1995) Predictors of cognitive change in middle-aged and older adults with memory loss. *Am. J. Psychiatry*, **152**: 1757–1764.
4. Lambe E.K. (1999) Dyslexia, gender, and brain imaging. *Neuropsychologia*, **37**: 521–536.
5. Kallmann F.J. (1953) *Heredity in Health and Mental Disorder*, Norton, New York.
6. Jarvik L.F. (1988) The future: some speculations. In *Treatments for the Alzheimer Patient: The Long Haul* (Eds L.F. Jarvik, C.H. Winograd), pp. 186–194, Springer, New York.

7. Schwartz J.M., Stoessel P.W., Baxter L.R. Jr., Martin K.M., Phelps M.E. (1996) Systematic changes in cerebral glucose metabolic rate after successful behaviour modification treatment of obsessive-compulsive disorder. *Arch. Gen. Psychiatry*, **53**: 109–113.

1.4

**Vascular Factors and Dementia**

Ingmar Skoog[1]

The review by Henderson and Jorm highlights the public health importance of dementia disorders, and the need for possible preventive strategies. As outlined in the review, several risk factors and possible protective factors have been suggested for Alzheimer's disease (AD), the most common form of dementia. Vascular risk factors were just mentioned briefly. However, several vascular disorders have been found to affect cognitive function in the population [1], and stroke increases the risk for dementia several-fold [2]. In addition, despite the findings that cerebrovascular diseases are generally exclusionary for the clinical diagnosis of AD, several epidemiological studies have recently reported an association between AD and vascular risk factors, such as hypertension, coronary heart disease, atrial fibrillation, diabetes mellitus, generalized atherosclerosis, smoking, anemia, and alterations in hemostasis [3,4]. The association between blood pressure and AD may be rather complicated, as illustrated by a longitudinal study [5] which reported that both systolic and diastolic blood pressure was increased 10–15 years before the onset of AD. However, blood pressure decreased the years before onset of dementia, and subjects who had manifest dementia had lower blood pressure levels than the non-demented [6]. The well-established association between inheritance of the apolipoprotein ε4 allele and AD may also suggest a vascular etiology in AD, as this allele has been implicated as a susceptibility factor for cardiovascular disease.

Neuropathological studies also suggest an association. Non-demented individuals with coronary heart disease [7] and hypertension [8] exhibit increased amounts of Alzheimer changes in their brains. Additionally, it has since long been recognized that AD is associated with profound changes in the cerebral microvessels [9]. Ischemic white matter lesions, associated with lipohyalinosis and narrowing of the lumen of the small perforating arteries and arterioles which nourish the deep white matter, have been

---

[1] *Department of Psychiatry, Sahlgrenska University Hospital, S–413 45 Göteborg, Sweden*

described in both clinical and autopsied cases of AD [10]. These lesions have consistently been associated with a history of hypertension.

It is not entirely clear how peripheral vascular disease may increase the risk of AD, but even if it only increases the risk by a small amount it may have a strong impact on the incidence of dementia, as cardiovascular disorders are very common in old age. Cerebrovascular disease and AD may thus often coincide, and it is often difficult to differentiate between AD and vascular dementia (VD). The use of different criteria for VD may thus result in substantial differences in the proportion of demented individuals diagnosed as having VD or AD [11]. The findings of an association between AD and vascular factors may thus reflect an overdiagnosis of AD in individuals with silent cerebrovascular disease. Indeed, a considerable proportion of subjects from the general population will have mixed pathologies [12]. The importance of this overlap has been emphasized by the 'Nun Study', which demonstrated that cerebrovascular diseases may increase the possibility that individuals with Alzheimer lesions in their brains will express a dementia syndrome [13]. Cerebrovascular disease may thus be the event that finally overcomes the brain's compensatory capacity in a subject whose brain is already compromised by Alzheimer pathology, and in many instances minor manifestations of both disorders which individually would be insufficient to produce dementia may produce it together [14]. Therapy against the cerebrovascular component could therefore ameliorate the symptoms of dementia in individuals with AD. For example, treatment of hypertension or atrial fibrillation to prevent new ischemic infarcts may be a rational approach to treating AD.

The association between AD and vascular factors may also reflect that similar mechanisms, e.g. disturbances of the blood–brain barrier (BBB), apolipoprotein E, oxidative stress the renin–angiotensin system, apoptosis and psychological stress, may be involved in both disorders [3,4]. These mechanisms may also interact, so that one disorder stimulates the other.

AD pathology may also cause or stimulate vascular diseases. It was reported that elderly individuals without previous stroke and with very low cognitive ability (which may represent a clinical diagnosis of AD) were at increased risk for later development of stroke [15]. AD pathology may also lead to lesions in the cerebral microvasculature. Thomas *et al* [16] reported that the interaction of β-amyloid with endothelial cells of the rat aorta produced excess of superoxide radicals, which caused endothelial damage.

It seems clear that there is a connection between AD and vascular factors. The exact mechanism behind this association, and how it will affect treatment, is not clear. In cases with concomitant cerebrovascular disease and AD, treatment of the vascular component may affect the clinical expression of AD. If vascular factors are involved in the pathogenesis of AD, it may have large implications for primary and secondary prevention.

## ACKNOWLEDGEMENT

The work was supported by a working grant from the Swedish Medical Research Council.

## REFERENCES

1. Breteler M.M.B., Claus J.J., Grobbee D.E., Hofman A. (1994) Cardiovascular disease and distribution of cognitive function in elderly people: the Rotterdam study. *Br. Med. J.*, **308**: 1604–1608.
2. Tatemichi T.K., Desmond D.W., Mayeux R., Paik M., Stern Y., Sano M., Remien R.H., Williams J.B., Mohr J.P., Hauser W.A. *et al* (1992) Dementia after stroke: baseline frequency, risks, and clinical features in a hospitalized cohort. *Neurology*, **42**: 1185–1193.
3. Skoog I. (1999) The interaction between vascular disorders and Alzheimer's disease. In *Alzheimer's Disease and Related Disorders: Etiology, Pathogenesis and Therapeutics* (Eds K. Iqbal, D.F. Swaab, B. Winblad, H.M. Wisniewski), pp. 523–530, Wiley, Chichester.
4. Skoog I., Kalaria R.N., Breteler M.M. (1999) Vascular factors and Alzheimer disease. *Alz. Dis. Assoc. Disord.*, **13** (Suppl. 3): S106–S114.
5. Skoog I., Lernfelt B., Landahl S., Palmertz B., Andreasson L.-A., Nilsson L., Persson G., Odén A., Svanborg A. (1996) A 15-year longitudinal study on blood pressure and dementia. *Lancet*, **347**: 1141–1145.
6. Skoog I., Andersson L.-A., Palmertz B., Landahl S., Lernfelt B. (1998) A population-based study on blood pressure and brain atrophy in 85-year-olds. *Hypertension*, **32**: 404–409.
7. Sparks D.L., Hunsaker J.C. III, Scheff S.W., Kryscio R.J., Henson J.L., Markesbery W.R. (1990) Cortical senile plaques in coronary artery disease, aging and Alzheimer's disease. *Neurobiol. Aging*, **11**: 601–607.
8. Sparks D.L., Scheff S.W., Liu H., Landers T.M., Coyne C.M., Hunsaker J.C. III (1995) Increased incidence of neurofibrillary tangles (NFT) in non-demented individuals with hypertension. *J. Neurol. Sci.*, **131**: 162–169.
9. Kalaria R.N. (1996) Cerebral vessels in ageing and Alzheimer's disease. *Pharmacol. Ther.*, **72**: 193–214.
10. Skoog I., Palmertz B., Andreasson L.-A. (1994) The prevalence of white matter lesions on computed tomography of the brain in demented and non-demented 85-year olds. *J. Geriatr. Psychiatry Neurol.*, **7**: 169–175.
11. Wetterling T., Kanitz R.-D., Borgis K.-J. (1996) Comparison of different diagnostic criteria for vascular dementia (ADDTC, DSM-IV, ICD-10, NINDS-AIREN). *Stroke*, **27**: 30–36.
12. Lim A., Tsuang D., Kukull W., Nochlin D., Leverenz J., McCormick W., Bowen J., Teri L., Thompson J., Peskind E.R. *et al* (1999) Clinico-neuropathological correlation of Alzheimer's disease in a community-based case series. *J. Am. Geriatr. Soc.*, **47**: 564–569.

13. Snowdon D.A., Greiner L.H., Mortimer J.A., Riley K.P., Greiner P.A., Markesbery W.R. (1997) Brain infarction and the clinical expression of Alzheimer disease. The Nun Study. *JAMA*, **277**: 813–817.
14. Erkinjuntti T., Hachinski V. (1993) Dementia post stroke. In *Physical Medicine and Rehabilitation: State of the Art Reviews*, vol. 7 (Ed. W. Teasell), pp. 195–212, Hanley & Belfus, Philadelphia.
15. Ferrucci L., Guralnik J.M., Salive M.E., Pahor M., Corti M.-C., Baroni A., Havlik R.J. (1996) Cognitive impairment and risk of stroke in the older population. *J. Am. Geriatr. Soc.*, **44**: 237–241.
16. Thomas T., Thomas G., McLendon C., Sutton T., Mullan M. (1996) β-amyloid-mediated vasoactivity and vascular endothelial damage. *Nature*, **380**: 168–171.

1.5
# Dementia: Known and Unknown
Eric D. Caine[1]

The review by Henderson and Jorm is especially compelling when one considers the fundamental ignorance and professional disinterest in dementia a mere 25–30 years ago, when many of us were beginning medical careers. One might well argue that the study of the neurodegenerative diseases that cause dementia now is the forefront of psychiatry, involving genetics, molecular biology and neuropathology, clinical phenomenology and therapeutics. This work can be considered from multiple perspectives.

There are no other conditions to be found in the psychiatric landscape where one can establish a diagnosis in life with as high accuracy (i.e. validity) as Alzheimer's disease (AD). While this is a diagnosis of exclusion, careful evaluation and follow-up yield remarkably robust results. The confidence that one derives from valid case definition serves as a powerful bulwark for the type of epidemiological work reviewed by Henderson and Jorm. At the same time, one must remain cautious about many current conclusions or assertions. This does not arise from any lack of scientific rigor; rather, a fair reading of the review and other work suggests that AD is not a unitary entity, as we have stated confidently during the past 20 years, despite its common neuropathology.

Throughout the past 150 years, physicians and other scientists regarded histopathology as the gold standard for correlative diagnosis. Focusing on characteristic stainable changes in brain cellular structure served, during the 1970s, to abolish any doubts about the unity of AD, such that apparently

[1] *University of Rochester Medical Center, 300 Crittenden Boulevard, Rochester, NY 14649-8409, USA*

arbitrary distinctions about age of onset disappeared. However, recent clinical, genetic and pathological research suggests that AD is an array of pathobiological disorders, characterized by genetic heterogeneity and ill-defined neuropathological and clinical borders. Included in the current "soup," one may find a variety of conditions such as "Lewy-body dementia", "frontotemporal dementia", and at least some vascular disease-based dementing conditions. It is ironic. Brain pathology had been the gold standard; now it must be viewed as an intermediate manifestation of fundamental molecular dysfunctions. Until we have developed valid molecular diagnostic tests, however, we will not know how to group true kin and separate phenocopies, where the phenotype is as much histopathological as it is clinical.

Henderson and Jorm's review also invites one to view the borderland between dementia and "normal aging" (perhaps one should say "normative aging"). At present we do not consider "aging" as a disease diagnosis. That was a practice of a bygone era. However, there is no doubt that normative aging processes are associated with definable and substantial cognitive losses in most people. While there are, as yet, no explanations for the fundamental nature of such declines, it is highly probably that, as we discern their molecular basis(-es), there will be substantial pressure from patients and their families, physicians, and industry to compensate for them therapeutically. Indeed, given the large aging populations in the USA, Europe and Japan, we may need such interventions just to maintain an effective work force into later years of life. So-called "age-related cognitive decline" (the DSM-IV "V" code name for "normative aging") may be as common a target for treatment (perhaps more common, given its greater apparent proportion in the population) as diseases that cause dementia.

While some might argue that such "patients" ought not to receive treatment, given their "benign" condition, one can imagine a scenario in which a very mildly impaired or at-risk individual enters the doctor's office, concerned about cognitive complaints. Molecular testing may show one or several risk factors warranting intervention. Under optimal circumstances, there will have been no significant, functionally impairing deterioration, and therapy can be initiated before any irreversible neuronal damage has supervened. Whether the patient has incipient AD, "z-factor" vasculopathy, or, the most common, "partial neuronal senescence due to mitochondrial depletion" (futuristic jargon, perhaps, for "normal aging"), the clinician will be challenged to provide effective interventions. Henderson and Jorm, and others in the field, today provide the necessary epidemiological database to assess whether newly developing therapies will make a difference in population-based rates of dementia. But at this time we have scant data regarding the case definition, epidemiology, natural history or functional outcome of aging-affected individuals. The best research has been in the "cognitive psychology of aging" literature, but it is not readily transported to the epidemiological and medical perspectives needed for establishing baseline data upon which to build a better understanding of targets for clinical interventions.

Another dimension: the diseases that cause the clinical presentation that we label "dementia" also lead to a variety of other manifestations, including changes in mood and emotion, disordered perception, and profound alterations in personality. Often the most troubling challenges for families and caregivers are behavioural problems such as wandering or aggression, not cognitive complaints. During this past decade, a literature addressing this topic has grown steadily, albeit slowly [1,2]. Unfortunately, there are few systematic studies of the epidemiology or natural history of the behavioural, mood, emotional or perceptual symptoms and signs of patients suffering neurodegenerative diseases. We desperately need such work to guide therapeutic interventions. No doubt, psychotropic medications can influence the behaviour or depressive symptoms of patients with AD. When and for how long are they indicated? Is there a predictable course for such symptoms? Are symptoms and signs stable or do they change over time? Does the depression or psychosis that is so commonly encountered in such patients remit spontaneously? Do distinctive signs and symptoms relate to fundamentally different molecular neuropathological mechanisms or specific changes in brain function?

Henderson and Jorm point to a wealth of data that emphasizes extraordinary progress during the past 30 years. Their review, as well, underscores the opportunities for new research during the decades ahead.

## REFERENCES

1. Finkel S. (1996) Behavioral and psychological symptoms of dementia. *Int. Psychogeriatrics*, **8** (Suppl. 3): 215–552.
2. Hope T., Keene J., Fairburn C.G., Jacoby R., McShane R. (1999) Natural history of behavioural changes and psychiatric symptoms in Alzheimer's disease. *Br. J. Psychiatry*, **174**: 39–44.

1.6
## Dementia: a Public Health Emergency and a Scientific Challenge
Laura Fratiglioni[1]

Due to the worldwide "greying" of the populations, dementia has emerged as a major public health problem for both developed and developing

[1] *The Kungsholmen Project, Stockholm Gerontology Research Centre, Box 6401, S-113 82 Stockholm, Sweden*

countries [1]. Due to the diagnostic difficulties and the multifactorial aetiology, a large effort from different disciplines is required to understand the aetiopathogenetic mechanisms of the dementias. This constitutes one of the main scientific challenges for the future.

Dementia is a syndrome due to progressive disorders, all characterized by high costs at both individual and societal levels. These costs have a great economical impact. *The individual costs* can be summarized in the following points:

1. Dementia shortens life expectancy, even in the very old. In a population-based, longitudinal study ongoing in Stockholm since 1987 (the Kung-sholmen Project), the risk of death for demented subjects was twice higher than the risk for non-demented people, after adjustment for sociodemographic variables and comorbidity [2].
2. Dementia patients deteriorate progressively over several years in both cognitive and physical functioning. In the Kungsholmen Project, the cognitive decline was constant during the two follow-up periods, with an annual average decrease of 2.8 in a 30-point cognitive scale. Complete functional dependence was found in 30% of the demented persons at baseline, and in 50% of the 7-year survivors [3].
3. Dementia subjects need care and constant surveillance, even during the initial mild stages. In these phases the assistance is usually provided by a family member. Psychological and physical consequences due to the burden experienced as the main caregiver of a demented person have been reported [4].

The *social costs* linked to dementia are due to the following epidemiological characteristics of this disorder:

1. Both incidence and prevalence of dementia are high, increasing exponentially with increasing age, as documented by Henderson and Jorm in their comprehensive review. In a cohort that included a large sample of nonagenarians, von Strauss *et al* [5] reported that dementia prevalence continues to increase even in the most advanced ages, supporting the hypothesis that dementia is an ageing-related process.
2. Dementia is associated with high mortality. In population-based studies, the mortality rate specific for dementia in 75+ year old subjects is 2–3 cases per 100 persons every year [2,6]. In spite of this high value, death certificates often do not report dementia as the cause of death. The consequence of such under-reporting is that dementia is usually neglected as a malignant condition.
3. Dementia is a major cause of functional dependence and institutionalization. In the Kungsholmen Project, dementia and cognitive impair-

ment make the strongest contribution to the development of long-term functional dependence and to functional decline [3].

As both degenerative and vascular mechanisms may contribute to the appearance of dementia symptoms, the differentiation between Alzheimer's disease (AD) and vascular dementia may be difficult in several cases, especially in the very old. Studying dementia as a whole, instead of specific dementing disorders, is a relatively new research line that reflects an orientation towards intervention. The detection of any risk factor that can be prevented/modified can help to decrease the occurrence of the dementia syndrome.

Until now, the main findings from this approach are the detection of a group of "vascular risk factors" that are strongly associated with dementia [7]. Apart from stroke, these factors include: diabetes mellitus, atrial fibrillation, atherosclerosis index, electrocardiographic evidence of ischaemia, alcohol, severe systolic hypertension, and high saturated fat and cholesterol intake. In addition, it has been reported that there is an inverse relationship between use of antihypertensive medication, especially diuretics, and risk of dementia, suggesting that the use of diuretics may protect against dementia in elderly persons [8].

Finally, the recent availability of drugs that improve cognition in AD has increased the interest in research on predictors and/or prodromal phases of dementia. In the last few years, many articles on mild cognitive impairment (MCI) have been published [9]. Among 75+ year old subjects, the prevalence of this condition is 15–16%. The identification of those subjects with MCI who will develop dementia is the aim of much current research.

Although the application of the epidemiological method to the dementias is relatively recent, three main contributions may be identified. First, the distribution pattern of the dementing disorders has been described in sufficient detail to be utilized for planning medical and social services, at least in all Western countries. Second, some risk factors have been clearly detected, and interesting working hypotheses have been suggested, giving the impression that we are not far away from the time when preventive interventions can be implemented. Third, some aspects of the natural history of the dementias have been sufficiently outlined to be useful at the community level for allocating medical and social resources, and at the individual level for counselling patients and relatives.

## REFERENCES

1. Fratiglioni L., De Ronchi D., Aguero-Torres H. (1999) World-wide prevalence and incidence of dementia. *Drugs Aging*, **15**: 365–375.

2. Aguero Torres H., Fratiglioni L., Guo Z., Viitanen M., Winblad B. (1999) Mortality from dementia in advanced age. A 5-year follow-up study of incident dementia cases. *J. Clin. Epidemiol.*, **52**: 737–743.
3. Aguero Torres H., Fratiglioni L., Guo Z., Viitanen M., von Strauss E., Winblad B. (1998) Dementia is the major cause of functional dependence in the elderly. Three-year follow-up data from a population-based study. *Am. J. Public Health*, **88**: 1452–1456.
4. Schulz R., Beach S.R. (1999) Caregiving as a risk factor for mortality. *JAMA*, **282**: 2215–2219.
5. von Strauss E., Viitanen M., De Ronchi D., Winblad B., Fratiglioni L. (1999) Ageing and the occurrence of dementia. Findings from a population-based cohort with a large sample of nonagenarians. *Arch. Neurol.*, **56**: 587–592.
6. Witthaus E., Ott A., Barendregt J., Breteler M., Bonneux L. (1999) Burden of mortality and morbidity from dementia. *Alz. Dis. Assoc. Disord.*, **13**: 176–181.
7. Fratiglioni L. (1998) Epidemiology. In *Health Economics of Dementia* (Eds B. Winblad, A. Wimo, B. Jönsson, G. Karlsson), pp. 13–31, Wiley, London.
8. Guo Z., Fratiglioni L., Li Z., Fastbom J., Winblad B., Viitanen M. (1999) The occurrence and progression of dementia in a community population aged 75 years and over, in relation to use of antihypertensive medication. *Arch. Neurol.*, **56**: 991–996.
9. Frisoni G.B., Fratiglioni L., Viitanen M., Fastbom J., Winblad B. (1999) Mortality in non-demented elderly with cognitive impairment: the influence of health-related factors. *Am. J. Epidemiol.*, **150**: 1031–1044.

1.7
## Dementia: Plenty of Questions Still to Be Answered
Robin Jacoby[1]

No persons are better qualified to address the topic of the review than Henderson and Jorm. Their contribution to research into the epidemiology of dementia has been of the highest order. Here, their opening sentence ("Dementia is a disorder of the brain") is a challenging statement, not because *what they mean* is false, but because it redefines the term. Most clinicians would prefer to state that dementia is a *syndrome* of mental state phenomena that is caused by one or more disorders of the brain. This is not mere semantic nit-picking, but a syndrome is the only way to arrive at an operational definition of dementia suitable for clinical practice, which is all important. Were we able to biopsy the brain with 100% safety and the certainty of establishing a pathological diagnosis, then dementia as a term would acquire a similar status to heart failure. Nevertheless, it is clear that Henderson and Jorm are seeking to make the point that a disorder of the brain is a *sine qua non* for dementia. This is true or false, depending on

[1] *Department of Psychiatry, Warneford Hospital, Oxford OX3 7JX, UK*

whether or not you subscribe to Mahendra's view [1] that if cognitive impairment due to depressive illness fulfils the criteria for dementia, then it must be called dementia. However, this is not a line I shall pursue further because it probably would amount to nit-picking.

More controversial is the authors' statement that "there is no evidence for a discrete break between [normal ageing and dementia]". This is certainly a view held by some psychologists but not all (see [2] for a review of this contentious question). Craik and Rabinowitz [3], for instance, argue that there are qualitative differences in the type of cognitive impairment afflicting patients with Alzheimer's disease (AD) as compared with unaffected elderly people. It is proposed that the latter show some impairment of mental processing, but differ from the former, who have more specific deficits of episodic memory which indicate involvement of limbic pathways. Is the continuum between normal ageing and dementia more apparent than real? Also, are Henderson and Jorm confusing dementia here with AD? For example, patients who present with primary progressive aphasia and develop sufficient global impairment to justify a diagnosis of dementia, seem to have a distinct zone of rarity between themselves and the normal elderly. The same might apply to some people who develop dementia after cerebrovascular accidents, to fronto-temporal dementia and to dementia caused by numerous other rarer conditions.

Henderson and Jorm discuss Berg's Clinical Dementia Rating Scale (CDR). Like almost all dementia researchers, they take it for granted that dementia can be staged, the implication being that the disorder follows a predictable course. However, this assumption should perhaps be challenged. Our own group [4] reported on a longitudinal study of 100 people with dementia, the majority due to AD, followed up until death. The patients were assessed at 4-monthly intervals using the Present Behavioural and Mini-Mental State Examinations. Whilst cognitive decline is inexorable and followed a more or less predictable course, the same was not true of behavioural and psychiatric symptoms (BPSD). The pattern of BPSD could be classified into three groups: (1) a single episode ending before death; (2) a single episode ending in death; (3) multiple discrete episodes which could or could not end in death. There was no fixed relationship between BPSD and cognitive decline, and behavioural changes could occur not only in one of the three patterns described, but also at more or less any stage in the disease. The authors concluded that "it may be of more value to characterize patients in terms of specific behavioural problems than by their 'stage' of dementia".

Henderson and Jorm quite rightly end their review dealing with the prospects for prevention of dementia. They are also entirely correct to focus on prevention rather than cure, for history has taught us that clean water and immunization have done far more to rid the world of disease than penicillin. Nevertheless, as far as AD is concerned, the exciting advances in laboratory research do give cause to hope for more specific treatment in the forthcoming century. We have already discovered a great deal about the pathogenesis of AD, specifically how amyloid is deposited and how tau-protein is hyperphosphorylated to form plaques and tangles, respectively. It is surely not too fanciful to conceive that a pharmaceutical way to prevent these processes will be found in due course. The challenge will then be to find out which people to treat. In other words, how can we discover who will develop plaques and tangles so that we can shut the stable door before the horse bolts?

## REFERENCES

1. Mahendra B. (1984)   *Dementia: A Survey of the Syndrome of Dementia*, MTP Press, Lancaster.
2. Luszcz M.A., Bryan J. (1999)   Toward understanding age-related memory loss in late adulthood. *Gerontology*, **45**: 2–9.
3. Craik F.I.M., Rabinowitz J.C. (1984)   Age differences in the acquisition and use of verbal information: a tutorial review. In *Attention and Performance. X. Control of Language Processes* (Eds X.H. Bouma, D.G. Bowhuis), pp. 471–499, Erlbaum, Hillsdale, NJ.
4. Hope T., Keene J., Fairburn C.G., Jacoby R., McShane R. (1999)   Natural history of behavioural changes and psychiatric symptoms in Alzheimer's disease. *Br. J. Psychiatry*, **174**: 39–44.

**1.8**
## Rates and Risk Factors for Dementia: Evidence or Controversy?

Per Kragh-Sørensen, Kjeld Andersen, Annette Lolk and Henry Nielsen[1]

Dementia is one of the most common diseases in the elderly, and a major cause of disability and mortality in old age. In their paper, Henderson and Jorm provide a useful overview of this disorder of the brain. This commentary will focus on two essential topics: (1) the impact of very mild and mild dementia on the rates of dementia; (2) risk factors for dementia: the comparison between prevalence and incidence data.

The prevalence of dementia in people aged 65 years or more has been estimated in several countries and is between 4% and 6%. However, pre-

[1] *Department of Psychiatry, Odense University Hospital, J.B. Winslowvej 20, DK–5000 Odense C, Denmark*

valence estimates of mild dementia have varied considerably, ranging from less than 3% to more than 50%. The fact that some studies made no distinction between mild and moderate severity of dementia, and that the characteristics of the examined populations varied from study to study, has probably contributed to the variance in prevalence estimates of mild dementia [1]. Many screening instruments fail to identify a considerable proportion of cases with mild dementia. A fixed cut-off score is often applied when the Mini-Mental State Examination (MMSE), the section for assessment of cognition of the Cambridge Examination for Mental Disorders of the Elderly (CAMCOG), or other instruments are used as a screening for dementia. These fixed cut-off scores, however, may not be warranted as scores on cognitive tests depending on age and education. This implies that a given cut-off score that is optimal for persons in their 60s is probably not optimal for those in their 80s and 90s. When one of the purposes of a study is to identify persons with very mild and mild dementia, these persons could be expected to score higher than the defined cut-off score. To circumvent this obstacle, a predicted score, on the screening instrument in use, for each person has to be calculated from a regression equation [2]. In our opinion, the use of individualized cut-off score, together with local validated normative data for neuropsychological tests, could result in more precise estimates of prevalence rates when very mild and mild dementia are included [3]. Furthermore, as discussed by Henderson and Jorm, the impact of various diagnostic criteria for dementia used in different population-based studies should also be taken into consideration.

The incidence of dementia has only been estimated in a limited number of population-based studies [3]. The problem of identification of very mild and mild dementia is even more important in incidence studies, as these studies offer an important insight into risk factors and thereby the etiology of the main subtypes of dementia, Alzheimer's disease (AD) and vascular dementia (VD).

In 1988, investigators working on European studies formed the European Studies of Dementia (EURODEM) network to harmonize the protocols used in their newly initiated, population-based follow-up studies on incident dementing diseases. Results of analyses based on pooling the data from the studies conducted in Denmark, France, the Netherlands and the UK were published in 1999 [4]. The analyses were based on 528 incident cases of mild to severe dementia, representing 28 768 person-years of follow-up. These collaborative analyses included the largest number of patients identified in population-based follow-up studies reported to date. A long row of risk factors have been reported to increase the risk of AD: old age, family history, head trauma, female gender, low levels of education, etc. Smoking, on the other hand, has been reported to reduce the risk of AD. The estimates of risk factors, however, are mostly based on data from prevalence studies, and might be flawed. Information about risk factors may be systematically different between patients and control subjects. Information data may come from a proxy, who may recall the patient's medical history differently than a proxy of a control subject or the control subject himself/herself. In incident population-based studies, it is possible to follow a person from a non-demented to a demented state. Thereby information about suggested risk factors is given from the patient and/or a proxy before the onset of dementia.

The results from the EURODEM study [4] confirmed that age is a risk factor for AD. One important finding was that women had a increased risk of AD. Recently, a significant gender difference in the risk of AD was also found in a Swedish study [5], which had a relatively older sample than other published studies.

Family history of dementia is considered to be a marker for genetic susceptibility. Compared with the risk reported in prevalence studies, the risk of AD in the EURODEM study is lower. Persons with a history of dementia in two or more first-degree family members had a non-significantly increased risk of AD. On the other hand, it was found that head trauma was not a risk factor for AD, and that smoking did not protect against AD.

In summary, the identification of very mild and mild dementia is crucial, not only to obtain more precise estimates of the rates of dementia, but also to get new insights into the risk factors and etiology of the main subtypes of dementia, AD and VD.

## REFERENCES

1. Ritchie K., Kildea D., Robine J.M. (1992)   The relationship between age and the prevalence of senile dementia: a meta-analysis of recent data. *Int. J. Epidemiol.*, **21**: 763–769.
2. Jorm A. (1994)   A method for measuring dementia as a continuum in community surveys. In *Dementia and Normal Ageing* (Eds F. Huppert, C. Brayne, D. O'Conner), pp. 244–253, Cambridge University Press, Cambridge.
3. Andersen K., Nielsen H., Lolk A., Andersen J., Becker I., Kragh-Sørensen P. (1999)   Incidence of very mild to severe dementia and Alzheimer's disease in Denmark. The Odense Study. *Neurology*, **52**: 85–90.
4. Launer L.J., Andersen K., Dewey M.E., Letenneur L., Ott A., Amaducci L.A., Brayne C., Copeland J.R.M., Dartiques J.-F., Kragh-Sørensen P. *et al* (1999)   Rates and risk factors for dementia and Alzheimer's disease. Results from EURODEM pooled analyses. *Neurology*, **52**: 78–84.
5. Fratiglioni L., Viitanen M., von Strauss E., Tontodonati V., Herlitz A., Winblad B. (1997)   Very old women at highest risk of dementia and Alzheimer's disease: incidence data from the Kungsholmen Project, Stockholm. *Neurology*, **48**: 132–138.

1.9
## Dementia: the Public Health Challenge
Kenneth I. Shulman[1]

In their review, Henderson and Jorm have set the stage for a full discussion of the multi-faceted nature of the disorders we call "dementia". Reliable and valid definitions of the syndrome and its sub-groups are essential in order to understand the scope and impact of these disorders on the world population. As much as a 10-fold difference in prevalence is dependent on the diagnostic criteria for dementia. Moreover, with significant therapeutic advances on the horizon, differentiation of subgroups is essential in order to match target specific treatments.

ICD-10 seems to have a much stricter definition for the syndrome than the American DSM-IV classification system. However, other widely used classification systems for Alzheimer's disease (AD) include the National Institute of Neurological and Communicative Disorders–Alzheimer's Disease and Related Disorders Association (NINCDS–ADRDA) workgroup [1] and the Consortium to Establish a Registry for Alzheimer's disease (CERAD) [2]. For vascular dementia, the National Institute of Neurological Disorders and Stroke–Association Internationale pour la Recherche et l'Enseignement en Neurosciences (NINDS–AIREN) international workshop established diagnostic criteria for research studies which have been widely utilized [3]. Growing interest in dementia of the Lewy body type has been effectively developed by McKeith et al [4]. Increasing interest has also focused on the subgroup of frontotemporal dementias (FTD) as described by the Lund–Manchester group [5]. In contrast to AD, FTD is differentiated by loss of personal awareness, abnormal eating, perseverative behaviour and decreased speech [5].

Henderson and Jorm provide an excellent summary of meta-analyses that have examined prevalence studies from across the world. The figures show a breakdown by age subgroups. However, a single figure for dementia prevalence for the elderly aged 65 and over would be helpful for health planners. An emerging figure based in part on the Canadian Study of Health and Aging [6] shows an overall prevalence of roughly 8% for dementia for over-65s. Most importantly, the authors note that the prevalence doubles for every 5-year age group up to age 85. Exceptions are the frontotemporal dementias, which peak in prevalence between ages 55 to 70 and do not seem to increase with advancing age [7]. From a public health perspective, this reveals an exponential increase in dementias in both developing and developed countries in the coming decades. The very old are the portion of the population increasing most rapidly, and it is

[1] *Sunny Brook Medical Centre, 2075 Bayview Avenue, Toronto N4N 3MS, Canada*

within that subpopulation that the prevalence is indeed highest, reaching over 25% in the over 85-year old age group. Hence, the inevitable conclusion that the dementias will represent one of the greatest public health challenges world-wide in the coming decades.

In light of such a daunting prospect, issues related to prevention achieve an even greater urgency. The authors identify old age, family history of dementia, Down's syndrome and the presence of the apolipoprotein E gene as clearly established risk factors for dementia. Unfortunately, as a society there is little we can do at this stage in our scientific knowledge and development to alter these factors. We must stand by helplessly and watch the projected prevalence without a realistic prospect of a reduction for the foreseeable future.

The association of dementia with previous head trauma is intriguing, but in order to be substantiated really requires larger prospective studies in an elderly population. One risk factor that might improve the identification of prospective cases is delirium [8]. The incidence of dementia for an elderly cohort without delirium was 5.6% per year, whereas those with delirium had an incidence of over 18% per year. The unadjusted relative risk for developing dementia in those with delirium was 3.23.

Promising pharmacological strategies, such as the use of anti-inflammatory drugs, estrogen and vitamin E also seem to offer some potential for prevention. But we must temper our enthusiasm until better data are available. Perhaps the most realistic and practical approach to prevention is for the vascular dementias, where we already possess the capability to alter vascular risk factors such as hypertension, diet, exercise, smoking and hyperlipidemias.

The comorbidity of depression and dementia is now well established and has been an intriguing area of investigation. Alexopoulos et al [9] have shown how even the reversible forms of dementia associated with depression are predictors of permanent cognitive decline. However, it is only after 3 years of follow-up that this association becomes apparent. Devanand et al [10] have also highlighted the importance of depressive symptoms as indicators of a future irreversible dementia in a community population. Henderson and Jorm rightly encourage clinicians to look for clinically significant depression when memory complaints of cognitive impairment are prominent. However, depressive symptoms and syndromes may also be risk factors for dementia in the long term.

In conclusion, Henderson and Jorm's review provides a cautious and sobering approach to the epidemiological perspective of dementia. This approach is essential in order to avoid the temptation to lurch towards quick "solutions" for such a massive and complex public health concern.

# REFERENCES

1.  McKhann G., Drachman D., Folstein M., Katzman R., Price D., Stadlan E.M. (1984) Clinical diagnosis of Alzheimer's disease: report of the NINCDS–ADRDA work group under the auspices of Department of Health and Human Services Task Force on Alzheimer's Disease. *Neurology*, **34**: 939–944.
2.  Mirra S.S., Heyman A., McKeel D., Sumi S.M., Crain B.J., Brownlee L.M., Vogel F.S., Hughes J.P., van Belle G., Berg L. (1991) The consortium to establish a registry for Alzheimer's Disease (CERAD). Part II. Standardization of the neuropathologic assessment of Alzheimer's disease. *Neurology*, **41**: 479–486.
3.  Roman G.C., Tatemichi T.K., Erkinjuntti T., Cummings J.L., Masdeu J.C., Garcia J.H., Amaducci L., Orgogozo J.-M., Brun A., Hofman A. *et al* (1993) Vascular dementia: diagnostic criteria for research studies. Report of the NINDS–AIREN international workshop. *Neurology*, **43**: 250–260.
4.  McKeith I.G., Galasko D., Kosaka K., Perry E.K., Dickson D.W., Hansen L.A., Salmon D.P., Lowe J., Mirra S.S., Byrne E.J. *et al* (1996) Consensus guidelines for the clinical and pathologic diagnosis of dementia with Lewy bodies (DLB): report on the consortium on DLB international workshop. *Neurology*, **47**: 1113–1124.
5.  Miller B.L., Ikonte C., Ponton M., Levy M., Boone K., Darby A., Berman N., Mena I., Cummings J.L. (1997) A study of the Lund–Manchester research criteria for frontotemporal dementia: clinical and single-photon emission CT correlations. *Neurology*, **48**: 937–942.
6.  Canadian Study of Health and Aging Working Group (1994) Canadian Study of Health and Aging: study methods and prevalence of dementia. *Can. Med. Assoc. J.*, **150**: 899–913.
7.  Cummings J.L. (1998) Fronto-temporal dementias vs. Alzheimer's disease: distinctions in life. *Neurobiol. Aging*, **19** (Suppl. 2).
8.  Rockwood K., Cosway S., Carver D., Jarrett P., Stadnyk K., Fisk J. (1999) The risk of dementia and death after delirium. *Age Ageing*, **28**: 551–556.
9.  Alexopoulos G.S., Meyers B.S., Young R.C., Mattis S., Kakuma T. (1993) The course of geriatric depression with "reversible dementia": a controlled study. *Am. J. Psychiatry*, **150**: 1693–1699.
10.  Devanand D.P., Sano M., Tang M.-X., Taylor S., Gurland B.J., Wilder D., Stern Y., Mayeux R. (1996) Depressed mood and the incidence of Alzheimer's disease in the elderly living in the community. *Arch. Gen. Psychiatry*, **53**: 175–182.

## 1.10
## Definition and Epidemiology of Dementia: Some Issues that Need Clarification

Peter J. Whitehouse[1]

Henderson and Jorm offer us a comprehensive review of dementia from the perspective of epidemiology. After considering current definitions of dementia itself and its subtypes, the authors review studies and meta-analyses

[1] *Alzheimer Center, University Hospital of Cleveland, 2074 Abington Road, Cleveland, Ohio 44106, USA*

that purport to demonstrate the prevalence of disease in different regions of the world. They point out that incidence studies are harder to conduct and thus rarer to find, but nevertheless review the information that is available to us. They conclude by reviewing epidemiological evidence, which suggest that certain factors may increase or decrease the risk of an individual suffering from Alzheimer's disease (AD) during his life.

The authors address many complex issues, including the many challenges of epidemiological studies. They raise the important issue of how significant regional and population variation is to be interpreted in epidemiological studies. As they point out, one interpretation is that this may reflect different balances of risk and protective factors in different populations. They review briefly the studies of apolipoprotein E (APOE) 4, but do not specifically discuss them in relationship to these geographic and population/ethnic variations. A key question is whether variations in APOE 4 gene frequency can explain some of the prevalence and incidence rate variations in different studies. The answer to this question may have profound implications in terms of interpreting population studies, but also affect the clinical utility of tests based on APOE 4 and other susceptibility loci that will be identified in the future. Without a knowledge of individuals' exposure to various risks and protective factors in the environment over time, as well as the rest of their relevant risk modifying genetic make-up, it is difficult to know how to use APOE information wisely. The variations in APOE 4 risk associated with having dark skin in the United States are a case in point. For example, African-Americans may have immigrated from various ports of Africa, as well as the Caribbean. Different groups have intermarried with these forced migrant populations during their history, so that the full genotypes of individuals of any skin colour are difficult to establish. Thus, genetic counselling becomes difficult if one cannot rely on phenotype such as skin colour to necessarily predict consistent patters of modifying gene or environmental factors. The authors, however, cannot be faulted for not discussing the complex interactions between genes and environment that may modify the risk of AD in individuals in different populations.

In the middle ground of Henderson and Jorm's review, the field is well covered. However, in the beginning and ending of their paper, there are some conceptual issues that need further clarification. The authors begin with the statement that "Dementia is a disorder of brain. This is an important assertion to make because many members of the general public and even some health professionals still believe something else". Dementia has a biology but it has broad clinical and cultural aspects as well [1]. It would be helpful to have some epidemiological data about this particular assertion, since I believe that most individuals who understand the word "dementia" as a linguistic label likely believe that dementia is a disorder of brain. That is not to say that other disorders of memory have not been associated with psychic trauma, but to my knowledge not seriously dementia. Moreover, the sentence "some attribute the cognitive and behavioural changes to senility" is not entirely consistent with later portions of the paper that claim that dementia is on a continuum with normal aging.

The authors rightfully point out that behavioural changes are a consistent feature of dementia, but they assert that they are not under conscious control. It is not clear what conscious control means in this case. Does it mean that the day after I am diagnosed with dementia my irritability with my wife is no longer under my conscious control? Perhaps the behaviour was not under such control even before the disease started.

Finally, the conclusion section is organized with an interesting structure of certain, possible and unknown categories. The first conclusion is that it is methodologically possible to estimate the prevalence of dementia, particularly AD and vascular dementia (VD), although a great challenge is the definition of the latter. The complexity of this diagnostic entity is only increasing. Conclusion number three in the certainty category may not be correct. Dementia, as the definitions offered in the paper often include, is frequently a progressive disorder, but there are in fact dementias that are static, such as an individual who has multiple cognitive impairments associated with a single head trauma. The unknown category calls for more epidemiological and preventive research. No clinician or scientist would argue with those recommendations.

## REFERENCE

1. Whitehouse P., Mauer K., Ballenger J. (2000) *Concepts of Alzheimer Disease: Biological, Clinical and Cultural Aspects*, The Johns Hopkins Press, Baltimore, MD.

1.11
### Dementia: the Challenge for the Next Decade
Anthony Mann[1]

After a long career in psychiatric research, it is remarkable to note how dementia is now in the forefront of biological, clinical and epidemiological interest rather than remaining an unmentioned, untreatable condition that

[1] *Institute of Psychiatry, Kings College London, De Crespigny Park, London SE5 8AF, UK*

made some older people senile. Its importance as a source of disability and cost in the developed world has been amply shown in Henderson and Jorm's tables. Even more alarming is the projected increase of prevalence in low-income countries, as the population ages there. At the moment, just under 50% of all world dementia cases are in low-income countries, but by the year 2020 the proportion will rise to approximately 70% [1]. The need for education for families, health care agencies and governments about this potential burden is of paramount importance.

The subclassification of dementia by categorical diagnosis has proved useful, as it has allowed internationally agreed consensus criteria for each diagnosis to be developed [2,3]. This has led to standardization in research methodology and international comparisons. However, the disadvantage of this system is its encouragement of clinicians to seek maximal points of difference between clinical cases, so that they may be clearly diagnosed. If two sub-diagnoses are thought to be present, then a diagnosis of "mixed" etiology has to be made. The separation of vascular from Alzheimer's dementia is the most common of these distinctions made in clinical practice. However, this distinction may no longer be valid. Evidence that a wide range of vascular risk factors and vascular disease itself is associated with the onset of Alzheimer's disease (AD) is growing [4]. Furthermore, post mortem examination of a consecutive sample of community-drawn cases on a dementia register indicated that "mixed" pathology, particularly vascular and Alzheimer's in type, is more likely than the carefully applied research criteria *in vivo* had suggested [5]. If vascular risk factors are associated with AD as well as vascular dementia, and if the two pathologies occur more frequently together than we had thought, then a categorical distinction between the two may be misleading and a spectrum or dimensional view more useful. The mechanism of action of vascular risk factors in promotion of AD is currently speculative: they could act as a trigger in the pathological process itself or to bring forward a clinically manifest dementia syndrome by adding vascular damage to a different area of the brain to that affected by the Alzheimer pathology. The more vascular risk factors are shown to be important in AD, though, the more opportunities arise for prevention. An interesting project will be to track the incidence of dementia in older age in those populations where cardiovascular health status has been improved in mid-life through initiatives to change diet, reduce smoking and screen for hypertension.

The discovery of the importance of apoliproprotein E (ApoE) gene as a risk factor has been important, although many questions about the extent of its role remain. Is the effect of the possession of the ApoE4 variant equally powerful in all ethnic groups and at all ages of onset? How strong is the evidence that it is E2 that is protective rather than E4 that produces risk? Most important is the need to know the effect of possession of E2, E3, and E4 upon survival. Most population studies of the gene have been of older populations who, by definition, are survivors. For example, if E4-based dementia were associated with a longer course compared to the others, then the associations could have a different explanation. The ability to obtain genetic material simply through cheek scrapes has made it possible to include the genotype as a variable within epidemiological studies. Until now, investigation of a "biological" variable has required tests, often not possible in the home, leading to a fall in response rate because a visit to a hospital was involved.

Most importantly, Henderson and Jorm address prevention, commenting upon the interesting reports of a potential beneficial effect of anti-inflammatory drugs and estrogens upon the chances of dementia. As they comment, a random controlled trial will be necessary, as the evidence so far is *post hoc*. It is, therefore, pleasing to report that the UK's Medical Research Council has recently funded a cognitive/dementia substudy within its WISDOM trial, in which very large samples of women in their 50s are being recruited from primary care for a random controlled trial of hormone replacement regimes. The dementia substudy begins at entry, but of course it will be a decade or more before any semblance of a result will be manifest, in view of the likely low incidence of dementia in the next decade for this cohort. The evidence of a protective factor of some form of "innate ability" has contributed to the "brain reserve theory", which hypothesizes that the more one has of some as yet undefined cognitive function, the more it seems that one can compensate for neuronal loss.

Henderson and Jorm have produced a careful review of current knowledge. The basis for a multifactorial etiological model of dementia is becoming clear, with genetic substrate, innate abilities, exposure to risk factors and protective factors during life all playing a part in the prediction of the onset of the clinical dementia syndrome.

## REFERENCES

1. Prince M. (1997) The need for research on dementia in developing countries. *Trop. Med. Int. Health*, **2**: 993–1000.
2. McKhann G., Drachman D., Folstein M., Katzman R., Price D., Stadlar M. (1984) Clinical diagnosis of Alzheimer's disease. Report of the NINCDS–ADRDA Work Group under the auspices of the Department of Health and Human Services Task Force on Alzheimer's Disease. *Neurology*, **34**: 939–944.
3. Roman G.C., Taemichi T.K., Erkinjuntti T., Cummings J.L., Masdeu J.C., Garcia J.B., Amaducci L., Orgogozo J.-M., Brun A., Hofman A. *et al* (1993) Vascular dementia: diagnostic criteria for research studies. Report of the NINDS–AIREN International Workshop. *Neurology*, **43**: 250–260.

4. Prince M.J. (1995) Vascular risk factors and atherosclerosis as risk factors for cognitive decline and dementia. *J. Psychosom. Res.*, **39**: 525–530.
5. Holmes C., Cairns N., Lantos P., Mann A. (1999) Validity of current clinical criteria for Alzheimer's disease, vascular dementia and dementia with Lewy bodies. *Br. J. Psychiatry*, **174**: 45–50.

**1.12**
## Recent Progress in the Definition and Epidemiology of Dementia
Alistair Burns[1]

Dementia is one of the major diseases of our times. The burden of the disorder is immense in terms of direct costs of care for sufferers, but the cost in terms of stress and strain imposed on carers is impossible to measure. It is well recognized that psychological and psychiatric diseases are more feared than some physical afflictions, and dementia is the archetypal example of this, because the symptoms lead to loss of independence and the inability of a person to be in control. Henderson and Jorm provide an unrivalled summary of the salient points in current thinking around dementia in terms of disease definition and epidemiology. There are seven aspects of the disorder which this commentator would like to emphasize.

The symptoms of dementia present a continuum between normal ageing and disease [1]. This fact has led people to believe that the syndrome is therefore the inevitable consequence of normal ageing and so nothing can or should be done to mitigate its effects. As a result, therapeutic nihilism has held back clinical innovations for decades, but now this is being slowly reversed. The classic pathological investigations in the early 1970s from Newcastle, with subsequent observations by others, demonstrating that the pathological changes seen in the brain at post-mortem correlate with the severity of the clinical picture, confirmed the close relationship between clinical and morphological findings. The contemporaneous neurochemical studies emphasized the importance of the cholinergic deficit, which formed the basis for current treatments [2].

The consideration of dementia is a two-stage process. First, the syndrome of dementia needs to be distinguished from normal ageing, the effects of drugs on cognitive function, learning disability, impoverished education or environment, delirium and depression. Second, the aetiology of the dementia needs to be established—Alzheimer's disease (AD), vascular dementia, dementia of frontal lobe type and Lewy body dementia being the commonest. Dementia is still regarded by some as a diagnosis in its own

[1] *University Department of Psychiatry, Withington Hospital, West Didsbury, Manchester M20 8LR, UK*

right, but this is as erroneous as considering jaundice or heart failure as a definitive diagnosis.

Epidemiology has been hugely successful in documenting the precise nature of the problem in terms of numbers of people affected by dementia, and this has been invaluable in helping to plan services. In developing countries, the increase in the numbers of older people is going to be particularly great in the future, and it is in those societies that preventive strategies might have the maximum benefit [3].

Risk factors have been clearly identified and their results validated from epidemiological studies. Risk factors are useful in that they can give insights into the mechanisms of dementia but, from the point of view of prevention, only those risk factors which can be manipulated are of importance. Hence, factors such as age, ancestry, family history of dementia, presence of Down's syndrome and possession of an apolipoprotein ε4 allele are essentially unavoidable, while head injury, herpes simplex infection and presence of aluminium might be ameliorated at a public health level. Risk factors which can be easily attended to include physical illness, such as hypertension, diabetes and high cholesterol. The other side of the coin is protective factors, which include estrogens, vitamin E and anti-inflammatory agents, and trials have shown their benefit. Prevention of dementia should be a priority for the twenty-first century.

Diagnosis in dementia is largely based on cognitive deficits, but there has been increasing interest in the presence of psychiatric symptoms and behavioural disturbances as core features of the syndrome. Examples of the former include depression, delusions and hallucinations, while aggression, wandering and disinhibition are examples of the latter [4]. These symptoms are particularly distressing for carers (whose needs are increasingly being recognized, with interventions directed to alleviate stress), and often precipitate the need for admission to long-term care. Their expression differs across cultures. They can be helpful in the differential diagnosis of the aetiology of dementia: visual hallucinations and paranoid ideas are more common in people with Lewy body dementia; affective disorders are commoner in vascular dementia; personality change is common in frontal lobe dementia. A wider appreciation of the significance of these features (alternatively described as non-cognitive or neuropsychiatric features, or denoted as behavioural and psychological symptoms of dementia, BPSD) is important in fully appreciating the significance of dementia.

Measurement of dementia has enabled the natural history of the disease to be identified and described, and a large number of scales have been published and validated [5]. Coupled with the tests for detecting cognitive dysfunction (a universal experience in dementia), these have enabled accurate estimates of prevalence and incidence to be obtained. By developing simple measurements for the main expressions of dementia (neuropsychological deficits, neuropsychiatric features, and problems with activities of daily living), disease definition will be improved and diagnosis made with more certainty.

There is much in the study of dementia in general, and AD in particular, which is exciting and innovative but is outwith the scope of this commentary. Treatments for AD are becoming available and will sit alongside those existing for vascular dementia. Sophisticated brain imaging is allowing functional neuroanatomy to be described in incredible detail. Treatments will be altering the natural history of dementia and imaging sharpening up disease definition. The challenge of dementia is one of the greatest facing medicine.

## REFERENCES

1. Ritchie K., Touchon J. (2000)   Mild cognitive impairment: conceptual basis and current nosological status. *Lancet*, **355**: 225–228.
2. Burns A., Russell E., Page S. (1999)   New drugs for Alzheimer's disease. *Br. J. Psychiatry*, **174**: 476–479.
3. Kramer M. (1980)   The rising pandemic of mental disorders and associated chronic diseases and disabilities. *Acta Psychiatr. Scand.*, **62** (Suppl. 285): 383–396.
4. Burns A., Jacoby R., Levy R. (1990)   Psychiatric phenomena in Alzheimer's disease. *Br. J. Psychiatry*, **157**: 72–94.
5. Burns A., Lawlor B., Craig S. (1999)   *Assessment Scales in Old Age Psychiatry*, Dunitz, London.

1.13
**Dementia: Some Controversial Issues**
Miguel R. Jorge[1]

Esquirol began to distinguish between acute, chronic and senile dementia in 1814, and he regarded the last one as resulting from aging and consisting in a loss of the faculties of understanding. In 1906, Alois Alzheimer reported the case of a 51-year-old woman with cognitive impairment, hallucinations, delusions and focal symptoms, whose brain was found on post mortem to show plaques, tangles and arteriosclerotic changes. In the 8th edition of Kraepelin's Textbook, he coined the term "Alzheimer's disease" (AD), as "a senium praecox if not perhaps a more or less age-independent unique disease process". Many authors from that period criticized this new entity

[1] *Department of Psychiatry, Federal University of São Paulo, Rua Botucatu 740, 04023–900 São Paulo, Brazil*

(presenile dementia) as something different from classical senile dementia [1].

Henderson and Jorm's review addresses several issues concerning definition, diagnostic criteria, differential diagnosis, types, natural history, incidence/prevalence rates and risk factors of dementia that have theoretical and clinical importance. I will offer two short remarks on prevalence rates and risk factors, and focus on two issues that are at present controversial.

Prevalence rates vary according to distinct diagnostic criteria used in different epidemiological studies and probably across different populations. Nevertheless, the worldwide prevalence rates of dementia in people aged 65 years and over is approximately 4.5%; AD is almost twice more common than vascular dementia (VD) in Western nations, but the reverse situation is observed in Asian countries [2].

According to Henderson and Jorm's conclusions, there are four known and a number of possible risk factors for AD. Whereas hereditary factors play a major role in AD, environmental factors associated with stroke (hypertension, smoking, excessive drinking, diabetes, hyperlipidemia) also appear important for VD [3,4].

One important question still pending is whether cognitive decline is a dimensional phenomenon. According to different authors, cognitive decline in the elderly can be considered dimensionally, including benign senescent forgetfulness [5], aging-associated memory impairment [6], mild cognitive disorder [7] and senile dementia. Caine [8] prefers aging-associated cognitive decline (AACD) as a designation to be listed among conditions that are not attributable to a mental disorder but are a focus of clinical attention. AACD reflects "decrement in cognitive processing abilities, including an array of intellectual functions; these are not so severe as to impair personal or vocational functioning significantly". If we accept a dimensional model to explain cognitive decline, AD would be the endpoint in a continuum of a normal aging process. However, Ritchie [9], reviewing the literature, concludes that "there is perhaps more evidence in favor of a medical model of AD as a pathologic process that, although perhaps triggered by critical loss of neuronal reserves related to normal aging, would appear to be related to independent etiologic factors".

Another important question is whether VD really exists as a distinct disease or is just a matter of strokes. Chui [2] pointed out some biases that prompted this question: VD is more frequently observed in stroke clinical centers and rarely observed in dementia clinical centers; there is no consistent phenotype for VD; and it is difficult to link stroke to dementia excluding the possibility of AD in the background. According to Chui's point of view, there is a place for VD (or vascular cognitive impairment as proposed by Hachinski, [10]), if we admit a plurality of VD phenotypes and that chronic ischemia, alone or in concert with other factors, can trigger neuronal dysfunction and death.

It is clear that further research evidence is needed in order to clarify the above questions.

## REFERENCES

1. Berrios G.E. (1996) *The History of Mental Symptoms*, Cambridge University Press, Cambridge.
2. Chui H.C. (1998) Rethinking vascular dementia: moving from myth to mechanism. In *The Dementias* (Eds J.H. Growdon, M.N. Rossor), pp. 377–401, Butterworth-Heinemann, Boston.
3. Bergem A.L.M., Engedal K., Kringlen E. (1997) The role of heredity in late-onset Alzheimer disease and vascular dementia. *Arch. Gen. Psychiatry*, **54**: 264–270.
4. Skoog I. (1998) Status of risk factors for vascular dementia. *Neuroepidemiology*, **17**: 2–9.
5. Kral V.A. (1958) Neuropsychiatric observations in an old people's home: studies of memory dysfunction in senescence. *J. Gerontol.*, **13**: 169–176.
6. Crook T., Bartus R.T., Ferris S.H. (1986) Age-associated memory impairment: proposed diagnostic criteria and measures of clinical change. Report of a National Institute of Mental Health Workgroup. *Dev. Neuropsychol.*, **2**: 261–276.
7. World Health Organization (1992) *The ICD-10 Classification of Mental and Behavioural Disorders: Clinical Descriptions and Diagnostic Guidelines*, World Health Organization, Geneva.
8. Caine E.D. (1994) Should aging-associated memory decline be included in DSM-IV? In *DSM-IV Sourcebook*, vol. 1 (Eds T.A. Widiger, A.J. Frances, H.A. Pincus, M.B. First, R. Ross, W. Davis), pp. 329–337, American Psychiatric Association, Washington, DC.
9. Ritchie K. (1998) Is Alzheimer's disease just old age? In *The Dementias* (Eds J.H. Growdon, M.N. Rossor), pp. 403–413, Butterworth-Heinemann, Boston.
10. Hachinski V.C. (1994) Vascular dementia: a radical redefinition. *Dementia*, **5**: 130–132.

### 1.14
### Is the Prevalence Rate of Alzheimer's Disease Increasing in Japan?

Akira Homma[1]

Local governments in Japan have been greatly concerned with the various problems of the aged, because of the rapid increase in their number. They have conducted surveys to investigate their living conditions and the needs for welfare services for them. In the last two decades, approximately 30 surveys on dementia in the community have been conducted in Japan.

[1] *Department of Psychiatry, Metropolitan Institute of Gerontology, Tokyo, Japan*

The sites of the investigations were distributed all over the country. Surveys were conducted by the two-step method, that is, a screening survey and a secondary survey for diagnosis by a psychiatrist during door-to-door visits. The use of functioning in activities of daily living, behavioural symptoms, and the degree of care required as criteria to screen the elderly with suspected dementia was one of the features in the surveys. In a community survey conducted in 1992 [1], 5000 persons aged over 65 years, randomly selected from approximately 340 000 elderly persons in Kanagawa prefecture, were subjected to a screening survey without psychometric examinations. In addition, in order to examine whether elderly with dementia were present among those who were not screened, a randomly selected subsample of these people was examined by psychiatrists. No case of dementia was found in this subsample. These results suggest that the screening criteria were likely to be valid and practical, taking into account the reluctant attitude of Japanese elderly persons toward such surveys. Recently we conducted a screening survey in a rural area of central Japan. The Mini-Mental State Examination was used to screen the elderly with dementia among approximately 7800 subjects. The refusal rate was as high as 25%. These findings seem to support the idea that the use of a psychometric examination is not useful as a screening instrument in Japan.

A major disadvantage in Japan is that only prevalence studies have been conducted, mainly due to financial constraints. Incidence rate is a function of prevalence rate. It is usually difficult to estimate change of incidence by the results in the prevalence studies. However, if similar tendencies are recognized in the results of the prevalence studies in some areas, change of incidence may be worthwhile to be considered to a certain extent. In metropolitan Tokyo, large-scale epidemiological surveys were conducted in 1974, 1980, 1987 and 1995 [2]. The survey in 1974 was carried out before the DSM concept of dementia was incorporated. Thus, that survey was excluded from the comparison of prevalence rates. The overall prevalence rates of dementia were 4.6% in 870 000 persons aged 65 years and over in 1980, 4.0% in 1 110 000 aged people in 1987 and 4.1% in 1 490 000 elderly persons in 1995. There were no significant differences in the distribution of the total aged population by age groups, but the proportion of those aged over 80 years slightly increased.

Remarkable findings were obtained in the disease-specific prevalence rates. It has been maintained that vascular dementia (VD) is more common than Alzheimer-type dementia (AD) in Japan. However, in the survey of 1995, the prevalence of AD was 1.8% and that of VD was 1.2%, with a ratio AD:VD almost identical to that reported in other countries. In Japan, the prevalence rate of AD increased from 1980 to 1995, while there was a decrease of the rates of other dementias and unspecified dementia. In the comparison of age and disease-specific prevalence rates in Tokyo and in the

Kame project conducted among Japanese-Americans in Seattle [3], the pattern of increasing prevalence of AD and VD with age seems almost identical, except for the finding that the prevalence rate of AD in extremely old people in Seattle is higher than that in Tokyo.

In addition to the increased visibility of AD, sociomedical factors should be considered as a reason for the increased prevalence rate of AD. The ratio of nursing home beds to the elderly population increased from 0.9 to 1.3 in 8 years. In 1987 and 1995, the institutionalized elderly were surveyed by psychiatrists to examine the prevalence of dementia. Prevalence rates of AD decreased from 23.8% to 19.8%. Also, the prevalence of VD increased from 19.2% to 28.9%. The total prevalence rate of dementia decreased from 56.9% to 54.3%. Although the increased prevalence of VD in nursing homes is not sufficient to explain its decreased prevalence in the community, the change of proportions of AD and VD in nursing homes might influence that in the community. The second problematic issue is that aged persons in medical facilities were not included in the study. A complete survey including medical facilities will be needed in the future.

It may seem that a predominant prevalence of VD is no longer a characteristic epidemiological feature of the demented elderly in the community of Japan. Recent results in other areas of Japan seem to support the tendency. Also, the higher prevalence of AD shown in the Kame study seems to coincide with the increasing prevalence rate of AD in Japan, possibly due to environmental factors.

## REFERENCES

1. Imai Y., Homma A., Hasegawa K., Hirakawa Y., Kosaka A., Oikawa K., Shimogaki H. (1994) An epidemiological study on dementia in Kanagawa prefecture. *Jpn. J. Geriatr. Psychiatry*, **5**: 855–862.
2. Homma A. (1998) Epidemiological study on Alzheimer type dementia. *Dementia Japan*, **12**: 5–9.
3. Graves A., Larson E.B., Edland S., Bowen J.D., McCormick W.C., McCurry S.M., Rice M.M., Wenzlow A., Uomoto J.D. (1996) Prevalence of dementia and its subtypes in the Japanese American population of King county. *Am. J. Epidemiol.*, **144**: 760–771.

# 2

# Clinical Diagnosis of Dementia: A Review

## Barry Reisberg[1,2], Emile Franssen[1,2], Muhammad A. Shah[1], Jerzy Weigel[3], Maciej Bobinski[3] and Henryk M. Wisniewski[3]

[1]Aging and Dementia Research and Treatment Center, and [2]Zachary and Elizabeth M. Fisher Alzheimer's Disease Education and Resources Program, New York University School of Medicine, New York, NY 10016, USA; [3]Institute for Basic Research in Developmental Disabilities, 1050 Forest Hill Road, Staten Island, NY 10314, USA

## CLINICAL DIAGNOSIS OF DEMENTING DISORDER

"Dementia" is a term which refers to "a general mental deterioration" [1]. The term has Latin roots. "*De*" is a prefix derived from Latin, signifying "separation, cessation or contraction", and "*mens*" denotes mind [1,2]. Consequently, in dementia there is "a contraction of the mind".

Chronicity has generally been implicit in the term "dementia". Although legal implications of what we now term dementia can be traced to Greek writings of Solon and Plato, the earliest known usage of the term dementia comes from Aurelius Cornelius Celsus, a Roman writer and encyclopedist [3–6]. In a work entitled *De Medicina*, in the first century A.D., Celsus distinguished "delirium" and "dementia". Roman writers, beginning with Celsus, used the word "delirium" more or less interchangeably with the Greek-derived term "phrenesis" ("phrenitis", or "frenzy"), which designated a temporary mental disorder occurring in the course of illness, and featuring excitement and restlessness [7].

Although dementia and delirium continue to be distinguished in current diagnostic nomenclature, the extent to which chronicity is implied in the usage of the terminology "dementia" is very variable. For example, the term "acute dementia" has been used in recent times [1]. Similarly, in terms of the distinction of delirium from dementia, there is universal recognition

*Dementia, Second Edition.* Edited by Mario Maj and Norman Sartorius.

that various medical disorders can produce both conditions [8]. Also "excitement" and "restlessness" can occur in both delirium and dementia. In the context of dementia, "excitement" is most commonly referred to as "agitation" or as "catastrophic reaction", and "restlessness" is most commonly referred to as "activity disturbance" or as "pacing". Additionally, dementia is itself a risk factor for delirium and the occurrence of delirium is a risk factor for dementia. Consequently, the boundaries between dementia and delirium remain somewhat blurred, although the distinction between these conditions has been considered to be a useful one for two millennia.

Another implication of the terminology "dementia" which is applied frequently is of a progressive, deteriorating course. Although a deteriorating course is characteristic of many of the most important dementing conditions, clearly dementia is also a broader term which can be appropriately applied to a "general mental deterioration" produced by head trauma, heavy metal poisoning, or any of numerous other conditions which may, or may not, be progressive in nature.

One current authoritative nomenclature, the DSM-IV [8], operationalizes the diagnosis of the "general mental deterioration" characteristic of dementia as the development of multiple cognitive deficits. In this definition, the deficits must "include memory impairment" and "must be sufficiently severe to cause impairment in occupational or social functioning and must represent a decline from a previously higher level of functioning".

A variety of mental status, neuropsychologic, functional, and other measures have been developed which can assist in the diagnosis of dementia. Some of the most widely used assessments will be noted in the course of this brief overview. It is important to note that all of these measures must be utilized in conjunction with a careful clinical history which documents the occurrence of decline from a higher premorbid cognitive and functional level of capacity.

Once the occurrence of dementia has been established, the clinician must determine the specific origin of the dementia, i.e. the specific dementing diagnostic entity. Dementia can be caused by numerous conditions, including degenerative brain diseases, cerebrovascular factors, infectious conditions, hormonal abnormalities, immune disorders, electrolyte abnormalities, toxins, medications, hereditary disorders, neoplastic conditions, traumatic changes, metabolic changes, nutritional deficiencies, normal pressure hydrocephalus, Parkinson's disease, multiple sclerosis, and other conditions. Additionally, in clinical practice, many of these conditions commonly interact to produce dementia, increase the magnitude of dementia, or affect the course of dementia. Consequently, the differential diagnosis of dementia requires a history of onset and course, a medical history, including a psychiatric and neurologic history, a social and occupational history, and a relevant family history. In the context of this history, relevant examinations for dementia diagnosis include a physical examination, psychiatric and mental status examination, and neurologic examination. Laboratory evaluations which are conventionally applied in the differential and diagnostic work-up for dementia include comprehensive metabolic evaluation with studies of serum electrolytes, urea, glucose and liver function tests. A complete blood count is obtained, as well as serum $B_{12}$ and folate values and thyroid function tests [8,9]. In many settings, other laboratory evaluations are conventionally obtained as part of a dementia diagnostic work-up, such as syphilis serology, human immunodeficiency virus (HIV) testing, or serum Lyme disease antibody assessment. Neuroimaging evaluations are obtained in the dementia work-up: they include a magnetic resonance imaging (MRI) or computed tomography (CT) scan of the brain. Many other laboratory and diagnostic procedures may be useful: for example, genetic and chromosomal evaluations in assessing familial Alzheimer's disease (AD), dementia due to Huntington's disease, or dementia due to diverse other causes, such as spinocerebellar ataxia. However, these genetic evaluations are difficult to obtain at present in most diagnostic settings. The presence of $B_{12}$ and/or folate deficiency can presently be sensitively assessed with serum methylmalonic acid and serum homocysteine levels. Neuroimaging evaluations may be augmented by information from single photon emission tomography (SPECT) scans, positron emission tomography (PET) scanning, or, more traditionally, electroencephalographic (EEG) assessment.

It should be noted that all of these evaluations only serve to inform what is ultimately a clinical diagnosis of dementia categorically, or more specifically, of any particular dementia diagnostic entity. For example, a patient may fulfill all of the diagnostic criteria for dementia in the DSM-IV and have memory impairment together with multiple cognitive deficits, and these deficits may be sufficiently severe to cause impairment in occupational and social functioning, and this may represent a decline from a previously higher level of functioning. Furthermore, the impairments may be noted on mental status, neuropsychologic and functional evaluations, and meet the severity criteria on these evaluations for dementia. Nevertheless, a clinician may correctly conclude, on the basis of the comprehensive evaluation, and, especially, the psychiatric history, that the patient's symptoms are secondary entirely to anxiety disorder. In this case, the diagnosis of dementia would conventionally not apply, despite the patient's temporarily fulfilling all of the "criteria" for a dementia diagnosis.

Indeed, many of the major categories of mental disorder can produce an acute, recurring, chronic, or even progressive condition, which fulfills the DSM-IV criteria for dementia, but for which the diagnosis of dementia, as conventionally utilized, would not apply. For example, an acutely psychotic schizophrenic patient may operationally fulfill the criteria for dementia, with low test scores, poor functioning, etc. Furthermore, the onset of these

may have been gradual. Nevertheless, a diagnosis of schizo-
ᴉe appropriate for this patient, whereas a diagnosis of demen-
_e [8]. Similarly, the onset and development of a maniform
disorder may produce a clinical picture which nominally fulfills the
"dementia" criteria, but for which the diagnosis of dementia would not
apply. The so-called "dementia syndrome" of depression, what was for-
merly termed "pseudodementia", is well known: a depressed patient may
fulfill the criteria for dementia; however, the clinician may conclude, on the
basis of the clinical history, associated clinical symptomatology, etc., that the
patient suffers from major depressive disorder, not dementia.

Other major categories of mental disorder in which patients may nominally fulfill dementia diagnostic criteria, but in which other, non-dementia,
clinical diagnoses would apply include substance related disorders and
delirium. The DSM-IV, for example, specifically notes that "dementia is
not diagnosed if these symptoms occur exclusively during the course of a
delirium" [8].

In summary, the term dementia has been useful in medical categorization
and classification for approximately 2000 years. Medically, Galen (130–201
A.D.) added the term "morosis", meaning dementia, to the list of mental
diseases, defining a person thus afflicted as one "in whom the knowledge of
letters and other arts are totally obliterated, indeed they can't even remember their own names" [5,10]. Although the term "dementia" has remained
in usage over these past two millennia, in general, until the advent of the
Renaissance, physicians who have followed the Galenic medical tradition,
dating from the time of the Roman Emperor, Marcus Aurelius, have utilized
this term, whereas physicians who have followed the Hippocratic medical
tradition, dating from ancient Greek times (circa 400 B.C.), did not identify
dementing disorders.

Currently, the DSM-IV definition of dementia as a condition with "general
mental deterioration", including memory impairment and with functional
deficits, has relatively high specificity and relatively low sensitivity. Various
mental disorders which fulfill the inclusion criteria, by convention, are not
currently termed dementia, whereas others, especially those with a degenerative course and/or overtly identifiable "medical" etiology, are currently
termed dementia. For example, the decision to exclude dementia praecox
(currently termed schizophrenia) from the dementia DSM-IV categorization,
although some schizophrenic patients may meet the dementia inclusion
criteria, appears somewhat arbitrary from certain perspectives.

The net result of the current categorization is that it is essential for
clinicians to recognize the salient clinical features of the major dementia
and non-dementia mental disorders and to formulate a diagnosis based
upon these salient features. In the past several years, the salient clinical
characteristics of the most important of the dementing disorders, AD, have

been described in some detail. These sailent characteristics, their origins, and their differentiation and overlap with other dementing conditions, will be briefly reviewed in this paper.

## CLINICAL DIAGNOSIS OF ALZHEIMER'S DISEASE (AD)

AD is, epidemiologically, the leading cause of dementia [11]. It is a characteristic clinical and pathological process [9]. Pathologically, it is characterized by the presence in the brain of neurofibrillary tangles, comprised in part of the tau protein, and amyloid (senile) plaques which contain the β-amyloid protein. Although characteristic of AD, these major pathologic elements are not pathognomonic, and can be found both separately and together in both normal aged persons and in other, non-AD, pathologic disorders. The magnitude of occurrence of these major pathologic constituents, their localization in particular brain regions, such as the hippocampus, and the co-occurrence of tau-positive neurofibrillary tangles and senile plaques containing β-amyloid, all assist in the pathologic differentiation of AD from other clinical entities.

### The Functional Course of AD: The Most Robust Marker of AD Clinical Course

Clinically, AD is also a characteristic illness entity, which is recognizable by its onset and course. For several reasons, the characteristic clinical course of AD is most readily appreciated by charting the progressive changes in functioning and daily life activities which occur with the evolution of the disease process. The characteristic functional course of AD is most clearly outlined using the Functional Assessment Staging (FAST) procedure [12]. The FAST course of AD is shown in Table 2.1. Current evidence for the superiority of the FAST staging procedure in tracking the course of AD in dementia patients who are generally free of non-AD related physical pathology is summarized in Table 2.2.

The evidence for the superiority of the FAST in tracking AD course includes evidence from what are termed criterion validity studies, which compare the utility of a measure in charting a disease in comparison with a hypothesized "gold standard"; concurrent validity studies, which compare a particular measure in charting a disease with other measures; and utility investigations, which examine how well the measure does in uncovering new findings when used to chart the disease process. Each of these lines of evidence supporting the conclusion that the FAST identifies a characteristic process of deterioration in AD will be briefly reviewed.

**TABLE 2.1** The characteristic functional course of Alzheimer's disease (AD): functional assessment staging (FAST)

1. No difficulty, either subjectively or objectively
2. Complains of forgetting location of objects. *Subjective work difficulties*
3. Decreased job functioning evident to co-workers. Difficulty in travelling to new locations. *Decreased organizational capacity*[*]
4. *Decreased ability to perform complex tasks*, e.g. planning dinner for guests, handling personal finances (such as forgetting to pay bills), difficulty marketing, etc.[*]
5. *Requires assistance in choosing proper clothing* to wear for the day, season or occasion, e.g. patient may wear the same clothing repeatedly, unless supervised[*]
6. (a) *Improperly putting on clothes without assistance or cuing* (e.g. may put street clothes on over night clothes, or put shoes on wrong feet, or have difficulty buttoning clothing) occasionally or more frequently over the past weeks[*]
   (b) Unable to bathe properly (e.g. *difficulty adjusting bath-water temperature*) occasionally or more frequently over the past weeks[*]
   (c) *Inability to handle mechanics of toileting* (e.g. forgets to flush the toilet, does not wipe properly or properly dispose of toilet tissue) occasionally or more frequently over the past weeks[*]
   (d) *Urinary incontinence* (occasionally or more frequently over the past weeks)[*]
   (e) *Fecal incontinence* (occasionally or more frequently over the past weeks)[*]
7. (a) Ability to speak limited to approximately *six intelligible different words* or fewer, in the course of an average day or *in the course of an intensive interview*
   (b) Speech ability limited to the use of a *single intelligible word* in an average day or *in the course of an intensive interview* (the person may repeat the word over and over)
   (c) Ambulatory ability lost (*cannot walk without personal assistance*)
   (d) *Cannot sit up without assistance* (e.g. the individual *will fall over if there are no lateral rests (arms) on the chair*)
   (e) *Loss of ability to smile*
   (f) *Loss of ability to hold up head independently*, or the neck is contracted and immobile

[*] Scored primarily on the basis of information obtained from a knowledgeable informant and/or caregiver.

*Note*: Interviewers are instructed to check the highest consecutive level of disability. The FAST stage is the highest consecutive enumerated score. Adapted from Reisberg (1986) © 1984 by Barry Reisberg, MD [57].

## Criterion Validity

Criterion validity studies include two major lines of investigation. One gold standard criterion is the capacity of a particular measure to chart the prospective course of a degenerative disease, in this instance, the degenerative course of AD. The other criterion validity line of investigation is the relationship between a measure and neuropathologic changes in AD.

TABLE 2.2  Evidence for the superiority of the FAST staging procedure in charting the characteristic clinical course of Alzheimer's disease (AD)

*Criterion validity*

Longitudinal course of AD — Progression of AD on the FAST accounted for about twice the variance in temporal course of AD as that accounted for by the MMSE in a 5-year prospective study of course of patients with probable AD [16, 17]

Neuropathologic investigations of AD — Relationships between volumes of hippocampal formation subdivisions and FAST stage 7 substages (NB: in FAST stage 7, MMSE scores are virtually uniformly zero [bottom]) [24]:

| | |
|---|---|
| Cornu ammonis | $r = 0.70$ $(p \leq 0.05)$ |
| Subiculum complex | $r = 0.79$ $(p \leq 0.001)$ |
| Entorhinal cortex | $r = 0.62$ $(p < 0.05)$ |

Correlations between total number of neurons in hippocampal formation subdivisions and FAST stage 7 substages [26]:

| | |
|---|---|
| Cornu ammonis | $r = 0.90$ $(p \leq 0.01)$ |
| CA1 | $r = 0.88$ $(p \leq 0.01)$ |
| Subiculum | $r = 0.79$ $(p \leq 0.001)$ |

Percentages of remaining neurons in hippocampal brain regions with neurofibrillary changes [26]:

| | Control (%) | FAST 7a–7c (%) | FAST 7e–7f (%) |
|---|---|---|---|
| Cornu ammonis | | | |
| CA 1 | 5.5 | 43.2 | 71.0 |
| CA 2 | 5.2 | 22.4 | 32.7 |
| CA 3 | 0.6 | 9.5 | 26.4 |
| CA 4 | 0.8 | 10.3 | 27.8 |
| Subiculum | 2.3 | 21.4 | 52.4 |

*Concurrent validity*

Neurologic reflexes and release signs — Correlations with a summary measure of neurologic reflexes and release signs [33–35] In 480 subjects at all severity levels with dependent variables [35]:

| | Correlation | Variance (%) |
|---|---|---|
| MMSE | $r = 0.74$ | 55 |
| FAST | $r = 0.80$ | 64 |

*(continues overleaf)*

**TABLE 2.2** (*continued*)

|  | In 37 subjects with MMSE scores of zero [35]: | |
|---|---|---|
|  | *Correlation* | *Variance (%)* |
|  | FAST    $r = 0.80$ | 64 |

Cognitive change — Correlations with cognitive change assessments [37–39, 41, 43]:

|  | *FAST correlations* |
|---|---|
| Concentration | 0.88 |
| Recent memory | 0.90 |
| Remote memory | 0.83 |
| Orientation | 0.94 |
| MMSE | 0.83 |
| M-OSPD (stages 6 and 7) | 0.77 |

*Utility*

| | |
|---|---|
| Identification of major physical disabilities in AD which could not be charted with traditional assessments | Contractures occur in approximately a quarter of a million AD patients in the USA alone [36]. 95% of AD patients with contractures have MMSE scores of zero. FAST correlation with contracture occurrence in AD is 0.70 [36] |
| Identification of a physical, neurologic marker of AD course | Neurologic reflexes distinguished early stage 6 AD patients (FAST 6a–6c) from early stage 7 AD patients (FAST 7a and 7b), with a specificity, sensitivity and overall accuracy of > 85% [54]. This differentiation corresponds to the point of emergence of incontinence in AD |

FAST, Functional Assessment Staging; MMSE, Mini-Mental State Examination; M-OSPD, Modified Ordinal Scales of Psychological Development

*Utility in tracking the longitudinal course of AD.* The course of AD is most often charted at the present time with the Mini-Mental State Examination (MMSE) [13]. This was originally proposed as a screening measure for dementia [14,15]. However, it is widely, even generally used at present, for assessing the magnitude of severity of AD and other dementia disorders at all severity levels. Consequently, the MMSE is an appropriate measure for comparison in terms of the utility of a measure in tracking the longitudinal course of AD.

In a prospective longitudinal study, the course of 103 community residing subjects with probable AD [16] at baseline was examined [17]. The mean MMSE score of these subjects at baseline was $15.4 \pm 5.6$. Subjects were followed over a mean interval of $4.6 \pm 1.4$ years. Follow-ups were conducted blind with respect to baseline measures. When necessary, they were conducted in residential and nursing home settings. At follow-up, eight subjects could not be located. Additionally, 30 subjects were deceased at the time of follow-up. Of the 65 surviving subjects who could be located, FAST stage distribution at baseline was as follows: FAST stage 4, $n = 34$; FAST stage 5, $n = 22$; FAST stage 6, $n = 8$; FAST stage 7, $n = 1$. The mean MMSE score at follow-up was $5.1 \pm 6.9$. Approximately half, 33 of the 65 surviving subjects, had MMSE scores of 0 at follow-up. The FAST stage distribution at follow-up was: FAST stage 4, $n = 2$; FAST stage 5, $n = 7$; FAST stage 6, $n = 27$; and FAST stage 7, $n = 29$.

The correlation between change in measures and temporal course (i.e. change in time) in this study was examined. There was a 0.32 correlation between change in MMSE scores and time elapsed in the 65 survivors ($p < 0.05$). Consequently, MMSE score change explained 10.2% of the variance in time elapsed.

The correlation between change in FAST scores and time elapsed in the 65 survivors was also examined. For these correlations, the major FAST stages were allotted corresponding integer values (i.e. FAST stage $1 = 1.0$, etc.), and the FAST substages were allotted proportional fractional values (i.e. FAST stage 6a $= 6.0$, 6b $= 6.2 \ldots$, 7a $= 7.0, \ldots$ 7f $= 8.0$, etc.). Using these procedures, the correlation between FAST score change and time elapsed in the 65 surviving subjects was 0.45 ($p < 0.001$). Therefore, FAST score change accounted for 20.3% of the variance in time elapsed in this longitudinal study. This was approximately twice the variance in time elapsed which was accounted for by the MMSE.

Reasons for the superiority of the FAST in tracking the characteristic course of AD in comparison with the MMSE include the wider temporal range of the FAST, which charts approximately twice the potential temporal duration of AD course as the MMSE (Figure 2.1) [18–20]. These floor effects of the MMSE (and many other measures which have been widely utilized in AD assessment) are well known [19–22].

Accordingly, several analyses were conducted in this longitudinal study to determine whether the superiority of the FAST in tracking the longitudinal course of AD was only associated with these floor effects [17]. In this longitudinal study, 33 of the 65 survivors followed had MMSE scores of zero (i.e. > 50%). Therefore, analyses were conducted to determine: (a) whether mean rate of change of MMSE scores per annum differed if subjects with MMSE floor (zero) scores were excluded; (b) whether MMSE correlations with temporal course improved if subjects with MMSE scores of zero were excluded, and (c) whether the relative superiority of the FAST in tracking the temporal course of AD would still be present if the least impaired cohort at baseline were analyzed separately.

Mean rates of change on the MMSE in this longitudinal study were $2.43 \pm 1.15$ points per annum, a result which is comparable with other published data with similar samples [23]. If the 33 subjects with MMSE scores of zero

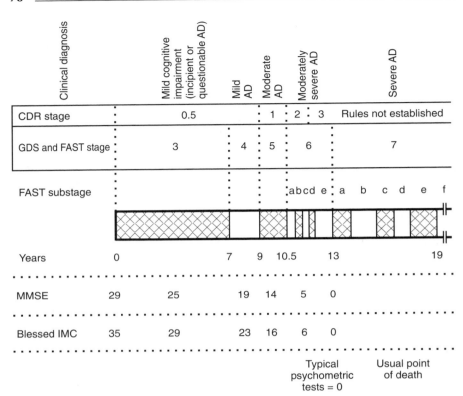

**FIGURE 2.1** Typical time course of Alzheimer's disease (AD). Stage range comparisons shown between CDR and GDS/FAST are based upon published functioning and self-care descriptors. CDR, Clinical Dementia Rating; GDS, Global Deterioration Scale; FAST, Functional Assessment Staging; MMSE, Mini-Mental State Examination; IMC, Information, Memory and Concentration test

*Source*: from Reisberg *et al* [19]

were excluded, the mean rate of change was virtually unchanged, i.e. 2.42 ± 1.32 points per year on the MMSE. An analysis of the variance in temporal course, accounted for by the MMSE if subjects with scores of zero were excluded, indicated that there was then no relationship between time elapsed and MMSE score change ($r = 0.00$). Consequently, eliminating subjects with bottom scores did not improve the relationship of MMSE to AD temporal course and, in fact, eliminated this relationship entirely.

Another analysis in this longitudinal study examined criterion validity in the least impaired cohort at baseline, i.e. 27 subjects followed whose Global Deterioration Scale (GDS) stage at baseline was 4. The mean MMSE score for these GDS stage 4 subjects was $20.5 \pm 3.4$. In this least impaired cohort, the correlation between MMSE change and temporal change in the longitudinally followed subjects was 0.35 ($p < 0.05$), accounting for 12.25% of variance. The correlation between FAST score change and time elapsed in these GDS stage 4 subjects followed was 0.51 ($p < 0.01$), accounting for 26.01% of temporal change variance.

Consequently, regardless of analytic strategies employed, the FAST staging procedure accounts for considerably more variance in the temporal course of AD in comparison with the MMSE. Therefore, using the criterion validity standard of longitudinal course, the FAST is a considerably more valid measure for assessing AD than the MMSE.

*Relationship to neuropathological markers of AD course.* Another criterion validity standard which has been widely proposed for AD is the relationship between change on a measure and neuropathologic markers of AD course. In AD these markers include: (a) degeneration in affected brain regions, (b) cell loss in affected brain regions, and (c) relationships to AD neuropathologic hallmarks. In each of these areas, currently published studies have supported the validity of the FAST staging procedure. Furthermore, the FAST compares favorably with any other *in vivo* markers in terms of neuropathologic relationships (i.e. in terms of neuropathologic assessment of criterion validity).

The relationship between hippocampal volumetric changes and FAST stage was examined in a study of 13 subjects with severe AD at GDS stage 7 who presented for post-mortem evaluation [24]. The FAST stages of these subjects at the time of demise ranged from 7a to 7f. Volumetric change in hippocampal brain regions was studied both in relationship to FAST stage and in comparison with 5 age-matched subjects who were free of symptoms of dementia. The results indicated robust linear relationships between atrophy of the hippocampus and its principal subdivisions and the evolution of AD assessed with the FAST. Overall, patients in the early portion of stage 7 (7a–7c) showed a 36% decrease in hippocampal volume in comparison with controls, and patients in late stage 7 (7e–7f) showed a 60% decrease in hippocampal volumes in comparison with controls. For the cornu ammonis, subicular complex, and entorhinal cortex, Pearson correlations of volumetric loss with FAST stage 7 ordinally enumerated substages were: $r = -0.70$, $-0.79$, and $-0.62$, respectively.

The hippocampal atrophy results using the FAST from the study of Bobinski *et al* [24] are among the strongest such relationships described in the current literature. These results strongly support the overall validity of the FAST staging procedure. More particularly, they also support the validity of the FAST staging procedure for AD in the final FAST 7 stage. FAST stage 7 is comprised of six distinct substages, all of which generally occur after the MMSE and other traditional measures which have been applied for AD assessment have reached floor values. The potential temporal duration of FAST stage 7 in persons who survive until and into the final 7f substage is 7 years or longer [19,20,25]. Consequently, FAST stage 7 represents more than half of the total potential temporal duration of AD. Therefore, demonstration of specific criterion validity for this major portion of AD course, where other measures which have been studied in comparison with neuropathologic data are not useful, is a major advance.

Subsequent studies have lent further weight to these findings of robust, even unprecedentedly strong, relationships between neuropathologically assessed brain changes and progression of AD assessed with the FAST. For example, in a subsequent study of the same severely impaired, 13 FAST stage 7 AD patients and five controls, the number of neurons in hippocampal formation subdivisions was examined by Bobinski et al [26]. Early FAST stage 7 subjects (FAST stages 7a–7c) had significantly ($p \leq 0.01$) more neuronal loss in the CA1 and subiculum regions of the hippocampus. In late FAST stage 7, significant neuronal loss relative to controls was found in all sectors of the cornu ammonis and in the subiculum ($p < 0.01$). Correlations between the total number of neurons in hippocampal formation subdivisions and FAST stage 7 substages were 0.90 in the cornu ammonis, 0.88 in the CA1 and 0.79 in the subiculum ($p \leq 0.01$). Similar linear relationships between the percentages of neurons with neurofibrillary tangles in hippocampal brain regions and the FAST staging procedures were noted (Figure 2.2).

Consequently, there is strong evidence from two forms of criterion validity studies, i.e. studies of the prospective course of AD, and studies of neuropathologic changes in AD, for the validity of the FAST staging procedure in marking the characteristic clinical course of functional losses in AD.

## Concurrent Validity

Another source of validity support for the utility of the FAST staging procedure and its superiority from various perspectives over traditional measures, such as the MMSE, in marking the characteristic course of AD comes from concurrent validity studies. Two separate lines of concurrent validity investigation have been pursued. One is the study of independent neurologic markers of deterioration in the AD patient and the other is the study of the concurrent relationship between cognition and functioning in AD.

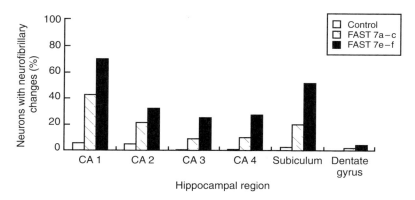

**FIGURE 2.2** Relationship between the percentages of neurons with neurofibrillary changes in hippocampal brain regions and FAST stages. FAST, Functional Assessment Staging

*Source*: from Bobinski *et al* [26]

*Correlation with neurologic reflex changes*. It has long been recognized that certain neurologic reflexes, which have been variously termed "frontal release signs" or "developmental reflexes" or "primitive reflexes" or "cortical disinhibition signs", emerge particularly in the course of what has been variously termed "late stage" or severe AD [27–32]. Franssen *et al* have studied these and other neurologic reflex and release sign markers of the emergence of AD in considerable detail [33,34]. Using published assessment procedures, Franssen and Reisberg examined 14 individual reflexes and two additional measures of muscle tone [35]. These were encompassed into five categories: (a) muscle stretch reflexes; (b) muscle tone; (c) the plantar extensor reflex; (d) nociceptive reflexes; and (e) prehensile reflexes. The total activity score for each of these five reflex categories consisted of the summed highest score of each of the constituent individual neurologic reflex variables. Pearson correlations were computed between combined scores of the reflex categories and clinical assessment variables. A total of 480 subjects spanning the severity spectrum from GDS stages 1 to 7 were assessed. Patients in FAST stages 7d–7f were excluded, because the high frequency of secondary joint contractures in these stages sometimes prevented the examination of all neurological reflexes [36]. All subjects studied fulfilled criteria for either normal aging (GDS stages 1 and 2, $n = 164$), mild memory impairment (GDS stage 3, $n = 46$) or AD (GDS stages $\geq 4$, $n = 270$). The relationships obtained provide an independent view of the concurrent validity of assessments in progressive aging and AD. The combined reflex category variable correlated with the MMSE at 0.74 and with the FAST at 0.80.

Consequently, 55% of the variance in neurologically assessed changes with the progression of AD was accounted for by MMSE scores, whereas 64% of this neurologic change variance was accounted for by FAST scores.

An analysis was also performed separately for those subjects in this neurologic change cohort whose MMSE scores were at bottom (zero) ($n = 37$). By definition, the correlation between MMSE score and neurologic change in this severely impaired AD cohort is zero. FAST scores correlated with neurologic changes in this cohort at 0.80, an identical magnitude of relationship to that seen in less impaired subjects.

Consequently, the neurologic concurrent validity studies support the apparent superior validity of the FAST staging procedure in comparison with the MMSE in tracking the course of AD.

*Relationship to cognitive changes.* Another form of concurrent validity which is applicable for procedures such as the FAST, which measure progressive functional deterioration, is the relationship between this deterioration and cognitive assessments of decline in AD. In a study of 50 subjects (25 men and 25 women) with normal aging ($n = 30$), mild cognitive impairment ($n = 4$), and AD ($n = 16$), the relationship of the major elements of the FAST to cognitive assessments from the Brief Cognitive Rating Scale (BCRS) was examined [37–40]. The functional stages correlated with progressive deterioration in concentration ($r = 0.88$), recent memory ($r = 0.90$), remote memory ($r = 0.83$), and orientation ($r = 0.94$). Consequently, there is a strong relationship between the FAST functional stages of AD and progressive cognitive deterioration. This relationship between the FAST and cognitive decline in AD is also seen in direct comparison with the MMSE. In a study of 566 subjects with normal aging, mild cognitive impairment and AD at all severity levels, the correlation between the FAST staging procedure and the MMSE was 0.83 (Figure 2.3) [41].

As previously noted, the MMSE and other cognitive tests which have been traditionally utilized for dementia assessment bottom out at the end of FAST stage 6. Even in the course of FAST stage 6, these measures are subject to floor effects and become less useful in charting the progressive course of AD. FAST stage 7, with six identifiable functional substages, represents more than half the potential temporal duration of AD. Therefore, it was important to demonstrate concurrent validity in the latter portion of the FAST, when traditional dementia assessment measures are subject to floor effects. Doing this required the development of psychological test measures which were capable of assessing cognition in severe dementia. Sclan *et al* [42] and Auer *et al* [43,44] developed these measures. They took psychological test measures which had originally been developed for infants and small children

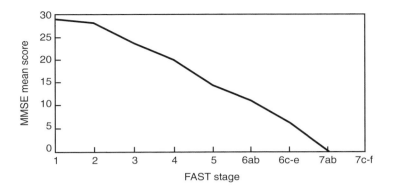

FIGURE 2.3 Scores on the MMSE with increasing functional impairment on the FAST in subjects with aging and Alzheimer's disease. MMSE, Mini-Mental State Examination; FAST, Functional Assessment Staging

*Source*: from Reisberg *et al* [41]

based upon Piagetian principles [45–48], and adapted these procedures for the assessment of the severely demented patient. The specific test procedures selected for adaptation were the Uzgiris and Hunt Ordinal Scales of Psychological Development [49]. The adapted version of these tests which were successfully applied for the assessment of severe dementia is termed the Modified Ordinal Scales of Psychological Development (M-OSPD) [43,44]. Studies demonstrated the same magnitude of robust correlation between these cognitive test assessments for severe dementia as had been noted in the early portion of AD course for the MMSE and other, theoretically functioning independent, dementia cognitive assessments. Specifically, in a study of 70 AD patients in FAST stages 6 and 7, the Spearman correlation coefficient between the M-OSPD total scores and the 11 FAST stage 6 and stage 7 substages represented was $-0.77$ ($p < 0.001$) (Figure 2.4) [43]. Consequently, it can be demonstrated throughout the entire course of AD, that there is a strong relationship between progressive and characteristic functional deterioration and progressive cognitive loss.

## Utility

An additional means of assessing the validity of a clinical procedure, apart from criterion validity and concurrent validity, is utility. In terms of the present discussion, can usage of the FAST procedure reveal relationships which would otherwise be difficult to discern? A few published studies which have demonstrated the utility of the FAST staging procedure in

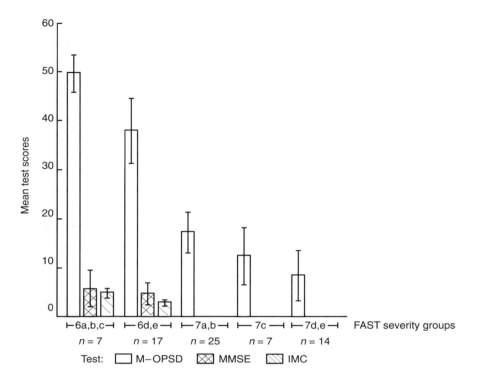

**FIGURE 2.4** Functioning and cognition in stage 6 and 7 Alzheimer's disease. Bars indicate 95% confidence limits above and below mean score. All comparisons between non-adjacent FAST severity groups are significant ($p < 0.001$); significant differences between adjacent groups were found between the 6d,e and the 7a,b FAST groups. FAST, Functional Assessment Staging; M-OSPD, Modified Ordinal Scales of Psychological Development; MMSE, Mini-Mental State Examination; IMC, Information, Memory and Concentration test

*Source*: from Auer *et al* [43]

uncovering previously obscure and difficult to discern relationships in AD will be discussed. These studies are an examination of physical changes in AD patients and a study of a specific neurologic marker of the advent of incontinence in AD.

*Utility in charting the emergence of physical disability.* Contractures are conditions in which joints become stiffened and immobile. They may be associated with structural changes in joints as well as muscle shorten-ing [50,51]. Contractures can result from various conditions, including nervous system pathology as well as disease of muscle or joints. Contractures are also known to be associated with immobilization and inactivity and can occur from such immobilizing central nervous system conditions as cerebral trauma and stroke [50–52]. Contractures had been known to be associated with immobility in nursing home patients, who are frequently frail and demented [53]. However, the precise relationship of contractures to AD had not been studied. Using the FAST staging procedure in conjunction with other measures in a longitudinally studied population, Souren *et al* studied the occurrence of joint contractures in AD [36].

For this study, a contracture was defined as a limitation of 50% or greater of the passive range of motion of the joint, secondary to permanent muscle shortening, ankylosis, or a combination of the two. Contractures were always associated with the involved joint in a position of flexion, with the exception of the ankle joint, where contractures also occurred in the extended joint.

The patients in this study represented a consecutive sample of all patients with AD in FAST stages 6 and 7, seen over a time period of 6 years. A total of 161 patients who ranged in age from 50 to 95 years were studied (mean age, 75.3 ± 8.6 years). The results of this study are illustrated in Figure 2.5. Approximately a quarter (24%) of the patients had a contracture involving at least one joint of one extremity. Of the 102 patients residing in the community, seven (7%) had contractures. Of the 59 institutionalized patients, 32 (54%) had contractures. The mean FAST substage for the community residing patients was 6c. The mean FAST substage for the nursing home residing patients was 7b.

The MMSE score was zero (bottom) in 95% of the patients with contractures (37 of the 39 patients). The FAST score (calculated as previously described), correlated with the occurrence of contractures ($r = 0.70, p < 0.001$). As can be seen in Figure 2.5, none of the patients in early stage 6 (FAST stages 6a–6c, corresponding to deficiency in activities of daily life), manifested contractures. Approximately 10% of patients in late FAST stage 6, i.e. FAST substages 6d and 6e, corresponding to incipient incontinence, manifested contractures. In FAST stage 7, about half of all patients had contractures.

The percentage of patients with these deformities increased throughout the course of the 7th stage. Specifically, approximately 40% of patients in FAST stages 7a and 7b, corresponding to an incipient non-verbal condition, about 60% of incipient non-ambulatory (FAST 7c) patients, and 95% of immobile (FAST stages 7d–7f) patients manifested contractures. When contractures were present, they involved all four extremities in ~ 70% of patients.

Therefore, strong relationships between these dramatic physical deformities, contractures, and the course of AD can be demonstrated using the FAST staging procedure for tracking the characteristic clinical course of AD. These relationships are obscure when viewed from the context of traditional measures such as the MMSE.

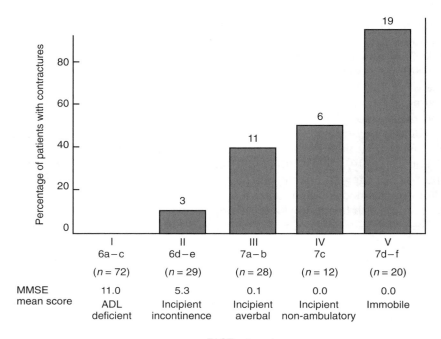

**FIGURE 2.5** Percentages of patients with contractures in stage 6 and 7 Alzheimer's disease. Significant differences: across the five categories, $p < 0.001$; between I and II, $p < 0.01$; between II and III, $p < 0.05$; between IV and V, $p < 0.01$. The prevalence of contractures was significantly correlated with FAST staging levels ($p < 0.001$). FAST, Functional Assesment Staging; ADL, Activities of Daily Living

*Source*: data and figure adapted from Souren *et al* [36]

*Utility in identifying independent physical (neurologic) markers of disease course.* Another dramatic example of the utility of the FAST staging procedure for marking the characteristic clinical course of AD is in demonstrating a specific physical, neurologic marker of AD course, corresponding to the advent of urinary incontinence in AD. As already noted, neurologic reflexes and release signs are strong correlates of the course of AD. A recent study of nearly 800 individuals with normal aging, mild cognitive impairment and progressive AD indicates that specific neurologic reflexes can serve as powerful markers distinguish-ing AD patients at FAST stages ≤ 6c from AD patients at FAST stages ≥ 7a, i.e. AD patients free of incontinence from AD patients who are doubly incontinent (Figure 2.6) [54]. Specifically,

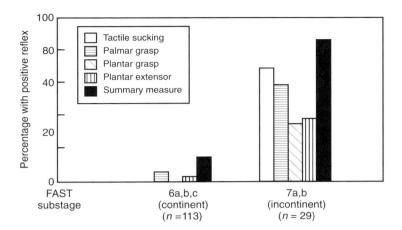

**FIGURE 2.6** Prevalence of five reflexes in continent and incontinent ambulatory Alzheimer's disease patients with deficits in activities of daily living (ADL). Differences in percentages of reflex measures between the groups of patients are significant for all measures ($p < 0.001$). FAST, Functional Assessment Staging

*Source*: from Franssen *et al* [54]

the so-called developmental reflexes, comprising the sucking reflex, hand and foot grasp reflexes and the plantar extensor (Babinski) reflex, were assessed in these subjects in accordance with the scale of Franssen [33,34, 55]. The four reflexes were scored as being present when they were prominent and persistent, as indicated by a rating of $\geq 5$ on this Franssen rating scale. A summary measure indicated the presence of any these reflexes at a rating of $\geq 5$.

Prevalence of all four individual reflexes and of the summary measure was more than 15 times higher in permanently doubly incontinent AD patients (i.e. patients at FAST stages $\geq$ 7a) compared to continent AD patients (i.e. patients at FAST stages $\leq$ 5) ($p < 0.001$). Prevalence of these reflexes was at least 6 times higher in FAST stage 7a and 7b patients in comparison with patients in early FAST stage 6 (i.e. 6a–6c) ($p < 0.001$). These differences in reflex prevalence remained very significant after age and gender were controlled for ($p < 0.001$). Comparing early stage 6 subjects (FAST stages 6a to 6c) to early stage 7 subjects (FAST stages 7a to 7b), the specificity of the summary neurologic measure in differentiating these FAST groups was 85.8%, the sensitivity was 86.2%, and the overall accuracy was 85.9% ($\chi^2 = 55.8$, $p < 0.001$). Consequently, the FAST staging procedure is useful in the identification of a physical, neurologic marker of the evolution of AD course. Traditional measures, such as the MMSE, would be much less useful in eliciting these relationships.

*The Characteristic Functional Course of AD: Conclusion*

Therefore, studies have demonstrated that the FAST course is a superior indicator of the characteristic clinical evolution of AD. Before a deeper understanding of this characteristic clinical course of AD can be achieved, a remarkable corollary observation must be noted. This observation relates directly to the etiopathogenic basis of the AD clinical process.

## The Etiopathogenic Basis of the Clinical Course of AD

The preceding discussion illustrated the utility of the characterization of the functional course of AD for longitudinally tracking the disease, identifying neuropathologic, neurologic, cognitive and physical correlates of AD, and revealing specific neurologic markers of AD course. Remarkably, this functional progression of AD is a precise reversal of the order of acquisition of the same functions in normal human development (Table 2.3) [56–58].

A general relationship between aging, dementia and normal development had been noted for millennia by playwrights and poets and is embodied in vernacular language [59,60]. For example, "dotage" has been defined in part as "childishness of old age" [2]. Clinicians and scientists have also recognized relationships between senescent dementia and normal development generally [61] and, in more recent times, more specifically [62–68]. However, the precise functional developmental reversal which was noted in the FAST staging considerably advanced clinical and scientific understanding of this relationship. Each FAST stage in AD can be usefully described in terms of a corresponding developmental age (DA). Studies indicated that the reversal of figure drawing (praxic) capacity, of feeding ability, and of other capacities in AD appeared to mirror the normal human developmental pattern and appeared to occur at the DA appropriate point based upon the FAST staging (Table 2.4) [69]. For example, neurologically, so-called "developmental" or "primitive" reflexes, which are present in the infant, re-emerge in the AD patient. Astoundingly, these reflexes appear to emerge at the DA-appropriate point, based upon the FAST/DA model [33,34,54].

A word for this process by which degenerative mechanisms reverse the order of acquisition in normal development, "retrogenesis", has recently been proposed [70,71]. Figure 2.7 illustrates this retrogenic process in terms of some of the developmental reflexes studied by Franssen *et al* [54]. For various reasons, it is difficult to compare AD patients with their DA peers precisely. For example, although retrogenesis applies to degenerative brain processes in AD, it does not apply to the body as a whole. AD patients don't shrink to the size of infants. One consequence of this is that a hand grasp reflex can be much stronger and more dramatic in a stage 7 AD patient in

TABLE 2.3  Functional stages in normal human development and Alzheimer's disease (from [12,57,58])

| Approximate age | Acquired abilities | Lost abilities | Alzheimer stage | |
|---|---|---|---|---|
| 12 + years | Hold a job | Hold a job | 3 | Incipient |
| 8–12 years | Handle simple finances | Handle simple finances | 4 | Mild |
| 5–7 years | Select proper clothing | Select proper clothing | 5 | Moderate |
| 5 years | Put on clothes unaided | Put on clothes unaided | 6a | Moderately severe |
| 4 years | Shower unaided | Shower unaided | b | |
| 4 years | Toilet unaided | Toilet unaided | c | |
| 3–4½ years | Control urine | Control urine | d | |
| 2–3 years | Control bowels | Control bowels | e | |
| 15 months | Speak 5–6 words | Speak 5–6 words | 7a | Severe |
| 1 year | Speak 1 word | Speak 1 word | b | |
| 1 year | Walk | Walk | c | |
| 6–10 months | Sit up | Sit up | d | |
| 2–4 months | Smile | Smile | e | |
| 1–3 months | Hold up head | Hold up head | f | |

TABLE 2.4  Select retrogenic* observations in Alzheimer's disease (AD) (from [70])

| Model | Observation |
|---|---|
| *Clinical* | |
| Cognitive | Order of changes in AD appear to reverse normal development [43,65,66,68] |
| Language | General pattern of loss in AD appears to reverse normal development [66,68] |
| Praxis | Order of loss, e.g. in ability to construct figures, appears to reverse normal developmental pattern [68,69] |
| Functioning | Loss of specific functions occurs in a reverse hierarchy from normal developmental functional acquisition [56,69] |
| *Physiologic* | |
| Electroencephalogram (EEG) observations | Progressive slowing of EEG activity with AD progression mirrors increments in brain wave activity in normal development [72,73] |
| Neurometabolic observations | Decrements in cerebral glucose metabolism measured with PET in AD reverse pattern of cerebral myelinization in normal development [74] |
| Neurologic reflexes | Normal human developmental reflexes emerge in the course of AD [33–35,54] |

(*continues overleaf*)

**TABLE 2.4** *(continued)*

| Model | Observation |
|---|---|
| *Neuropathologic and neuroanatomic* | |
| Neurofibrillary changes | Pattern of change in AD appears to reverse pattern of developmental myelinization [75,76,78] |
| Neuronal loss | Pattern of neuronal loss in AD appears to reverse pattern of myelin deposition in normal development [74,78] |

\* The process by which changes in AD occur in apparent reverse order to normal human developmental processes.

comparison with an infant. Also, the physical and social environment of the AD patient is very different from that of the infant and child at corresponding DAs. For example, AD patients, because of their age, are prone to various comorbidities. Also, unlike infants who are cuddled and "played with", stage 7 AD patients are often left in immobile positions and even prevented from

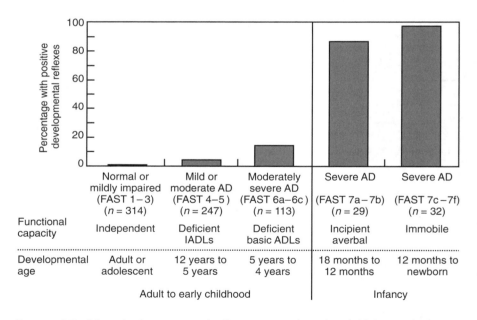

**FIGURE 2.7** Neurologic retrogenesis. Percentages of aged and Alzheimer's disease (AD) patients with developmental (primitive) neurologic reflexes. FAST, Functional Assessment Staging; IADL, Instrumental Activities of Daily Living; ADL, Activities of Daily Living

*Source*: data and figure adapted from Franssen *et al* [54]

moving by both physical and chemical restraints. These differences in care may predispose AD patients to contractures. The presence of contractures, in turn, confounds reflex assessment in the AD patient.

Given the differences in size, concomitant illnesses, social attention, etc., it is difficult to compare AD patients to DA peers precisely. However, as can be seen in Figure 2.7, the neurologic reflexes appear to emerge at the DA appropriate point in AD from the retrogenesis model.

As outlined in Table 2.4, there is evidence from numerous clinical and physiologic studies of the validity and applicability of the retrogenesis process in AD. For example, physiologically, the progressive slowing of EEG activity which occurs in the brain of the AD patient appears to reverse the normal developmental pattern [71–73]. The pattern of neurometabolic changes noted in the brain of the AD patient has also been observed to mirror specific developmental brain mechanisms [74].

Neuropathologic mechanisms which appear to account for the clinical and physiologic retrogenic observations in AD have been independently described by three groups of investigators [74–77]. These investigative groups have noted from different and independent perspectives that the order of pathologic involvement in the brain in aging and AD appears to reverse the temporal sequence of myelination of the brain. Studies indicate that myelination is a process which continues well into adult life [76–81].

In the early decades of the twentieth century, Flechsig [78] hypothesized that "the development of function follows the same sequence as myelination and is partly dependent on it. A corollary to that theory is that tardily myelinated areas engage in complex functions highly related to the organism's experience" [82]. Lecours [83] and Yakolev [84] extended these hypothesized developmental myelination relationships beyond the functional domains, including progressive behavioural and cognitive development. Lecours noted that "It is reasonable to assume that the cycles of myelination ... can be related to the emergence and gradual differentiation ... of behavioural patterns such as locomotion, manipulation of instruments, articulated speech, and language ... the development of myelin in the sheaths of a fiber system may be taken as an indication that the impulse conduction in this system has become space committed in an invariable path .. [and] reached functional maturity" [83].

There is a further element to the myelinogenic/functional and behavioural interrelationship which is of great relevance for the degenerative process of AD and, as will be discussed, other dementias as well. This is that myelination is a progressive process and the myelin appears to protect the axon against degenerative processes [71,85]. Therefore, regions of the brain which are myelinated early in development become progressively more thickly myelinated and areas which are myelinated late in development are the most vulnerable. The process of brain vulnerability has been described as "last in, first out". Therefore, the most recently acquired skills and, in general, the most recently acquired information is the most vulnerable, and is lost first. The order of degeneration mirrors the developmental pattern of acquisition.

## Further Implications of the Etiopathogenic Basis of AD for Clinical Diagnosis: Additional Clinical Diagnostic Markers of AD

As a retrogenic process with characteristic pathologic elements, notably manifested by the presence of β-amyloid and the progressive accumulation of tau-positive neurofilaments, AD has a characteristic temporal course as well as a characteristic order of clinical degeneration.

This temporal course of AD is most clearly charted in terms of the progressive pattern of functional deterioration as described using the FAST staging procedure. Table 2.5 shows the mean duration of the functional stages and substages of AD in patients who are free of significant confounding physical and non-dementia-related mental pathology. Several remarkable aspects of the functional progression of AD should be noted in the context of the retrogenic pattern of deterioration described in the preceding section. One of these remarkable features of AD course is that, in addition to mirroring the order of functional acquisition in normal development, the time course of functional deterioration in AD, until the final 7th stage, mirrors the time course of acquisition of the same functions in normal human development [57,58,86]. Consequently, AD patients lose the ability to manage a complex job and deteriorate to double incontinence over a mean period of approximately 13 years. This is approximately the same time which it takes for a child to progress from incipient control of bowel movements, at 2–3 years of age, to being able to manage competently in an executive level job at age 15 or 16.

Interestingly, the time course of loss of each of the successive functional levels, and even the temporal disparities between the successive levels in AD, is also mirrored by the time course of acquisition of functional capacities in normal development. For example, AD patients deteriorate from loss of ability to select proper attire, to double incontinence over approximately the same period (4 years, Table 2.5) as a child takes to advance from double incontinence at age 2–3, to being able to select clothing properly at approximately 5–7 years (Table 2.3). Additionally, just as the ability to bathe independently and to put on clothing independently are acquired at similar developmental ages and the sequence of acquisition of these capacities is not rigidly fixed, the same is true of the loss of these same capacities in the course of the degenerative process of AD [87]. To cite another example, just as the acquisition of fecal continence occurs in close temporal proximity to the acquisition of urinary continence in normal child development, and the

TABLE 2.5  FAST stages and time course of functional loss in normal aging and Alzheimer's disease (AD) (Adapted from [57])

| FAST stage | Clinical characteristics | Clinical diagnosis | Estimated duration of FAST stage or substage in AD[*] | Mean MMSE[**] |
|---|---|---|---|---|
| 1 | No decrement | Normal adult | | 29–30 |
| 2 | Subjective deficit in word finding or recalling location of objects | Normal aged forgetfulness | | 28–29 |
| 3 | Deficits noted in demanding employment settings | Mild cognitive impairment | 7 years | 24–28 |
| 4 | Requires assistance in complex tasks, e.g. handling finances, planning dinner party | Mild AD | 2 years | 19–20 |
| 5 | Requires assistance in selecting proper attire | Moderate AD | 18 months | 15 |
| 6a | Requires assistance in dressing | Moderately severe AD | 5 months | 9 |
| b | Requires assistance in bathing properly | | 5 months | 8 |
| c | Requires assistance with mechanics of toileting (such as flushing, wiping) | | 5 months | 5 |
| d | Urinary incontinence | | 4 months | 3 |
| e | Fecal incontinence | | 10 months | 1 |
| 7a | Speech ability limited to about a half-dozen words | Severe AD | 12 months | 0 |
| b | Intelligible vocabulary limited to a single word | | 18 months | 0 |
| c | Ambulatory ability lost | | 12 months | 0 |
| d | Ability to sit up lost | | 12 months | 0 |
| e | Ability to smile lost | | 18 months | 0 |
| f | Ability to hold head up lost | | 12 months or longer | 0 |

Copyright 1984 by Barry Reisberg MD.
  FAST, Functional Assessment Staging; MMSE, Mini-Mental State Examination
* In subjects without other complicating illnesses who survive and progress to the subsequent deterioration stage.
**  MMSE score from [13]. Estimates based in part on published data summarized in [20].

sequence of acquisition is not rigidly fixed, similarly, the losses of urinary and fecal continence in the degenerative course of AD occur in close temporal proximity and the sequence of deterioration is not rigidly fixed [87].

The course of normal development is best charted not only in terms of the attainment of functional landmarks, but also in terms of the attainment of cognitive and intellectual skills, as well as emotional maturity. Similarly, the degenerative course of AD is best charted not only in terms of the loss of functional landmarks, but also in terms of the loss of cognitive and intellectual skills, as well as emotional changes.

Longitudinal studies provide strong support for this observation in AD. The prospective longitudinal study reviewed in detail earlier in this chapter, in which 103 community-residing AD patients were followed over a 4.6-year mean interval, directly addressed the utility of various measurement modalities in the assessment of the longitudinal course of AD [17]. The "gold standard" criterion was longitudinal course. Operationally, this was defined as change in measure in comparison with change in time in survivors. The assessment measure which showed the strongest relationship to temporal change using this criterion was a global measure encompassing characteristic cognitive, functional and behavioural changes in AD, specifically the GDS.

In the 65 survivors studied, GDS correlated with time at 0.48, accounting for 23% of the variance. In a stepwise multiple regression analysis, the strongest correlation with temporal change was seen for GDS. Functional change as assessed with the FAST added significant additional variance to GDS. Together, the multiple $R$ with the GDS and FAST was 0.53. Therefore, the GDS and FAST together explained 28% of temporal course variance. The MMSE did not add significant additional variance to longitudinal course assessment beyond that explained by the GDS and FAST.

Therefore, just as the best marker of the course of normal development would be a global assessment of cognitive, functional and emotional maturity, the best marker of the degenerative course of AD is a global assessment of cognitive, functional and emotional deterioration, the GDS. Just as the course of normal development is also usefully marked by functional landmarks, the same functional landmarks are also useful in marking the degenerative course of AD. A comprehensive understanding of the course of normal development encompasses both global and functional development. Similarly, a comprehensive clinical diagnostic understanding of the degenerative course of AD encompasses both global and functional deterioration. Because of its diagnostic relevance, the course of global deterioration in AD as charted with the GDS is shown in Table 2.6.

The global changes described in the GDS have been dissected and reconstructed in terms of the constituent elements of the GDS. Specifically, concordant ordinal descriptions in terms of progressive changes in

TABLE 2.6   Global Deterioration Scale (GDS) for age-associated cognitive decline and Alzheimer's disease

| GDS stage | Clinical characteristics | Diagnosis |
|---|---|---|
| 1 | *No subjective complaints of memory deficit.* No memory deficit evident on clinical interview | Normal |
| 2 | *Subjective complaints of memory deficit,* most frequently in following areas:<br>(1)  Forgetting where one has placed familiar objects<br>(2)  Forgetting names one formerly knew well<br>No objective evidence of memory deficit on clinical interview<br>No objective deficit in employment or social situations<br>Appropriate concern with respect to symptomatology | Normal aging |
| 3 | *Earliest subtle deficits.* Manifestations in more than one of the following areas:<br>(1)  Patient may have gotten lost when traveling to an unfamiliar location<br>(2)  Co-workers become aware of patient's relatively poor performance<br>(3)  Word and name finding deficit become evident to intimates<br>(4)  Patient may read a passage or book and retain relatively little material<br>(5)  Patient may demonstrate decreased facility remembering names upon introduction to new people<br>(6)  Patient may have lost or misplaced an object of value<br>(7)  Concentration deficit may be evident on clinical testing<br>Objective evidence of memory deficit obtained only with an intensive interview<br>Decreased performance in demanding employment and social settings<br>Denial begins to become manifest in patient<br>Mild to moderate anxiety frequently accompanies symptoms | Mild memory impairment |
| 4 | *Clear-cut deficit on careful clinical interview.* Deficit manifest in following areas:<br>(1)  Decreased knowledge of current and recent events<br>(2)  May exhibit some deficit in memory of one's personal history<br>(3)  Concentration deficit elicited on serial subtractions | Mild Alzheimer's disease |

*(continues overleaf)*

TABLE 2.6 *(continued)*

| GDS stage | Clinical characteristics | Diagnosis |
|---|---|---|

(4)  Decreased ability to travel, handle finances, etc.
Frequently no deficit in following areas:
   (1)  Orientation to time and place
   (2)  Recognition of familiar persons and faces
   (3)  Ability to travel to familiar locations
*Inability to perform complex tasks*
Denial is dominant defense mechanism
Flattening of affect and withdrawal from challenging
     situations occur

**5**  *Patient can no longer survive without some assistance*   Moderate
Patient is unable during interview to recall a major   Alzheimer's
relevant aspect of his current life, e.g.   disease
   (1)  His address or telephone number for many years
   (2)  The name of close members of his family (such as
        grandchildren)
   (3)  The name of the high school or college from
        which he graduated
Frequently some disorientation to time (date, day of the
     week, season, etc.) or to place
An educated person may have difficulty counting back
     from 40 by 4s or from 20 by 2s
Persons at this stage retain knowledge of many major
     facts regarding themselves and others
They invariably know their own names and generally
     know their spouse's and children's names
They require no assistance with toileting or eating, but
     may have difficulty choosing the proper clothing to
     wear

**6**  May occasionally forget the name of the spouse upon   Moderately
     whom they are entirely dependent for survival   severe
Will be *largely unaware of all recent events and experiences*   Alzheimer's
     *in their lives*   disease
Retain some knowledge of their surroundings; the year,
     the season, etc.
May have difficulty counting by 1s from 10, both
     backward and sometimes forward
*Will require some assistance with activities of daily living:*
   (1)  May become incontinent
   (2)  Will require travel assistance but occasionally
        will be able to travel to familiar locations
Diurnal rhythm frequently disturbed
Almost always recall their own name
Frequently continue to be able to distinguish familiar
     from unfamiliar persons in their environment

TABLE 2.6 *(continued)*

| GDS stage | Clinical characteristics | Diagnosis |
|---|---|---|
| | Personality and emotional changes occur. These are quite variable and include:<br>(1) Delusional behaviour, e.g. patients may accuse their spouse of being an imposter; may talk to imaginary figures in the environment, or to their own reflection in the mirror<br>(2) Obsessive symptoms, e.g. person may continually repeat simple cleaning activities<br>(3) Anxiety symptoms, agitation, and even previously non-existent violent behaviour may occur<br>(4) Cognitive abulia, e.g. loss of willpower because an individual cannot carry a thought long enough to determine a purposeful course of action | |
| 7 | *All verbal abilities are lost over the course of this stage*<br>(1) Early in this stage words and phrases are spoken, but speech is very circumscribed<br>(2) Later there is no speech at all—only babbling<br>Incontinent of urine; *requires assistance toileting and feeding. Basic psychomotor skills* (e.g. ability to walk) are lost with the progression of this stage<br>The brain appears to no longer be able to tell the body what to do. Generalized and cortical neurologic signs and symptoms are frequently present | Severe Alzheimer's disease |

From [159]. Copyright 1983 Barry Reisberg, MD

concentration, recent memory, remote memory, orientation, functioning, language, motoric changes, mood and behaviour, praxic (figure drawing) capacity, calculation ability, and feeding abilities have been published and validated as part of an assessment tool known as the BCRS [18,86,88,89]. Each of these BCRS axes was designed to be optimally concordant, at any given level, with the corresponding GDS stage. Therefore, in summation, these procedures can describe the course of AD as powerfully as the GDS and the FAST from which they are derived (the FAST is an expanded version of the original BCRS functioning axis).

In a remarkable study conducted in Canada, a consecutive series of cases of putative dementia, but without clear ante-mortem clinical diagnoses, were assessed through informant interviews subsequent to the patient's demise [90]. Previous studies had demonstrated that with traditional dementia assessments an accurate diagnosis of the presence of dementia, but not the specific cause of dementia, could be made retrospectively with information from caregivers [91–96]. Since, as already noted, the GDS and the FAST track a characteristic clinical course of dementia associated with AD, this Canadian study was conducted to determine whether one could use the BCRS and FAST, specific derivatives of the GDS, to accurately diagnose AD retrospectively, post-demise. The BCRS and FAST were modified for retrospective, post-mortem informant interview. The resulting modification was entitled RetroBCRS. A consecutive series of 36 cases from the Maritime Brain Tissue Bank were studied for diagnostic concordance between the informant interview-based diagnosis and the post-mortem pathological diagnosis. The results indicated that "at a cutpoint of 4 or more, both the sensitivity and specificity of the RetroBCRS as a test of dementia compared with the pathologic diagnosis was 100%" [90]. The authors found that, using the informant-based RetroBCRS, the diagnosis of AD as the specific cause of dementia was confirmed in 27 of 27 cases. Overall, using the RetroBCRS, the specific cause of the dementia was identifiable by the clinicians in 92% of cases. The authors concluded that "the RetroBCRS used by an expert physician with a reliable informant is a valid method of detecting dementia and determining whether AD was present".

Additionally, in this study of Rockwood *et al* [90], the duration of dementia was assessed using the methods of Sano *et al* [97]. The correlation between the RetroBCRS score and the duration of dementia was 0.51. This result from this retrospective, Brain Bank-based, study is very consistent with the results obtained from the ante-mortem, prospective longitudinal study of the temporal course of AD in community-residing subjects [17] described earlier in this section. Specifically, in that study, the GDS and FAST measures together, in the multiple regression model, correlated with the prospective course of AD at 0.53. As already noted, the RetroBCRS procedure of Rockwood *et al* (which includes the FAST) would be expected to be virtually identical to the GDS and FAST procedures in dementia assessment. Consequently, the study of Rockwood *et al* adds further support to a very substantial body of evidence indicating that these procedures chart a characteristic course of dementia associated with AD.

## Differential Diagnostic Import of the Characteristic Clinical Course of AD

As indicated by the study of Rockwood *et al* and numerous other studies, including those reviewed in the preceding sections, AD has a characteristic ordinal and temporal course which can be differentiated from other dementing entities. This characteristic course of AD is charted most clearly with the

FAST staging procedure in terms of both its ordinal progression and the usual temporal course.

Some entities characterized by dementia, or in which dementia may occur, differ strikingly from the characteristic FAST progression of AD [57,86]. A few examples, which are familiar to all clinicians with a knowledge of brain disease, are stroke and normal pressure hydrocephalus (NPH). For example, a patient may have a stroke and the stroke may result in urinary incontinence. This urinary incontinence may be the only clinically manifest sequela of the cerebrovascular accident (CVA). Alternatively, the CVA with resultant urinary incontinence may also be accompanied by dementia. When this dementia occurs, it may be of *any* magnitude. For example, the dementia may be of sufficient magnitude to interfere with executive functions, such as organizational skills, and the ability to manage instrumental activities, such as management of personal finances, but *not* interfere with the ability to choose proper clothing, to put on clothing independently, to bathe without assistance, to toilet without assistance, to maintain fecal continence, to speak, to ambulate, to sit up independently, to smile, or to hold up one's head. Consequently, the presentation of a dementia associated with a stroke can be, and frequently is, vastly different from the characteristic functional presentation of AD as outlined in Table 2.1. These clinical differences in the presentation of a stroke with, or without, concomitant dementia, are of diagnostic and differential diagnostic relevance.

A stroke characteristically produces a dementia with an acute or, relatively acute, onset. As noted in the previous paragraph, the characteristic presentation of AD, as outlined with FAST staging procedure, is very different from the acute dementia which may result from a stroke. Importantly, the characteristic functional progression of AD also differs from the functional progression of more chronic dementing processes.

For example, NPH is an entity of gradual onset characterized in part by increased fluid in the cerebral ventricles. NPH is characteristically associated with dementia. However, the course of dementia presentation in NPH is dramatically different from the course of dementia presentation of AD as, for example, outlined in Table 2.1. In NPH, gait disturbance with difficulties in ambulation is characteristically the earliest presenting symptom. Subsequently, urinary incontinence characteristically occurs. Only later on do symptoms associated with the earliest dementia stages of AD occur, such as decreased executive and instrumental functioning. In AD, the functional presentation is in completely different order from that in NPH. As outlined in Table 2.2, AD patients first lose executive and instrumental functional capacities, such as the ability to function in a job setting and the ability to perform complex daily life tasks, and subsequently, years later, develop urinary incontinence and, years later, develop gait disturbances resulting in loss of ambulation.

The order of functional loss in prion dementias, in dementia associated with central nervous system (CNS) brain metastasis, in dementia associated with electrolyte disturbances, and in dementia associated with numerous other conditions, differ markedly from the characteristic functional presentation of AD as outlined with the FAST staging procedure [57,86].

## The Characteristic Clinical Course of Retrogenic Dementias

Although the characteristic clinical course of AD, as outlined most clearly with the FAST staging procedure, is very different from many other dementing conditions, it is also interesting and of diagnostic relevance that many dementias of diverse etiology occasionally, or more frequently, follow the characteristic FAST sequential progression of AD more or less precisely. The advances in understanding of the etiopathogenic mechanisms of AD provide an explanation for the observed clinical similarities between these ostensibly etiopathogenically diverse, but frequently clinically similar, dementia processes.

As described earlier in this review, in AD an etiopathogenic process termed retrogenesis accounts for the pattern of functional losses and of clinical symptomatology. The pathologic basis of this retrogenic process is that the most thinly (recently) myelinated brain regions are the most vulnerable, and the most thickly myelinated brain regions are affected last in the evolution of dementing disorder. The myelin is a major constituent of the so-called "white matter" of the brain. Therefore, any dementing disorder which progressively and diffusely affects the white matter of the brain is likely to produce a retrogenic-type dementia, similar to AD in its clinical progression.

Many conditions associated with dementia are known to produce white matter pathology as a prominent, or even pre-eminent, pathologic change. To the extent to which this white matter pathology is generalized and diffuse, these dementias are likely to mimic the clinical presentation of AD. For example, vitamin $B_{12}$ deficiency is known to be associated with dementia as well as signs of demyelination, especially in the spinal cord, but also in the brain [98]. More general white matter lesions have also been found to be associated with vitamin $B_{12}$ deficiency [99,100]. Treatment of the $B_{12}$ deficiency has been associated with resolution of both myelin and white matter changes as well as resolution of neurologic and cognitive disturbances [98–100].

White matter pathology, in contrast to primary neuronal pathology, has also been implicated in the etiopathogenesis of other potentially dementing conditions, for example, anoxia. Basic studies in rats have shown that occlusion of the common carotid artery combined with hypoxemia "causes white matter necrosis in the ipsilateral cerebral hemisphere originating and spreading from myelinogenic foci" [101,102].

Subsequent studies have supported these observations [103]. Azzarelli *et al* have studied this phenomenon in detail in neonates [102]. They concluded that, at the moment of insult, damaged brain areas are ones which have the greatest susceptibility to oxygen deprivation. Consequently, at any given developmental age, tissues having higher metabolic rates for glucose should be particularly sensitive to oxygen deprivation. Furthermore, they note that myelinization is related to increased neuronal oxidative activity in oligodendroglia. Hence, brain areas most involved in myelination are the most sensitive to hypoxic damage.

Others have noted that the highly specialized architecture of myelinated axons renders them vulnerable to injury [104]. During anoxia, myelin, in contrast to glial cell bodies and proximal processes, accumulates ionic calcium [105]. The result may be relative vulnerability of oligodendroglia and related myelin to free radical damage, glutamate toxicity and anoxia *per se* [106–110].

It is also possible that "myelin may play a role . . . in protection of the axon and in maintenance of the integrity of the oligodendroglia/myelin/axonal relationship" [71]. Therefore, the most recently and, as a result, thinly myelinated brain regions may be selectively vulnerable to anoxic and related insults. Anoxia and hypoxia, in turn, have been implicated in diverse brain and dementia-related pathologies, from hyponatremia [111] to cerebrovascular dementia and stroke.

Depression is a condition which has long been known to be associated with a potentially or frequently reversible dementia [112–114]. A series of recent studies have related late life depression to increased white matter hyperintensities in neuroimaging brain studies [115–121]. The cognitive impairment sometimes noted in late life depression can be difficult to distinguish from AD [112–114,122]. The reasons for these similarities appear to be explainable on the basis of the retrogenesis model. Specifically, the brain regions most vulnerable to the white matter insults would be the same as in AD, and hence the presentations of these conditions in the context of progressive dementia would be similar.

## AD Risk Factors and Retrogenesis

Many risk factors for the development of AD are now well recognized [11]. Some of these risk factors are the same conditions which may produce dementias of a retrogenic type which can be confused with AD, such as those described in the previous section.

For example, low levels of vitamin $B_{12}$ have been associated with increased risk of AD [123]. Other conditions, sometimes biochemically related to vitamin $B_{12}$ deficiency, have also been associated with increased risk for AD. These include folate deficiency and the biochemical markers of chemical $B_{12}$ deficiency, i.e. serum homocysteine and methylmalonic acid [123–126]. In addition to vitamin $B_{12}$ being associated with myelin disturbance, some of these risk factors for AD are independently associated with white matter cerebrovascular pathology [127] as well as peripheral atherosclerosis [128]. Depression also, apart from being associated with an occasionally reversible dementia, appears to be an independent risk factor for AD [129–132].

A broad variety of conditions which are known to be associated with either cerebrovascular or cardiovascular disease are now recognized as risk factors for AD. These include atherosclerosis *per se* [133] as well as indicators of cerebrovascular disease [134,135]. Cerebrovascular disease has also, in turn, been directly related to AD pathogenic elements and various well-recognized AD risk factors. For example, AD is now known to be characterized by cerebrovascular amyloid deposition, termed cerebral amyloid angiopathy (CAA) [136–138]. This CAA and related pathology have been considered to be of possible relevance in the etiopathogenesis of AD [136–141]. CAA involves intracortical arterioles and brain capillaries as well as the leptomeninges. Almost all AD patients studied exhibit CAA. CAA has been related to trauma and anoxia, known risk factors for AD and dementia more generally. Foremost among these factors is the magnitude of amyloid-$\beta$ (A $\beta$) deposition. Studies suggest that A$\beta$ may be the cause of CAA and of associated degeneration of cerebral microvasculature [138]. Degeneration of cerebral microvasculature associated with these CAA/A$\beta$ related processes "may have wider implications on cerebral perfusion and permeability" [138]. Resulting decrements in permeability would be expected to affect the most metabolically dependant and the most vulnerable myelin structures [101,102].

Interestingly, the occurrence of CAA adds insight into some of the reasons for the observed diversity in the clinical manifestations of dementing disorders. CAA is the principal lesion in some familial cerebral angiopathies, such as hereditary cerebral amyloidosis Dutch type [138,142]. In this dementing disorder, there are widespread brain hemorrhages, presumably associated with a more severe vascular CAA-related pathology than that which occurs in AD.

Another AD risk factor which is well established is the occurrence of the ε4 allelic genotype of the apolipoprotein E (APOE) gene [143]. Whereas the ε4 allele is associated with an increased risk of AD, the APOE ε2 allele is associated with decreased risk of AD. APOE has a major role in lipid and lipoprotein metabolism [144]. APOE polymorphism is associated with variations in the transport and clearance of lipids as well as other compounds [144, 145]. Furthermore, the APOE genotypes are associated with cerebrovascular disease, and with both cerebrovascular and cardiovascular disease risk factors, in a manner consistent with their role in association with increased AD risk. For example, persons with the APOE ε4 allele and persons with the APOE ε2 allele have, respectively, higher and lower low-density lipoprotein cholesterol levels [146]. Furthermore, the risk of myocardial infarction is increased in persons with an APOE ε4 allele and decreased in persons with an APOE ε2 allele [146]. Consequently, APOE genotypic risk for AD is readily related to cardiovascular and cerebrovascular pathology, as well as maintenance of brain lipids and, presumably, myelin integrity. These APOE-related risk factors apply to dementias other than AD, as well as to AD [144,147].

In summary, AD risk factors can assist in increasing clinician's understanding of both commonalities and differences between AD and other dementing disorders, as well as in improving understanding of the basic etiopathogenic nature of AD.

## Characteristic Behavioural Changes in AD

Apart from changes in functioning and cognition, characteristic behavioural changes also occur in the course of AD, which have been termed behavioural and psychological symptoms of dementia (BPSD) [148]. These BPSD symptoms are quite diverse, and include: (a) paranoid and delusional ideation; (b) hallucinatory disturbances; (c) activity disturbances; (d) aggressivity; (e) sleep rhythm disturbances; and (f) anxieties and phobias. Characteristic symptoms occurring at particular stages of AD can be identified. However, because they are the product of the psychological external and internal environment of the AD patient, as well as the neurochemical milieu in the brain of the AD patient, these BPSD symptoms, although to a greater or lesser extent characteristic of AD, are not pathognomonic.

For example, studies have shown that approximately 75% of AD patients at GDS stage 5 have suspiciousness and more than 40% of these patients have the specific delusion that people are stealing things [149]. Similarly, hallucinations are relatively uncommon in AD, and when they occur, they tend to be visual and not dramatic in nature. Less than 25% of AD patients at any stage appear to manifest these visual hallucinations [149]. Activity disturbances and aggressivity appear to peak in occurrence and magnitude in stages 5 and 6 of AD, where they occur in a majority of patients [149]. Sleep disturbance in AD is marked by disrupted sleep with frequent wakenings. This sleep disturbance peaks in occurrence in stage 5, affecting approximately 40% of AD patients [149]. AD patients have a characteristic affective disturbance in which they say "I wish I were dead" or an equivalent statement, as a morbid commentary on their situation, but without true suicidal ideation or intent. This statement is noted in 30–40% of AD patients in stages 4 and 5 [149].

Characteristic anxieties and phobias are noted in AD: nearly half of patients in stage 5 exhibit an anxiety regarding upcoming events and more than 40% of patients in stages 5 and 6 exhibit a fear of having being left alone [149].

Because the BPSD symptoms of AD appeared to be characteristic but not universally occurring or inevitable, their diagnostic utility was considered limited. However, Lewy body dementia and frontotemporal dementia are now considered major dementia entities which should be differentiated from AD. The nature of BPSD symptomatology is believed to be very different in these entities [151,152]. To cite one example, visual hallucinations are frequently much more vivid and frightening in Lewy body dementia in comparison with AD, and these visual hallucinations occur more frequently in Lewy body dementia than they do in AD [151]. Also, treatment issues are very different: for example, in Lewy body dementia, neuroleptics are believed to be deleterious and even possibly life-threatening, whereas in AD they appear to be useful [150,151,153].

Therefore, the characteristic nature of BPSD symptoms in AD does appear to be useful in differentiating AD from some other major forms of dementing disorders, and this differentiation can be of major importance for the health and well-being of patients.

## SUMMARY

### Consistent Evidence

There is abundant and consistent evidence that a characteristic clinical course of the dementia of AD can be described. In AD patients who are free of significant concomitant illness, this characteristic clinical course is most clearly charted in terms of the characteristic sequence of functional changes which occur [12]. Evidence for this characteristic functional course from available studies is overwhelming and appears to be as strong as for any psychiatric clinical process.

Briefly, this characteristic functional sequence of deficit in AD is supported by criterion validity studies, including both prospective longitudinal study [17] and neuropathologic studies of cellular [26], volumetric [24] and neurofibrillary changes [26] in the hippocampus. It is also supported by independent concurrent validity studies of neurologic reflex and release sign changes over the course of AD [34,35] and independent studies of the course of cognitive changes in AD [37–39,41,43]. Further support for the validity of this characteristic functional sequence of loss in AD comes from the utility of this characteristic sequence in uncovering and charting otherwise difficult to identify, or virtually entirely obscure, physical markers [54] and physical changes [36] in AD.

Because of the consistent evidence for this characteristic sequence of progressive functional loss over the course of AD, this sequence is presently being utilized as a criterion for care needs in the United States by the Medicare program [154]. This AD functional progression has also been utilized in various multicenter, consortia studies from the US National Institute of Aging of the National Institutes of Health [155,156] and in US national and worldwide antidementia trials of behavioural [150,157] and more general antidementia agents (for example, as part of the clinical global assessment in the recent worldwide rivastigmine trials [158]).

A corollary observation to the characteristic functional sequence of loss in AD is that this functional progression in AD mirrors or, more precisely, occurs in an inverse sequence to the order of acquisition of the same functions in normal human development [57,58,86].

Apart from a characteristic functional sequence of loss in AD, various clinical sequences of loss can also be described. These clinical sequences have been shown to add to information on the functional progression of AD, in prospectively charting the course of AD [17] and in the retrospective post-mortem diagnosis of AD [90].

## Incomplete Evidence

It is clear that the dementia of AD has a characteristic order of symptomatic loss. It is also clear that the time course of clinical loss of capacities is much more variable. Although factors such as concomitant cerebrovascular disease are known to produce a more rapid sequence of loss in AD patients, much more information is needed regarding factors influencing the temporal variability of AD.

Additionally, it is clear that other dementing disorders can sometimes follow a clinical sequence more or less similar to that of AD. On the other hand, other dementing disorders can sometimes, or as a general rule, present differently from the AD clinical sequence. The factors influencing the clinical course in these other dementia disorders need to be better understood. Also, much more information is needed regarding the similarities and differences between AD and other dementing processes in terms of clinical presentation and course.

## Areas Still Open to Research

A theory of the neuropathologic and biomolecular basis for the characteristic clinical sequence of loss in AD has been forwarded [71,74,75,77]. Although this theory might explain many observations regarding the known risk factors for AD, and the similarities and differences between the clinical presentation of AD and other dementing disorders, much more research needs to be conducted before these issues can be resolved. Improved etiopathogenic information regarding the dementia process in AD and in other dementias and improved neuroimaging and other investigative techniques should assist in resolving many of these issues in coming years.

The term dementia and the differentiation of delirium and dementia have been in wide usage for two millennia [7]. Rapid progress has been possible in recent years, by identifying and differentiating the most important dementing disorders. Study of these entities in coming years can be readily translated not only into improved diagnosis, but also into improved care [70] and into a continually narrowed gap between scientific understanding of the clinical presentation of the dementias and the molecular and pathologic presentation of these prevalent disorders.

## ACKNOWLEDGEMENTS

Supported by US Department of Health and Human Services grants AG03051, AG08051, and 90AR 2160, and through a grant from the Zachary and Elizabeth Fisher Alzheimer Center for Research Foundation.

## REFERENCES

1. *Stedman's Medical Dictionary*, 21st edn (1966)   Williams and Wilkins, Baltimore.
2. *Webster's New Twentieth Century Dictionary of the English Language*, Unabridged 2nd edn. (1977)   Collins World, USA.
3. Plutarch (1967 translation)   *Lives*, AMS Press, New York.
4. Plato (1921 translation, book IX)   *The Laws*, University Press, Manchester.
5. Torack R.M. (1983)   The early history of senile dementia. In *Alzheimer's Disease* (Ed. B. Reisberg), pp. 23–28, Free Press/Macmillan, New York.
6. Cohen G.D. (1983)   Historical views and evolution of concepts. In *Alzheimer's Disease* (Ed. B. Reisberg), pp. 29–33, Free Press/Macmillan, New York.
7. Lipowski Z.J. (1980)   *Delirium: Acute Brain Failure in Man*, Thomas, Springfield.
8. American Psychiatric Association (1994)   *Diagnostic and Statistical Manual of Mental Disorders*, 4th edn, American Psychiatric Association, Washington, DC.
9. Reisberg B., Burns A., Brodaty H., Eastwood R., Rossor M., Sartorius N., Winblad B. (1997)   Diagnosis of Alzheimer's disease: report of an International Psychogeriatric Association Work Group under the cosponsorship of Alzheimer's Disease International, the European Federation of Neurological Societies, the World Health Organization, and the World Psychiatric Association. *Int. Psychogeriatrics*, **9** (Suppl. 1): 11–38.

10. Galen (1821–1833 translation) De symptomatum differentiis liber, cap. VII, In *Opera Omnia*, vol. 7 (Ed. K. Kuhn), pp. 200–201, Knobloch, Leipzig.
11. Henderson A.S., Jorm A.F. (2000) Dementia: definition and epidemiology. In *Dementia* (Eds M. Maj, N. Sartorius), pp. 1–33, Wiley, Chichester.
12. Reisberg B. (1988) Functional assessment staging (FAST). *Psychopharmacol. Bull.*, **24**: 653–659.
13. Folstein M.F., Folstein S.E., McHugh P.R. (1975) Mini-Mental State: a practical method for grading the cognitive state of patients for the clinician. *J. Psychiatr. Res.*, **12**: 189–198.
14. Folstein M. (1983) The Mini-Mental State Examination. In *Assessment in Geriatric Psychopharmacology* (Eds T. Crook, S.H. Ferris, R. Bartus), pp. 47–51, Powley, New Canaan.
15. Anthony J.C., Le Resche L., Niaz U., Von Korff M.R., Folstein M.F. (1982) Limits of the Mini-Mental State as a screening test for dementia and delirium among hospitalized patients. *Psychol. Med.*, **12**: 397–408.
16. McKhann G., Drachman D., Folstein M., Katzman R., Price D., Stadlan E.M. (1984) Clinical diagnosis of Alzheimer's disease: report of the NINCDS–ADRDA work group under the auspices of Department of Health and Human Services Task Force on Alzheimer's disease. *Neurology*, **34**: 939–944.
17. Reisberg B., Ferris S.H., Franssen E., Shulman E., Monteiro I., Sclan S.G., Steinberg G., Kluger A., Torossian C., de Leon M.J. *et al* (1996) Mortality and temporal course of probable Alzheimer's disease: a five-year prospective study. *Int. Psychogeriatrics*, **8**: 291–311.
18. Reisberg B., Franssen E., Bobinski M., Auer S., Monteiro I., Boksay I., Wegiel J., Shulman E., Steinberg G., Souren L. *et al* (1996) Overview of methodologic issues for pharmacologic trials in mild, moderate, and severe Alzheimer's disease. *Int. Psychogeriatrics*, **8**: 159–193.
19. Reisberg B., Sclan S.G., Franssen E., Kluger A., Ferris S. (1994) Dementia staging in chronic care populations. *Alz. Dis. Assoc. Disord.*, **8**: S188–S205.
20. Reisberg B., Ferris S.H., de Leon M.J., Kluger A., Franssen E., Borenstein J., Alba R. (1989) The stage specific temporal course of Alzheimer's disease: functional and behavioural concomitants based upon cross-sectional and longitudinal observation. In *Alzheimer's Disease and Related Disorders: Progress in Clinical and Biological Research*, vol. 317 (Eds K. Iqbal, H.M. Wisniewski, B. Winblad), pp. 23–41, Liss, New York.
21. Mohs R., Kim G., Johns C., Dunn D., Davis K. (1986) Assessing changes in Alzheimer's disease: memory and language. In *Handbook for Clinical Memory Assessment of Older Adults* (Ed. L.W. Poon), pp. 149–155, American Psychological Association, Washington, DC.
22. Wilson R., Kaszniak A. (1986) Longitudinal changes: progressive idiopathic dementia. In *Handbook for Clinical Memory Assessment of Older Adults* (Ed. L. W. Poon), pp. 285–293, American Psychological Association, Washington, DC.
23. Tombaugh N., McIntyre J. (1992) The Mini-Mental State Examination: a comprehensive review. *J. Am. Geriatr. Soc.*, **40**: 922–935.
24. Bobinski M., Wegiel J., Wisniewski H.M., Tarnawski M., Reisberg B., Mlodzik B., de Leon M.J., Miller D.C. (1995) Atrophy of hippocampal formation subdivisions correlates with stage and duration of Alzheimer disease. *Dementia*, **6**: 205–210.

25. Reisberg B., Kluger A. (1988)   Assessing the progression of dementia: diagnostic considerations. In *Clinical Geriatric Psychopharmacology*, 3rd edn (Ed. C. Salzman), pp. 432–462, Williams and Wilkins, Baltimore.

26. Bobinski M., Wegiel J., Tarnawski M., Reisberg B., de Leon M.J., Miller D.C., Wisniewski H.M. (1997)   Relationships between regional neuronal loss and neurofibrillary changes in the hippocampal formation and duration and severity of Alzheimer disease. *J. Neuropathol. Exper. Neurol.*, **56**: 414–420.

27. Sjogren T., Sjogren H., Lindgren A.G.H. (1952)   Morbus Alzheimer and morbus Pick: a genetic, clinical and patho-anatomical study. *Acta Psychiatr. Scand.*, **27** (Suppl. 82): 69–115.

28. Galasko D., Kwo-on-Yuen P.E., Klauber M.R., Thal L.J. (1990)   Neurological findings in Alzheimer's disease and normal aging. *Arch. Neurol.*, **47**: 625–627.

29. de Ajuriaguerra J., Rego A., Tissot R. (1963)   Le reflexe oral et quelques activites orales dans les syndromes dementiels du grand age. Leur signification dans la desintegration psycho-motrice. *Encephale*, **52**: 179–219.

30. Huff F.J., Boller F., Luchelli F., Querriera R., Beyer J., Belle S. (1987)   The neurologic examination in patients with probable Alzheimer's disease. *Arch. Neurol.*, **44**: 929–932.

31. Huff F.J., Growdon J.H. (1986)   Neurological abnormalities associated with severity of dementia in Alzheimer's disease. *Can. J. Neurol. Sci.*, **13**: 403–405.

32. Paulson G., Gottlieb G. (1968)   Developmental reflexes: the reappearance of foetal and neonatal reflexes in aged patients. *Brain*, **91**: 37–52.

33. Franssen E.H., Reisberg B., Kluger A., Sinaiko E., Boja C. (1991) Cognition-independent neurologic symptoms in normal aging and probable Alzheimer's disease. *Arch. Neurol.*, **48**: 148–154.

34. Franssen E.H., Kluger A., Torossian C.L., Reisberg B. (1993)   The neurologic syndrome of severe Alzheimer's disease: relationship to functional decline. *Arch. Neurol.*, **50**: 1029–1039.

35. Franssen E.H., Reisberg B. (1997)   Neurologic markers of the progression of Alzheimer disease. *Int. Psychogeriatrics*, **9**: 297–306.

36. Souren L.E.M., Franssen E.M., Reisberg B. (1995) Contractures and loss of function in patients with Alzheimer's disease. *J. Am. Geriatr. Soc.*, **43**: 650–655.

37. Reisberg B., Schneck M.K., Ferris S.H., Schwartz G.E., de Leon M.J. (1983)   The Brief Cognitive Rating Scale (BCRS): findings in primary degenerative dementia (PDD). *Psychopharmacol. Bull.*, **19**: 47–50.

38. Reisberg B., Ferris S.H., Anand R., de Leon M.J., Schneck M.K., Crook T. (1985)   Clinical assessment of cognitive decline in normal aging and primary degenerative dementia: concordant ordinal measures. In *Psychiatry*, vol. 5 (Eds P. Pichot, P. Berner, R. Wolf, K. Thau), pp. 333–338, Plenum Press, New York.

39. Reisberg B., Ferris S.H., Anand R., de Leon M.J., Schneck M.K., Buttinger C., Borenstein J. (1984)   Functional staging of dementia of the Alzheimer's type. *Ann. N.Y. Acad. Sci.*, **435**: 481–483.

40. Reisberg B., Ferris S.H., de Leon M.J., Crook T. (1985)   Age-associated cognitive decline and Alzheimer's disease: implications for assessment and treatment. In *Thresholds in Aging* (Eds M. Bergener, M. Ermini, H.B. Stahelin), pp. 255–292, Academic Press, London.

41. Reisberg B., Ferris S.H., Torossian C.L., Kluger A., Monteiro I. (1992)   Pharmacologic treatment of Alzheimer's disease: a methodologic critique based upon

current knowledge of symptomatology and relevance for drug trials. *Int. Psychogeriatrics*, **4** (Suppl. 1): 9–42.

42. Sclan S.G., Foster J.R., Reisberg B., Franssen E., Welkowitz J. (1990) Application of Piagetian measures of cognition in severe Alzheimer's disease. *Psychiatr. J. Univ. Ottawa*, **15**: 221–226.
43. Auer S.R., Sclan S.G., Yaffee R.A., Reisberg B. (1994) The neglected half of Alzheimer disease: cognitive and functional concomitants of severe dementia. *J. Am. Geriatr. Soc.*, **42**: 1266–1272.
44. Auer S.R., Reisberg B. (1996) Reliability of the Modified Ordinal Scales of Psychological Development (M-OSPD): a cognitive assessment battery for severe dementia. *Int. Psychogeriatrics*, **8**: 225–231.
45. Piaget J. (1952) *The Origins of Intelligence in Children*, Routledge and Kegan Paul, London.
46. Piaget J. (1960) *The Psychology of Intelligence*, Littlefield, Adams and Co., Totowa.
47. Piaget J. (1970) *L'Epistemologie Genetique*, Presses Universitaires de France, Paris.
48. Piaget J. (1973) *The Child and Reality: Problems of Genetic Psychology*, Grossman, New York.
49. Uzgiris I., Hunt J.M. (1975) *Assessment in Infancy: Ordinal Scales of Psychological Development*, University of Illinois, Urbana.
50. Yarkony G.M., Vinod S. (1986) Contractures, a major complication of craniocerebral trauma. *Clin. Orthopaed. Relat. Res.*, **219**: 93–96.
51. Adams R.D., Victor M. (1993) Principles of clinical myology. Diagnosis and classification of muscle disease. In *Principles of Neurology*, 4th edn (Eds R.D. Adams, M. Victor), pp. 1184–1199, McGraw-Hill, New York.
52. Anderson T.P. (1990) Rehabilitation of patients with completed stroke. In *Krusen's Handbook of Physical Medicine and Rehabilitation*, 4th edn (Eds F.J. Kottke, J. Lehmann), pp. 656–678, Saunders, Philadelphia.
53. Selikson S., Damus K., Hamerman D. (1988) Risk factors associated with immobility. *J. Am. Geriatr. Soc.*, **36**: 707–712.
54. Franssen E.H., Souren L.E.M., Torossian C.L., Reisberg B. (1997) Utility of developmental reflexes in the differential diagnosis and prognosis of incontinence in Alzheimer disease. *J. Geriatr. Psychiatry Neurol.*, **10**: 22–28.
55. Franssen E.H. (1993) Neurologic signs in ageing and dementia. In *Aging and Dementia, a Methodological Approach* (Ed. A. Burns), pp. 144–174, Arnold, London.
56. Reisberg B., Ferris S.H., Franssen E.H. (1986) Functional degenerative stages in dementia of the Alzheimer's type appear to reverse normal human development. In *Biological Psychiatry 1985*, vol. 7 (Ed. C. Shagass), pp. 1319–1321, Elsevier, New York.
57. Reisberg B. (1986) Dementia: a systematic approach to identifying reversible causes. *Geriatrics*, **41**: 30–46.
58. Reisberg B., Franssen E.H., Souren L.E.M., Auer S., Kenowsky S. (1998) Progression of Alzheimer's disease: variability and consistency: ontogenic models, their applicability and relevance. *J. Neural Transm.*, **54** (Suppl.): 9–20.
59. Aristophanes (1938 translation) The Clouds. In *The Complete Greek Drama* (Eds W.J. Oates, E.J. O'Neil) p. 595, Random House, New York.
60. Shakespeare W. (1599/1988) As you like it, Act 2, Scene 7. In *William Shakespeare: The Complete Works* (Eds S. Wells, G. Taylor), p. 638, Oxford Press, Oxford.

61. Rush B. (1793)  An account of the state of mind and body in old age. In *Medical Inquiries and Observations* (Ed. B. Rush), p. 311, Dobson, Philadelphia.

62. Linden M., Courtney D. (1953)  The human life cycle and its interruptions. A psychologic hypothesis. Studies in gerontologic human relations I. *Am. J. Psychiatry*, **109**: 906–915.

63. Linden M. (1957)  Regression and recession in the psychoses of the aging. In *The Kirkpatrick Memorial Programs on Gerontology for 1955 and 1956*, p. 35.

64. de Ajuriaguerra J., Rey M., Bellet-Muller M. (1964)  A propos de quelques problems posees par le deficit operatoire des viellards atteints de demence degenerative en debut d'evolution. *Cortex*, **1**: 232–256.

65. de Ajuriaguerra J., Tissot R. (1968)  Some aspects of psychoneurologic disintegration in senile dementia. In *Senile Dementia* (Eds C.H. Mueller, L. Ciompi), pp. 69–79, Huber, Bern.

66. de Ajuriaguerra J., Tissot R. (1975)  Some aspects of language in various forms of senile dementia: comparisons with language in childhood. In *Foundations of Language Development*, vol. 1 (Eds E.H. Lennenberg, E. Lennenberg), pp. 323–339, Academic Press, New York.

67. Cole M.G., Dastoor D.P., Koszycki D. (1983)  The hierarchic dementia scale. *J. Clin. Exper. Gerontol.*, **5**: 219–234.

68. Cole M.G., Dastoor D.P. (1987)  A new hierarchic approach to the measurement of dementia. *Psychosomatics*, **28**: 298–304.

69. Reisberg B., Pattschull-Furlan A., Franssen E.H., Sclan S., Kluger A., Dingcong L., Ferris S.H. (1990)  Cognition-related functional, praxis and feeding changes in CNS aging and Alzheimer's disease and their developmental analogies. In *Molecular Mechanisms of Aging* (Eds K. Beyreuther, G. Schettler), pp. 18–40, Springer, Berlin.

70. Reisberg B., Kenowsky S., Franssen E.H., Auer S.R., Souren L.E.M. (1999)  President's report: towards a science of Alzheimer's disease management: a model based upon current knowledge of retrogenesis. *Int. Psychogeriatrics*, **11**: 7–23.

71. Reisberg B., Franssen E.H., Hasan S.M., Monteiro I., Boksay I., Souren L.E.M., Kenowsky S., Auer S.R., Elahi S., Kluger A. (1999)  Retrogenesis: clinical, physiologic and pathologic mechanisms in brain aging, Alzheimer's and other dementing processes. *Eur. Arch. Psychiatry Clin. Neurosci.*, **249** (Suppl. 3): 28–36.

72. Prichep L.S., John E.R., Ferris S.H., Reisberg B., Alper K., Almas M., Cancro R. (1994)  Quantitative EEG correlates of cognitive deterioration in the elderly. *Neurobiol. Aging*, **15**: 85–90.

73. Cioni G., Biagioni E., Cipolloni C. (1992)  Brain before cognition: EEG maturation in pre-term infants. In *Neurodevelopment, Aging and Cognition* (Eds I. Kostovic, S. Knezevic, H.M. Wisniewski, G.J. Spillich), pp. 75–98, Birkhauser, Boston.

74. McGeer P.L., McGeer E.G., Akiyama H., Itagaki S., Harrop R., Peppard R. (1990)  Neuronal degeneration and memory loss in Alzheimer's disease and aging. *Exp. Brain Res.*, **21** (Suppl.): 411–426.

75. Braak H., Braak E. (1996)  Development of Alzheimer-related neurofibrillary changes in the neocortex inversely recapitulates cortical myelogenesis. *Acta Neuropathol.*, **92**: 197–201.

76. Braak H., Braak E. (1997)  Aspects of cortical destruction in Alzheimer's disease. In *Connections, Cognition and Alzheimer's Disease* (Eds B.T. Hyman, C. Duyckaerts, Y. Christen), pp. 1–16, Springer, Berlin.

77. Raz N. (2000) Aging of the brain and its impacts on cognitive performance: integration of structural and functional findings. In *Handbook of Aging and Cognition* (Eds F.I.M. Craik, T.A. Salthouse), pp. 1–90, Erlbaum, Mahwah.
78. Flechsig P. (1920) *Anatomie des Menschlichen Gehirns und Ruckenmarks auf Myelogenetischer Grundlage*, Thieme, Leipzig.
79. Yakovlev P.I., Lecours A.-R. (1967) The myelogenetic cycles of regional maturation of the brain. In *Regional Development of the Brain in Early Life* (Ed. A. Minkowski), pp. 3–70, Davis, Philadelphia.
80. Benes F.M. (1989) Myelination of cortical hippocampal relays during late adolescence. *Schizophr. Bull.*, **15**: 585–593.
81. Arnold A.G., Trojanowski J.Q. (1996) Human fetal hippocampal development: I. Cytoarchitecture, myeloarchitecture and neuronal morphologic features. *J. Comp. Neurol.*, **367**: 274–292.
82. Fuster J.M. (1997) *The Prefrontal Cortex: Anatomy, Physiology, and Neuropsychology of the Frontal Lobe*, 3rd edn, Lippincott-Raven, Philadelphia.
83. Lecours A.R. (1975) Myelogenetic correlates of the development of speech and language. In *Foundations of Language Development: A Multidisciplinary Approach* (Eds E.H. Lennenberg, E. Lennenberg), pp. 121–135, Academic Press, New York.
84. Yakovlev P.I. (1962) Morphological criteria of growth and maturation of the nervous system in man. *Assoc. Res. Nerv. Ment. Dis.*, **39**: 3–46.
85. Yamada T., Tsuboi Y., Takahashi M. (1997) Interrelationship between beta-amyloid deposition and complement-activated oligodendroglia. *Dement. Geriatr. Cogn. Disord.*, **8**: 267–272.
86. Reisberg B., Ferris S.H., de Leon M.J. (1985) Senile dementia of the Alzheimer type: diagnostic and differential diagnostic features with special reference to functional assessment staging. In *Senile Dementia of the Alzheimer Type* vol. 2, (Eds J. Traber, W.H. Gispen), pp. 18–37, Springer, Berlin.
87. Sclan S.G., Reisberg B. (1992) Functional assessment staging (FAST) in Alzheimer's disease: reliability, validity and ordinality. *Int. Psychogeriatrics*, **14** (Suppl. 1): 55–69.
88. Reisberg B. Ferris S.H. (1988) The Brief Cognitive Rating Scale (BCRS). *Psychopharmacol. Bull.*, **24**: 629–636.
89. Reisberg B., London E., Ferris S.H., Borenstein J., Scheier L., de Leon M.J. (1983) The Brief Cognitive Rating Scale: language, motoric, and mood concomitants in primary degenerative dementia. *Psychopharmacol. Bull.*, **19**: 702–708.
90. Rockwood K., Howard K., Thomas V.S., Mallery L., MacKnight C., Sangalang V., Darvesh S. (1998) Retrospective diagnosis of dementia using an informant interview based on the Brief Cognitive Rating Scale. *Int. Psychogeriatrics*, **10**: 53–60.
91. Blessed G., Tomlinson B.E., Roth M. (1968) The association between quantitative measures of dementia and senile change in the cerebral gray matter of elderly subjects. *Br. J. Psychiatry*, **114**: 797–811.
92. Jorm A.F. (1988) Assessment of cognitive decline in the elderly by informant interview. *Br. J. Psychiatry*, **152**: 209–213.
93. Jorm A.F., Korten A.E. (1994) A short form of the Informant Questionnaire on Cognitive Decline in the Elderly (IQCODE): development and cross-validation. *Psychol. Med.*, **24**: 145–153.
94. Jorm A.F., Scott R., Jacomb P.A. (1989) Assessment of cognitive decline in dementia by informant questionnaire. *Int. J. Geriatr. Psychiatry*, **4**: 35–39.

95. Jorm A.F., Scott R., Cullen J.S., MacKinnon A.J. (1991) Performance of the Informant Questionnaire on Cognitive Decline in the Elderly (IQCODE) as a screening test for dementia. *Psychol. Med.*, **21**: 785–790.
96. Thomas L.D., Gonzales M.F., Chamberlain A., Beyreuther K., Masters C.L., Flicker L. (1994) Comparison of clinical state, retrospective informant interview and the neuropathologic diagnosis of Alzheimer's disease. *Int. J. Geriatr. Psychiatry*, **9**: 233–236.
97. Sano M., Devanand D.P., Richards M., Miller L.W., Marder K., Bell K., Dooneief G., Bylsma F.W., Lafleche G., Albert M. *et al* (1995) A standardized technique for establishing onset and duration of symptoms of Alzheimer's disease. *Arch. Neurol.*, **52**: 961–966.
98. Lovblad K., Ramelli G., Remonda L., Nirkko A.C., Ozdoba C., Schroth G. (1997) Retardation of myelination due to dietary vitamin $B_{12}$ deficiency: cranial MRI findings. *Pediatr. Radiol.*, **27**: 155–158.
99. Chatterjee A., Yapundich R., Palmer C.A., Marson D.C., Mitchell G.W. (1996) Leukoencephalopathy associated with cobalamin deficiency. *Neurology*, **46**: 832–834.
100. Stojsavljevic N., Levic Z., Drulovic J., Dragutinovic G. (1997) A 44-month clinical–brain MRI follow-up in a patient with $B_{12}$ deficiency. *Neurology*, **49**: 878–881.
101. Rice J.E., Vannucci R.C., Brierley J.B. (1981) The influence of immaturity on hypoxic ischemic brain damage in the rat. *Ann. Neurol.*, **9**: 131–141.
102. Azzarelli B., Caldemeyer K.S., Phillips J.P., DeMyer W.E. (1996) Hypoxic–ischemic encephalopathy in areas of primary myelination: a neuroimaging and PET study. *Pediatr. Neurol.*, **14**: 108–116.
103. Tomimoto H., Akiguchi I., Wakita H., Kimura J. (1997) White matter lesions after occlusion of the bilateral carotid arteries in the rat—temporal profile of cerebral blood flow (CBF), oligodendroglia and myelin [in Japanese] *No to Shinkei—Brain and Nerve*, **49**: 639–644.
104. Stys P.K. (1998) Anoxic and ischemic injury of myelinated axons in CNS white matter: from mechanistic concepts to therapeutics. *J. Cerebr. Blood Flow Metab.*, **18**: 2–25.
105. LoPachin R.M., Stys P.K. (1995) Elemental composition and water content of rat optic nerve myelinated axons and glial cells: effects of *in vitro* anoxia and reoxygenation. *J. Neurosci.*, **15**: 6735–6746.
106. Wender M., Szezech J., Godlewski A., Grochowalska A. (1998) Karyometric and cytophotometric studies of the oligodendroglia in the corpus callosum of the rat after hypoxia. *Exp. Pathol.*, **33**: 249–255.
107. Oka A., Belliveau M.J., Rosenberg P.A., Volpe J.J. (1993) Vulnerability of oligodendroglia to glutamate: pharmacology, mechanisms, and prevention. *J. Neurosci.*, **13**: 1441–1453.
108. Husain J., Juurlink B.H. (1995) Oligodendroglial precursor cell susceptibility to hypoxia is related to poor ability to cope with reactive oxygen species. *Brain Res.*, **698**: 86–94.
109. Juurlink B.H. (1997) Response of glial cells to ischemia: roles of reactive oxygen species and glutathione. *Neurosci. Biobehav. Rev.*, **21**: 151–166.
110. McDonald J.W., Althomsons S.P., Hyra K.L., Choi D.W., Goldberg M.P. (1998) Oligodendrocytes from forebrain are highly vulnerable to AMPA/Kainate receptor-mediated excitotoxicity. *Nature Med.*, **4**: 291–297.
111. Knochel J.P. (1999) Hypoxia is the cause of brain damage in hyponatremia *JAMA*, **281**: 2342–2343.

112. Kiloh L.G. (1961) Pseudo-dementia. *Acta Psychiatr. Scand.*, **37**: 336–351.
113. Wells C.E. (1979) Pseudodementia. *Am. J. Psychiatry*, **136**: 895–900.
114. Reifler B.V., Larson E., Hanley R. (1982) Coexistence of cognitive impairment and depression in geriatric outpatients. *Am. J. Psychiatry*, **139**: 623–626.
115. Coffey C.E., Figiel G.S., Djang W.T., Weiner R.D. (1990) Subcortical hyper intensity on magnetic imaging: a comparison of normal and depressed elderly subjects. *Am. J. Psychiatry*, **147**: 187–189.
116. Zubenko G.S., Sullivan P., Nelson J.P., Belle S.H., Wolf G. (1990) Brain imaging abnormalities in mental disorders of late life. *Arch. Neurol.*, **47**: 1107–1111.
117. Lesser I.M., Miller B.L., Boone K.B., Hill-Gutierrez E., Mehringer C.M., Wong K., Mena I. (1991) Brain injury and cognitive function in late-onset psychotic depression. *J. Neuropsychiatry Clin. Neurosci.*, **3**: 33–40.
118. Rabins P.V., Pearlson G.D., Aylward E., Kumar A.J., Dowell K. (1991) Cortical magnetic resonance imaging changes in elderly inpatients with major depression. *Am. J. Psychiatry*, **148**: 617–620.
119. Howard R.J., Beats B., Forstl H., Graves P., Bingham J., Levy R. (1993) White matter changes in late-onset depression: a magnetic resonance imaging study. *Int. J. Geriatr. Psychiatry*, **8**: 183–185.
120. Krishnan K.R., McDonald W.M., Doraiswamy P.M. (1993) Neuroanatomical substrates of depression in the elderly. *Eur. Arch. Psychiatry Clin. Neurosci.*, **243**: 41–46.
121. Hickie I., Scott E., Mitchell P., Wilhelm K., Austin M.B., Bennett B. (1995) Subcortical hyperintensities on magnetic resonance imaging: clinical correlates and prognostic significance in patients with severe depression. *Biol. Psychiatry*, **37**: 151–160.
122. Caine E.D. (1981) Pseudodementia. *Arch. Gen. Psychiatry*, **38**: 1359–1364.
123. Clark R., Smith D., Jobst K.A., Refsum H., Sutton L., Ueland P.M. (1998) Folate, Vitamin $B_{12}$, and serum total homocysteine levels in confirmed Alzheimer disease. *Arch. Neurol.*, **55**: 1449–1455.
124. Stabler S.P., Lindenbaum J., Allen R.H. (1996) The use of homocysteine and other metabolites in the specific diagnosis of vitamin B-12 deficiency. *J. Nutrition*, **126**: 1266S–1272S.
125. Kristensen M.O., Gulmann N.C., Christensen J.E.J., Ostergaard K., Rasmussen K. (1993) Serum cobalamin and methylmalonic acid in Alzheimer dementia. *Acta Neurol. Scand.*, **87**: 475–481.
126. Diaz-Arrastia R. (1998). Hyperhomocysteinemia: a new risk factor for Alzheimer disease? *Arch. Neurol.*, **55**: 1407–1408.
127. Fassender K., Mielke O., Bertsch T., Nafe B., Fröschen S., Hennerici M. (1999) Homocysteine in cerebral macroangiopathy and microangiopathy. *Lancet*, **353**: 1586–1587.
128. Ridker P.M., Manson J.E., Buring J.E., Shih J., Matias M., Hennekens C.H. (1999) Homocysteine and risk of cardiovascular disease among postmenopausal women. *JAMA*, **281**: 1817–1821.
129. Agbayewa O. (1986) Earlier psychiatric morbidity in patients with Alzheimer's disease. *J. Am. Geriatr. Soc.*, **34**: 561–564.
130. Baker F.M., Kokmen E., Chandra V., Schoenberg B.S. (1991) Psychiatric symptoms in cases of clinically diagnosed Alzheimer's disease. *J. Geriatr. Psychiatry Neurol.*, **4**: 71–78.
131. Kral V.A. (1982) Depressiv Pseudodemenz und senile Demenz von Alzheimer-type: eine Pilot-studie. *Nervenarzt*, **53**: 284–288.

132. Kral V.A., Emery O.B. (1989) Long-term follow-up of depressive pseudode-mentia of the aged. *Can. J. Psychiatry*, **34**: 445–446.
133. Hofman A., Ott A., Breteler M.M.B., Bots M.L., Slooter A.J.C., van Harskamp F., van Duijn C.N., van Broeckhoven C., Grobbee D.E. (1997) Atherosclerosis, apolipoprotein E, and prevalence of dementia and Alzheimer's disease in the Rotterdam Study. *Lancet*, **349**: 151–154.
134. Snowdon D.A., Greiner L.H., Mortimer J.A., Riley K.P., Greiner P.A., Markesbery W.R. (1997) Brain infarction and the clinical expression of Alzheimer's disease. The Nun Study. *JAMA*, **277**: 813–817.
135. Esiri M.M., Zsuzsanna N., Smith M.Z., Barnetson L., Smith A.D. (1999) Cere-brovascular disease and threshold for dementia in the early stages of Alzhei-mer's disease. *Lancet*, **354**: 919–920.
136. Kalaria R.N. (1992) The blood–brain barrier and cerebral microcirculation in Alzheimer's disease. *Cerebrovasc. Brain Metab. Rev.*, **4**: 226–260.
137. Kalaria R.N. (1996) Cerebral vessels in ageing and Alzheimer's disease. *Phar-macol. Ther.*, **72**: 193–214.
138. Kalaria R.N. (1997) Cerebrovascular degeneration is related to amyloid-$\beta$ protein deposition in Alzheimer's disease. *Ann. N.Y. Acad. Sci.*, **826**: 263–271.
139. De La Torre J.C. (1994) Impaired brain microcirculation may trigger Alzhei-mer's disease. *Neurosci. Biobehav. Rev.*, **18**: 397–410.
140. Premkumar D.L., Cohen D.L., Hedera P., Friedland R.P., Kalaria R.N. (1996) Apolipoprotein E-epsilon 4 alleles in cerebral amyloid angiopathy and cerebrovascular pathology in Alzheimer's disease. *Am. J. Pathol.*, **148**: 2083–2095.
141. Hofman A. (1996) Epidemiology of Alzheimer's disease: the interplay of nature and nurture. *Neurobiol. Aging*, **17** (Suppl.): S5.
142. Haan J., Hardy J.A., Roos R.A.C. (1991) Hereditary cerebral hemorrhage with amyloidosis-Dutch type: its importance for Alzheimer's disease. *Trends Neu-rosci.*, **14**: 231–234.
143. Strittmatter W.J., Saunders A.M., Schmechel D., Pericak-Vance M., Enghild J., Salvesen G.S., Roses A.D. (1993) Apolipoprotein E: high-avidity binding to $\beta$-amyloid and increased frequency of type 4 allele in late-onset familial Alzhei-mer disease. *Proc. Natl. Acad. Sci. USA*, **90**: 1977–1981.
144. Amouyel P., Richard F., Lambert J.-C., Chartier-Harlin M.-C., Helbecque N. (1999) Apolipoprotein E, vascular factors and Alzheimer's disease. In *Alzhei-mer's Disease and Related Disorders* (Eds K. Iqbal, D.F. Swaab, B. Winblad, H.M. Wisniewski), pp. 53–58, Wiley, Chichester.
145. Weisgraber K.H., Mahley R.W. (1996) Human apolipoprotein E: the Alzhei-mer's disease connection. *Fed. Am. Soc. Exp. Biol. J.*, **10**: 1485–1494.
146. Luc G., Bard J.M., Arveiler D., Evans A., Cambou J.P., Bingham A., Amouyel P., Schaffer P., Ruidavets J.B., Cambien F. (1994) Impact of apolipoprotein E polymorphism on lipoproteins and risk of myocardial infarction. The ECTIM Study. *Arteriosclerosis Thrombosis*, **14**: 1412–1419.
147. Namba Y., Tomonaga M., Kawasaki H., Otomo E., Ikeda K. (1991) Apolipo-protein E immunoreactivity in cerebral amyloid deposits and neurofibrillary tangles in Alzheimer's disease and kuru plaque amyloid in Creutzfeldt–Jakob disease. *Brain Res.*, **541**: 163–166.
148. Finkel S.I., Costa e Silva J.C., Cohen G.D., Miller S., Sartorius N. (1998) Beha-vioral and psychological symptoms of dementia: a consensus statement on current knowledge and implications for research and treatment. *Am. J. Geriatr. Psychiatry*, **6**: 97–100.

149. Reisberg B., Franssen E., Sclan S.G., Kluger A., Ferris S.H. (1989) Stage specific incidence of potentially remediable behavioural symptoms in aging and Alzheimer's disease: a study of 120 patients using the BEHAVE-AD. *Bull. Clin. Neurosci.*, **54**: 95–112.

150. Katz I.R., Jeste D., Mintzer J.E., Clyde C., Napolitano J., Brecher M. (1999) Comparison of risperidone and placebo for psychosis and behavioural disturbances associated with dementia: a randomized, double-blind trial. *J. Clin. Psychiatry*, **60**: 107–115.

151. McKeith I.G. (2000) Behavioral and psychological symptoms of dementia and dementia with Lewy bodies. *Int. Psychogeriatrics*, **12** (Suppl. 1): 189–193.

152. Kertesz A. (2000) Behavioral and psychological symptoms and frontotemporal dementia (Pick's disease). *Int. Psychogeriatrics*, **12** (Suppl. 1): 183–187.

153. McKeith I., Fairbairn A., Perry R., Thompson P., Perry E. (1992) Neuroleptic sensitivity in patients with senile dementia of Lewy body type. *Br. Med. J.*, **305**: 673–678.

154. Health Care Financing Administration (HCFA) (1998) Hospice-determining terminal status in non-cancer diagnoses-dementia. *The Medicare News Brief/ Empire Medical Services*, **98**: 45–47.

155. Ferris S.H., Mackell J.A., Mohs R., Schneider L.S., Galasko D., Whitehouse P., Schmitt F.A., Sano M., Thomas R., Ernesto C. *et al* (1997). A multicenter evaluation of new treatment efficacy instruments for Alzheimer's disease clinical trials: overview and general results. *Alz. Dis. Assoc. Disord.*, **11** (Suppl. 2): S1–S12.

156. Teresi J.A., Morris J., Mattis S., Reisberg B. (2000). Cognitive impairment among SCU and non-SCU residents in the United States: prevalence estimates from the National Institute on Aging collaborative studies of special care units for Alzheimer's disease. *Res. Pract. Alz. Dis.*, **4**: 117–138.

157. De Deyn P.P., Rabheru K., Rasmussen A., Bocksberger J.P., Dautzenberg P.L., Eriksson S., Lawlor B.A. (1999) A randomized trial of risperidone, placebo, and haloperidol for behavioural symptoms of dementia. *Neurology*, **53**: 946–955.

158. Corey-Bloom J., Anand R., Veach J. (1998) A randomized trial evaluating the efficacy and safety of ENA 713 (rivastigmine tartrate), a new acetylcholinesterase inhibitor, in patients with mild to moderately severe Alzheimer's disease. *Int. J. Geriatr. Psychopharmacol.*, **1**: 55–65.

159. Reisberg B., Ferris S.H., de Leon M.J., Crook T. (1982) The Global Deterioration Scale for assessment of primary degenerative dementia. *Am. J. Psychiatry*, **139**: 1136–1139.

# Commentaries

## 2.1
## The Value of Inclusive Diagnostic Thinking and Appreciating Developmental Variance

### Eric B. Larson[1]

The clinical diagnosis of dementia is usually not a problem. As Reisberg *et al* note in their elegantly referenced review, the term "dementia" has been both used and useful for over two millennia. The existence of two related phenomena with their own equally useful names, "delirium" and "depression", is noteworthy for clinicians. They alert us to the fact that, although clinical diagnosis of dementia is not usually a problem, patients, especially elderly patients, often have more than one condition. Dementia and delirium, dementia and depression, commonly coexist, thus the job of reductionist classification of a patient's condition to a single entity in everyday practice often is not possible.

We have traditionally taught that parsimony is a reasonable goal when diagnosing or classifying a patient's condition into a disease or syndrome. In geriatrics, however, reality suggests an alternative approach. In fact, the "problem" in clinical diagnosis of all three related phenomena, dementia, depression and delirium, is one of detection, not diagnosis. All three are well known to be under-recognized by providers, patients and families. Yet, if well-trained clinicians simply consider the possibility of, for example, dementia, I believe that a diagnosis of dementia based on a routine mental status exam or use of a simple, brief cognitive screening test (like the Mini-Mental State Examination) is not a problem in most cases. If anything, one can argue that the reductionist goal of a single explanatory diagnosis could create a problem if clinicians fail to recognize the presence of related, frequently coexistent conditions, like dementia and delirium or depression, occurring in the same patient.

The same argument can be advanced regarding differential diagnosis. While I agree that the goal of differential diagnosis is to determine a single, most probable cause, the facts are that multiple causes of dementia frequently coexist in the same patient. Furthermore, if a patient has coexistent delirium and dementia, each of those syndromes typically has its own cause

[1] *University of Washington Medical Center, 1959 North East Pacific Street, Box 356330, Seattle, WA 98195, USA*

or causes. Treatment and prognosis, of course, are determined by cause(s), and thus an inclusive rather than a reductionistic approach is important. As the severity of dementia progresses over time, the likelihood that more than one cause exists in the same person increases. For example, Lim *et al* [1] recently reported that only 34 of 94 cases in a community-based Alzheimer's disease (AD) patient registry had pure AD at neuropathology. The remainder frequently had coexisting vascular or Parkinson's disease lesions along with AD.

For me, the most intriguing concept of Reisberg's review is the parallelism he describes between the characteristic loss of function in AD and the inverse sequence of acquisition of the same functions in normal human development. This reminded me that P. I. Yakovlev, one of the pioneers in describing the process of brain maturation, described a similar parallelism between paraplegia in flexion (the end stage of untreated degenerative brain disease, seen in state institutions for the insane in the past) and the fetal position. He described the trajectory of this disintegration of behaviour as an evolution occurring from without inward, in the reverse order of its developmental evolution. These extreme behavioural stages were correlated with neuroanatomic findings [2]

What further intrigues me about the parallelism between development of function and the inverse sequence in the order of loss of function is the characteristic phenomenon of variability in growth and development. Reisberg and colleagues properly point out that the sequence of change is characteristic. It is equally noteworthy, however, that variability is considerable, both in development and decline. Indeed, population variability is highest at these two opposite stages in the life cycle. I believe that where there is variability, we may find clues to pathogenesis and, eventually, treatment or prevention of degenerative diseases. In this context, it is interesting to note that risk for a chronic disease like AD may be a function of early life development. For example, Moceri *et al* [3] recently observed that social and economic markers of adequacy in early life correlate with risk of AD in late life. That is, using birth and census records, linked with an AD patient registry, she found that larger family size, later birth order and a paternal occupation in the lower economic strata were associated with increased risk of AD late in life. Moceri's hypothesis is that this increased risk is related to less complete brain development in early life, presumably related to the process of axonal myelination of the central nervous system, and thereby decreased brain reserve to withstand age-related decline.

In geriatrics, as in life, there is both intrigue and potential, as we recognize the complexity and variability of human phenomena.

## REFERENCES

1. Lim A., Tsuang D., Kukull W.A., Nochlin D., Leverenz J., McCormick W., Bowen J., Teri L., Thompson J., Peskind E. *et al* (1999)   Clinico-neuropathological correlation of Alzheimer's disease in a community-based case series. *J. Am. Geriatr. Soc.*, **47**: 564–569.
2. Yakovlev P.I. (1954)   Paraplegia in flexion of cerebral origin. *J. Neuropathol. Exp. Neurol.*, **3**: 267–295.
3. Moceri V. M., Kukull W.A., Emanuel I., van Belle G., Larson E.B. (2000)   Early-life risk factors and the development of Alzheimer's disease. *Neurology*, **54**: 415–420.

2.2
## Reflections on Retrogenesis

John O'Brien[1]

Reisberg *et al*'s excellent review on the clinical diagnosis of dementia presents a very powerful and lucid account of the idea of "retrogenesis" that he and his colleagues have developed over the last few years. In essence, this highlights the similarities between progression in Alzheimer's disease (AD) and reversal of development, such that in cognitive function, functional impairment, behaviour and social interactions, the more severely demented a patient becomes, the more similar he appears to an earlier developmental phase. Apart from being purely observational, this has extended into a theory regarding neurodegenerative processes in AD (particularly reversal of the myelination process) which may have an important bearing on our understanding of dementia and its progression. In particular, Reisberg *et al* make a very strong case for the use of the particular rating scale there group has championed (the Functional Assessment Staging, FAST) and how this corresponds to severity of dementia and neuropathology.

Professor Reisberg's theory is indeed eloquent and the weight of evidence supporting this view is impressive. In my commentary, I can do little to present alternative evidence or disagree with the weight of his argument. However, it does remain just one perspective of dementia and it might be worth commenting on issues which the review is unable to accommodate. The emphasis on the diagnosis of dementia is in regard to the discussion of DSM-IV, though it is important to remember that there are other definitions of dementia. In particular, the DSM-IV definition has been heavily criticized because of its undue emphasis on memory impairment. Memory impair-

[1] *Wolfson Research Centre, Institute for Health of the Elderly, Newcastle General Hospital, Westgate Road, Newcastle upon Tyne NE4 6BE, UK*

ment is essential for the diagnosis and so dementia cannot be diagnosed in its absence. This creates a number of problems. It is possible to have early AD without the severity of memory impairment necessary for a DSM-IV diagnosis of dementia. This means that someone can have AD without dementia. There are many other causes of what is usually accepted to be dementia which would not fulfil DSM-IV criteria. Frontotemporal dementias, such as Pick's disease, commonly cause behavioural and social irregularities, in conjunction with severe language difficulties and semantic problems, often with memory relatively well preserved until later. Thus, it might be possible to be institutionalized because of one's Pick's disease, but not fulfil DSM-IV criteria for dementia. Similarly, several other disorders, particularly dementia with Lewy bodies and vascular dementia, may well fulfil the general rubric for dementia (being a progressive impairment in several cognitive domains affecting occupational and social functioning) but still not involve memory. This has been suggested by some to be an inherent weakness and limitation of the DSM-IV criteria and it might be expanding the discussion to include other definitions of dementia which exist in ICD-10 and elsewhere. In addition, although the FAST is comprehensively covered, it is important to remember that there are several other rating scales in dementia, such as the Mini-Mental State Examination, Cambridge Cognitive Examination and others which deserve mention.

In the face of the strength of the argument made by Reisberg *et al* regarding retrogenesis, it is perhaps worth reflecting on the possible counterarguments to the notion that the progression of AD is, in effect, the reversal of the developmental process. Here are just a few suggestions which may merit further discussion and debate. First, brain changes. Progression in AD may reflect reversal of myelination, but several characteristic brain changes associated with AD have been described. These include generalized cerebral atrophy, specific atrophy of the temporal lobes and hippocampus, magnetic resonance imaging (MRI) spectroscopic changes indicating neuronal loss, blood flow changes indicating temporal and parietal hypoperfusion, and abnormalities in the acetylcholine and dopamine systems. Although earlier developmental processes have not been subjected to investigation with the same degree of scrutiny, it does not appear that similar degrees of generalized or temporal lobe atrophy or transmitter changes occur in early development. Second, the pattern of cognitive dysfunction associated with early development in late stage dementia may not be compatible. Children often have excellent memory in the space of quite marked higher cognitive executive and mathematical problems. In contrast, memory is one of the earliest functions lost in AD even when other functions and social and occupational function are well preserved. Third, as AD progresses, characteristic behavioural and psychological symptoms of dementia (BPSD) become frequent. As discussed by Reisberg *et al*, these include depression, psychosis, aggression, wandering, incontinence and sleep disturbance. While some of these (one particularly thinks of temper tantrums, night-time disturbance and incontinence) are characteristic of early developmental phases, others, such as depression, psychosis, persistent aggression, sexual disinhibition and wandering, are arguably never seen at early developmental stages. Fourth, one has to ask whether the relationship between cognitive decline and functional decline seen in dementia is the same as that in reverse during the course of development. Anecdotal observation by the author suggests this may not always be the case. Finally, the proof of the pudding may well be in the eating. Ultimately, the test of whether retrogenesis is a useful concept in terms of our thinking about patients with AD might depend on how we approach and manage them. Should we give a patient with dementia cuddly toys and cuddles? Perhaps we should, although again the lack of social concern and feeling observed in many patients with dementia seems at variance with the great need for physical affection seen early on in development.

This commentary does not want in any sense to detract from the cogent persuasive argument made by Reisberg *et al* regarding retrogenesis. It is more, as the title implies, to reflect on some of the broader implications and highlight some factors which might need to be reconciled within the theory of retrogenesis for it to become widely accepted and, much more importantly, practically useful in the management of patients with dementia.

### 2.3
### Dementia: Diagnosis, Progression and Retrogression
Perminder S. Sachdev[1]

Prof. Reisberg has addressed a number of concepts in relation to dementia in his review. He begins with a history of the term "dementia", from its Latin roots about 2000 years ago, and goes on to discuss the clinical progression of Alzheimer's disease (AD), in particular the functional decline as charted by the Functional Assessment Staging (FAST) procedure. He argues that the pattern of decline in AD is a reversal of neurodevelopment in childhood and refers to it as "retrogenesis", implicating demyelination in the pathogenesis, just as myelination plays a role in development. He puts forward the intriguing concept of "the retrogenic dementias".

[1] *Neuropsychiatric Institute, McNevin Dickson Building, Prince of Wales Hospital, Randwick, NSW 2031, Australia*

*Dementia.* The term dementia has seen may vicissitudes in its long history, and it is quite recently that it acquired its current conceptualization of multifaceted cognitive decline in clear consciousness [1]. Even though the concept of dementia is now firmly established in psychiatric taxonomy, it continues to have many limitations. It lacks operationalized diagnostic criteria, introducing considerable subjectivity to its definition. There is no consensus on what constitutes memory "impairment", "disturbance in executive functioning" or "significant impairment in social or occupational functioning". As an example, a 70-year old man with cognitive impairment who is still employed will receive a diagnosis of dementia, whereas his retired counterpart who is similarly impaired may escape the diagnosis. The lack of operational criteria has compromised the reliability of the diagnosis of dementia between raters and across sets of criteria, without which the validity of the concept can become elusive. In a recent report from the Canadian Study of Health and Aging [2], the proportion of subjects with dementia varied from 3.1% by ICD-10 criteria to as high as 29.1% using DSM-III, a 10-fold difference!

The emphasis on memory impairment in most criteria for dementia is understandable for AD but is restrictive when applied to dementia from other causes, e.g. vascular dementia (VD) and frontotemporal dementia (FTD). The application of the criteria for dementia results in the situation that, when patients are diagnosed with VD, they are at relatively advanced stages of their illness, precluding any efforts at prevention [3]. There are other arguments as well which suggest that dementia may be an arbitrary categorical imposition on a continuous construct of cognitive impairment, and there has even been a call for its abandonment as a diagnosis [4], to be replaced by "cognitive impairment" or "cognitive disorder" [5]. While this seems unlikely to happen, given the vast medical-industrial and socioeconomic complex that now surrounds this term, the limitations of the term deserve serious consideration.

*Progression.* Prof. Reisberg has presented his FAST procedure for staging AD and argued for its superior validity over other measures of progression, such as the Mini-Mental State Examination (MMSE). Since the MMSE measures only the cognitive dimension, it is not difficult to appreciate its limitations in predicting functional change and the impact of floor effects. The FAST procedure itself has many limitations, which may explain why it has not been more generally accepted by clinicians and researchers worldwide. First, it is again an arbitrary staging of a continuous process, and it is not clearly apparent why a new stage has been reached if a particular function is impaired. Second, in its early stages, it emphasizes frontal-executive dysfunction rather than memory impairment, which many regard as the early and more salient disturbance, at least in the clinic population. Third, too fine a categorization of the later stages of dementia may not have major practical implications. In fact, the application of a seven-stage (with substages) classification lacks the simplicity that a clinician may need for routine use. Fourth, it is not free of cultural bias in the choice of the items. It seems likely that researchers and clinicians will continue to use a combination of scales to map the progression of AD and other dementias, which will include a brief cognitive battery, an activities of daily living scale and some other measure(s).

*Regression.* The retrogenesis hypothesis of AD is intriguing, even though it is based on a superficial similarity between the sequence of skills acquisition in childhood and their loss in the course of AD. The important question is whether it reflects the neurobiological processes involved. The focus by Prof. Reisberg on myelination is in accordance with the "sensitivity" hypothesis of Braak and Braak [6], which explains the topography of AD lesions on differences in myelination. There are competing hypotheses, however, such as the "inactivity" hypothesis [7], and the "connectivity" hypothesis [8], among others. The myelination stage sensitivity hypothesis needs further empirical support. Neurodevelopment involves many processes, which include dendritic proliferation and pruning, synaptic exuberance and their loss as well as myelination, with the latter continuing well into the third decade of life for intracortical connections [9]. The myelination process cannot explain postnatal neurodevelopment in its entirety. Further research is necessary to determine why some brain regions are more sensitive to AD pathology than others, and animal models, as they become available, may help determine this. If retrogenesis is indeed a valid concept and mimics development, the role of environmental influences on neurodegeneration may be as important as they are for neurodevelopment, which will be a hopeful finding for the treatment of AD.

## REFERENCES

1. Berrios G.E. (1996) *The History of Mental Symptoms*, Cambridge University Press, Cambridge.
2. Erkinjuntti T., Ostye T., Steenhuis R., Hachinski V. (1997) The effect of differential diagnostic criteria on the prevalence of dementia. *N. Engl. J. Med.*, **337**: 1667–1674.
3. Looi J.C.L., Sachdev P. (1999) Differentiation of vascular dementia from AD on neuropsychological tests. *Neurology*, **53**: 670–678.
4. Sachdev P. (2000) Is it time to retire the term "dementia"? *J. Neuropsychiatry Clin. Neurosci.*, **12**: 276–279.
5. Hachinski V.C., Bowler J.V. (1993) Vascular dementia. *Neurology*, **43**: 2159–2160.
6. Braak H., Braak E. (1996) Development of Alzheimer-related neurofibrillary changes in the neocortex inversely recapitulates cortical myelinogenesis. *Acta Neuropathol.*, **92**: 197–201.

7. Swaab D.F., Salehi A. (1997)  The pathogenesis of Alzheimer disease: an altern-ative to the amyloid hypothesis. *J. Neuropathol. Exp. Neurol.*, **56**: 216.
8. Hyman B.T., Duyckaerts C.D., Christen Y. (1997)  *Connection, Cognition and Alzheimer Disease. Research and Perspective in Alzheimer Disease*, Springer, Berlin.
9. Albert M.S., Diamond A.D., Fitch R.H., Neville H.J., Rapp P.R., Tallal P.A. (1999)  Cognitive development. In *Fundamental Neuroscience* (Eds M.J. Zigmond, F.E. Bloom, S.C. Landis, J.L. Roberts, L.R. Squire), pp. 1313–1338, Academic Press, San Diego.

## 2.4
## Staging of Severe Alzheimer's Disease and the Concept of Retrogenesis: Doors to be Opened for Research and Clinical Practice

Reinhard Heun[1]

Among others, there are two most exciting aspects in the paper by Reisberg *et al*. First, the authors present consistent evidence for the fact that severe Alzheimer's disease (AD) can be precisely described cross-sectionally and during disease progression using the Functional Assessment Staging (FAST). Second, they present the concept of retrogenesis, which implies that subjects with dementia develop backwards, i.e. in the opposite direc-tion to the development during childhood. These two aspects are briefly dealt with in this commentary.

Reisberg *et al* present a comprehensive data set showing the validity of the FAST to assess the severity and, even more importantly, to follow the course of dementia. This is more than can be expected from the Mini-Mental State Examination (MMSE [1]), which to some extent is still the gold standard in epidemiology and clinical practice for the assessment of the severity of cognitive decline. The fact that there are more severe stages which cannot be adequately described by this and other cognitive tests is well known. The MMSE, like most other cognitive scales, has not been developed for staging and measuring the disease course. The special merit of Reisberg and his group is the extensive research and careful description of these severe stages of dementia which, up to now, have not yet received the scientific interest they need. The precise description of all stages of dementia including the most severe stages is a hallmark in gerontopsychiatry, because it allows the complete natural course of AD to be investigated. This has already been performed to some extent by Reisberg *et al*. More importantly, it will enable the development and improvement of therapeutic interventions for the most disabled patients.

[1] *Department of Psychiatry, University of Bonn, Venusberg, D-55105 Bonn, Germany*

The second major issue to be mentioned is the concept of retrogenesis. It implies that the progression of AD follows a fixed course which is the opposite of the development during childhood. Functional landmarks, such as double continence, are lost in the opposite sequence to the one observed during child development. This is an interesting scientific concept, even though this analogy is not totally new. Some observations have already been published in the lay press, i.e. demented subjects are like children, higher cognitive abilities which develop late are lost first. However, Reisberg *et al* present more than that. They provide adequate tools to examine this analogy in the clinical setting. The value of an analogy is not its truth; the analogy that ontogenesis is a repetition of phylogeny was not the absolute truth, and, as I suppose, it was even not meant to represent the truth, but to be a useful theory, allowing the deduction of new testable hypotheses. If the same applies to the concept proposed by Reisberg *et al*, it will definitely help to stimulate the research for these most demented subjects. There is a lot of knowledge on child cognitive development and on instruments to improve learning which might be used for the development of cognitive training programs for AD subjects. The concept might also be used to develop and test hypotheses on the structure of cognitive dysfunction in AD. New results of research in this respect might enable us to teach patients and their relatives what to do to improve the use of cognitive abilities when the patients already lack metacognitive knowledge, and, last but not least, to accept that certain things cannot be achieved in different stages of disease because it is beyond the limits. Acceptance of the patient's limits does not necessarily mean resignation, but realism which might help to end long-term intrafamilial controversies on the patient's abilities, disabilities and his corresponding insight. We all know of highly motivated relatives complaining of aggressive demented patients who are unable, but not unwilling, to accept their enthusiastic help. Thus, more research on the cognitive abilities of demented patients is required for clinical purposes. Additionally, one might wish more research analysing the hypothesis proposed by Reisberg that AD is a retrogenic disorder which can be differentiated from other dementias by its course. It remains to be proven that retrogenic disorders are characterized by a specific aetiopathogenic process. Reisberg *et al* have provided the tools to investigate these issues by developing scales and by providing an exciting theoretical framework.

A major obstacle to research on and for the most severely disabled patients still is the increasing need for informed consent, which subjects to be included in therapeutic research have to provide. The scientific community and society have to develop the tools to improve the general welfare of subjects who cannot decide for themselves. This might be done by permanently evaluating the interventions currently performed to treat the demented patients as proposed by quality-of-care assessments. An alternative would be to find possibilities to allow and encourage research for these severely demented patients who are in need of improved treatment. As far as I am aware, there are different approaches in different countries, depending on their cultural background, to solve these problems [2, 3]. However, there are still many obstacles which have to be overcome before the impressive work by Reisberg can be used for practical improvements. A dogma that research can only be done with fully informed subjects cannot hold without compromise.

## REFERENCES

1. Folstein M.F., Folstein S.E., McHugh P.R. (1975) "Mini-Mental State". A practical method for grading the cognitive state of patients for the clinician. *J. Psychiatr. Res.*, **12**: 189–198.
2. Helmchen H. (1990) The problem of informed consent in dementia research. *Med. Law*, **9**: 1206–1213.
3. High D.M., Whitehouse P.J., Post S.G., Berg L. (1994) Guidelines for addressing ethical and legal issues in Alzheimer disease: a position paper. National Institute on Aging. *Alz. Dis. Assoc. Disord.*, **8** (Suppl. 4): 66–74.

2.5
### When Diagnosis is Certain, Functional Scores are Robust and Recommendable Markers of the Progression of Alzheimer's Disease

Gerhard Ransmayr[1]

Barry Reisberg and co-workers have been studying extensively the natural history and course of dementia of the Alzheimer type (DAT). On their search for robust markers for disease progression, they have been evaluating clinical neurological signs, cognitive tests, microscopic quantitative parameters (hippocampus) and secondary musculoskeletal changes, such as contractures, and the order of loss of functions as the reversal of acquisition of functions during normal development. Using the Functional Assessment Staging (FAST) procedure, they found that functional course is the best marker of disease progression. Two other scales conceived by Reisberg *et al*, the GDS (Global Deterioration Scale) and the BCRS (Brief Cognitive Rating Scale), also explain a substantial proportion of the variance of cognitive decline in DAT patients. Combination of the scales may improve the significance of the assessed functional stages [1–5].

[1] *Department of Neurology, University of Innsbruck, Anichstrasse 35, A-6020 Innsbruck, Austria*

The concepts and findings of Reisberg are of major clinical and scientific relevance. In clinical practice, assessment of the course of the disease is essential. Robust markers are required to help the clinician to assess the degree of disability for various purposes, such as the decision to start or to finish a treatment, or how to manage the care of the patient or to plan costs or social support or legal questions. Moreover, these scales provide insight in the natural course of DAT, including the mean duration of the specific stages of functional decline.

FAST, GDS and BCRS have been validated and proved to be useful tools for the staging of DAT, in particular in advanced DAT, when other scales, such as the Mini-Mental State Examination (MMSE), are no more suitable. However, FAST, GDS and BCRS should be used with caution and only by people with experience in the fields of neurology, psychiatry, geriatric medicine and medical psychology. The functional scores are applicable to the assessment of the progression of DAT, but contribute little to the diagnosis of dementia.

The most widely used diagnostic criteria for dementia in general and for DAT are mainly clinical (memory impairment, aphasia, apraxia, agnosia and impairment of executive functions) [6,7]. The indispensable diagnostic criterion "functional decline" of the DSM-IV and ICD-10 is vaguely defined and may therefore cause diagnostic uncertainties, for instance in early dementia, when there is severe concomitant physical or sensory impairment, or in persons deprived of routine activities of daily living and social contacts (e.g. residents in old people's homes). The FAST and GDS stage 4, corresponding to mild DAT, is also vaguely defined with respect to decline in occupational and social functions and therefore also contributes little to this diagnostic issue. Mild cognitive impairment, irrespective of origin and prognosis, corresponding to FAST and GDS stages 2 and 3, may convert to DAT, but may also remit or continue as "benign senescent forgetfulness". On the other hand, symptoms of mild cognitive impairment may indicate the onset of a depressive episode or other types of dementia, such as frontotemporal dementia, dementia with Lewy bodies and vascular dementia (e.g. "small vessel dementia"). The user of FAST and GDS should be aware of this variability.

For the detection of minor changes of DAT, such as improvement in response to drug treatment, the FAST, GDS and BCRS may not be sensitive enough. Recent clinical pharmacological trials in DAT have been showing improvements in the cognitive subscale of the Alzheimer's Disease Assessment Scale (ADAS-cog) and the Clinician Interview Based Impression of Change-plus (CIBIC-plus) scales, in MMSE and in the Activities of Daily Living (ADL) scales [8–11]. With respect to applicability for therapeutic trials, FAST, GDS and BCRS need to be evaluated in future studies. The functional scales should also be used with caution in patients with severe concomitant depression (pseudodementia) and lack of social stimulation.

# REFERENCES

1. Reisberg B. (1988) Functional Assessment Staging (FAST). *Psychopharmacol. Bull.*, **24**: 653–659.
2. McKhann G., Drachman D., Folstein M., Katzman R., Price D., Stadlan F.M. (1984) Clinical diagnosis of Alzheimer's disease: report of the NINCDS–ADRDA Work Group under the auspices of Department of Health and Human Task Force on Alzheimer's Disease. *Neurology*, **34**: 939–944.
3. Reisberg B., Ferris S.H., Franssen E., Shulman E., Monteiro I., Sclan S.G., Steinberg G., Kluger A., Torossian C., de Leon M.J. *et al* (1996) Mortality and temporal course of probable Alzheimer's disease: a five-year prospective study. *Int. Psychogeriatrics*, **8**: 291–311.
4. Bobinski M., Wegiel J., Wisniewski H.M., Tarnawski M., Reisberg B., Mlodzik B., de Leon M.J., Miller D.C. (1995) Atrophy of hippocampal formation subdivisions correlates with stage and duration of Alzheimer's disease. *Dementia*, **6**: 205–210.
5. Selkinson S., Damus K., Hamerman D. (1988) Risk factors associated with immobility. *J. Am. Geriatr. Soc.*, **36**: 707–712.
6. American Psychiatric Association (1994) *Diagnostic and Statistical Manual of Mental Disorders*, 4th edn, American Psychiatric Association, Washington, D.C.
7. World Health Organization (1993) *The ICD–10 Classification of Mental and Behavioural Disorders: Diagnostic Criteria for Research*, World Health Organization, Geneva.
8. Knapp M.J., Knopman D.S., Solomon P.R., Pendlebury W.W., Davis C.S., Gracon S.I. for the Tacrine Study Group (1994) A 30-week randomized controlled trial of high dose tacrine in patients with Alzheimer's disease. *JAMA*, **271**: 985–991.
9. Rogers S.L., Farlow M.R., Doody R.S., Mohs R., Friedhoff L.T. and the Donepezil Study Group (1998) A 24-week, double-blind, placebo-controlled trial of donepezil in patients with Alzheimer's disease. *Neurology*, **50**: 136–145.
10. Corey-Bloom J., Anand R., Veach J. for the ENA 713 B352 Study Group (1998) A randomized trial evaluating the efficacy and safety of ENA 7113 (rivastigmine tartrate), a new acetylcholinesterase inhibitor, in patients with mild to moderate Alzheimer's disease. *Int. J. Geriatr. Psychopharmacol.*, **1**: 55–65.
11. Rosler M., Anand R., Cicin-Sain A., Gauthier S., Agid Y., Dal-Bianco P., Stahelin H.B., Hartman R., Gharabawi M. (1999) Efficacy and safety of rivastigmine in patients with Alzheimer's disease: international randomised controlled trial. *Br. Med. J.*, **318**: 633–638.

2.6
## Findings with the Aid of Functional Assessment Staging (FAST)
Sir Martin Roth[1]

Professor Reisberg and his colleagues have developed the Functional Assessment Staging (FAST) schedule over many years and applied it in a

[1] *Department of Surgery, University of Cambridge, Box 202, Addenbrooke's Hospital, Hills Road, Cambridge CB2 2QQ, UK*

range of studies, a number of which are summarized in their review. Part of those studies in recent years have been undertaken with investigators from other disciplines, using brain imaging and other techniques.

The evaluation in the FAST commences with a careful clinical history from patients and relatives. When this suggests a recent decline from a higher level of mental functioning, enquiries are directed towards associated cerebral disease and other physical conditions. Full psychiatric, neurological and general examinations are undertaken and relevant laboratory investigations initiated. Imaging studies such as a magnetic resonance imaging (MRI) scan are arranged when mental decline seems possible. The FAST technique is, therefore, interpreted against a rich background of medical, neurobiological, familial and social investigations.

Information is elicited from the patient (as far as possible), relatives and friends regarding the patient's ability to manage his daily life, and his main impediments. Prof. Reisberg states that relevant observations can be made and evidence elicited with the aid of the FAST instrument over a period of some two-thirds of the total course of Alzheimer's disease (AD) or other dementias.

*A clinical follow-up study.* The approach of Prof. Reisberg and his group is exemplified by the account of a prospective longitudinal study of 103 community resident individuals with probable AD [1]. The mean Mini-Mental State Examination (MMSE) score at the outset was $15.4 \pm 5.6$. Follow-up was conducted over a mean interval of $4.6 \pm 1.4$ years. The investigators were blind in respect of the baseline measures of MMSE scores.

The FAST assessment was made before the study commenced, but follow-up was conducted blind in relation to such baseline measurements. At the end of the trial, the measurements were repeated in the 65 patients who survived at the end of the follow-up period. A special technique was applied to arrive at their FAST schedule. Patients were set out in hierarchical order in accordance with their staging status. The correlation between the change in these FAST scores and the variance in time elapsed during the period in which the 65 survivors were under observations was 0.45 ($p <$ 0.001). All possible confounding factors that might have contributed to the results were eliminated by special calculations. The figure accounted for 20.3% of the variance in score during the time elapsed.

The 65 survivors were also re-tested with the MMSE. The score at follow-up was $5.1 \pm 6.9$ as against $15.4 \pm 5.6$ at the outset. The correlation of 0.32 between the change in MMSE scores and the variance in time elapsed in the 65 survivors was found to explain 10.2% of the variance in the change in scores.

The authors concluded that the FAST staging procedure had accounted for twice the variance in the record of progress in respect of MMSE scores. FAST was therefore superior to MMSE for measuring the progression of AD.

*Decrease of hippocampal volume and FAST measures.*    A decrease in the size of hippocampus in AD and to some extent in normal subjects of advanced age has been established for some years. The studies by Bobinski *et al* [2, 3] carry this knowledge forward with a number of new observations. Brains of 13 subjects with severe AD and of five age-matched normal controls were compared. A number of significant differences emerged. Those graded in the lower part of stage 7 of FAST showed a 36% decrease in hippocampal volume; those in higher stages of degeneration a 60% decrease. There was a similar situation in relation to Ammon's horn and the entorhinal cortex. All the correlations of volume of hippocampus and related structures with gradation of the dementia by FAST proved highly significant [2,3]. An enquiry into the differences in neuronal outfall between AD patients and controls, and their correlations with the staging derived from use of the FAST technique, yielded a similar picture.

*Conclusions.*    The body of observations reported in the review paper by Reisberg *et al* is of considerable interest. His methods of evaluation of clinical phenomenology, course and adaptation differ from the techniques of assessment undertaken with the standardized scales of diagnostic assessment and prediction which are widely employed by most investigators in this field. Some of these instruments contain quantified scales for such dimensions as cognitive impairment, "depression", "vascular" features, "organicity", and scales for depicting conditions of mixed aetiology. But, as Prof. Reisberg's review indicates, the reported achievements of FAST are considerable. There would therefore be merit in undertaking diagnostic exercises and follow-up studies which utilize both the FAST method in operationalized form and one of the established standardized schedules. Both instruments would need to be administered to all patients, and the results compared.

   Tracing the origins of any differences could be informative; the information jointly provided might well prove complementary. They could well pave the way for the development of new hybrid instruments, and promote more extensive knowledge and understanding of the FAST and its findings by investigators who employ the standardized forms of evaluation for diagnosis, assessment of severity and prediction.

# REFERENCES

1.  Reisberg B., Ferris S.H., Franssen E., Shulman E., Monteiro I., Sclan S.G., Steinberg G., Kluger A., Torossian C., de Leon M.J. *et al* (1996)  Mortality and temporal course of probable Alzheimer's disease: a five-year prospective study. *Int. Psychogeriatrics*, **8**: 291–311.

2. Bobinski M., Wegiel J., Wisniewski H.M., Tarnawski M., Reisberg B., Mlodzik B., de Leon M.J., Miller D.C. (1995) Atrophy of hippocampal formation subdivisions correlates with stage and duration of Alzheimer's disease. *Dementia*, **6**: 205–210.
3. Bobinski M., Wegiel J., Tarnawski M., Reisberg B., de Leon M.J., Miller D.C., Wisniewski H.M. (1997) Relationships between regional neuronal loss and neurofibrillary changes in the hippocampal formation and duration and severity of Alzheimer disease. *J. Neuropathol. Exp. Neurol.*, **56**: 414–420.

2.7
# Two Decades of Longitudinal Research in Alzheimer's Disease
Sanford I. Finkel[1]

In their review, Prof. Reisberg and colleagues succinctly summarize more than two decades of intensive longitudinal research on patients with Alzheimer's disease [AD]. Reisberg's earliest work involved the progression and staging of AD and resulted in the widely used Global Deterioration Scale (GDS) [1]. As a result of reviewing the clinical course of the illness with significant detail, it became clear that patients spent as much as a third to half of the course of the illness in the most advanced stages. Accordingly, Reisberg and colleagues developed the Brief Cognitive Rating Scale (BCRS) [2] and subsequently the Functional Assessment Staging (FAST) [3].

The FAST has been an extremely useful clinical and research tool that allows professionals and caregivers to understand the sequence of lost functions. Further, Prof. Reisberg and colleagues were able to subdivide these stages of advancing functional loss into 11 categories, with norms of duration which have proved clinically accurate. The sequence has allowed caregivers and health care professionals to prepare for the advances of the illness, while allowing for additional opportunities for research. The FAST criteria cover a much broader temporal range than the Mini-Mental State Examination (MMSE) and are not limited by the floor effects. Accordingly, it is not surprising that the FAST staging procedure is a superior way of measuring the temporal course of the illness. Subsequent work has demonstrated that functional losses occur exactly in reverse order of developed functions in childhood. This not only allows health care professionals and caregivers to anticipate losses, but also allows researchers to study the effects of pharmacologic and non-pharmacologic interventions on functioning. Finally, the physical deformities of AD are also highly correlated with the FAST.

[1] *Council for Jewish Elderly, 3003 W. Touhy Avenue, Chicago, IL 60645, USA*

Reisberg *et al*'s paper also summarizes the behavioural and psychological symptoms of dementia (BPSD), describing the clinical symptomatology commonly seen in AD patients [4, 5]. The BEHAVE-AD, which derives from Reisberg's work, has been used extensively in clinical drug trials and has been demonstrated to be a valid and reliable measurement of these symptoms [6, 7].

Subsequent work focused on neuroradiologic and neuropathologic markers. These revealed that loss of hippocampal volume progresses as the illness itself progresses [8]. Further, these radiologic/pathologic changes correspond with functional changes seen on the FAST [9]. This is particularly so in the more advanced stages of the illness. Further, neurologic reflex changes have been documented, corresponding with the progression of the illness [10–12].

Further research has demonstrated the correlation between biochemical and neuropathological changes in the central nervous system and functional loss. This includes demyelinization in addition to the more commonly described neuropathological changes. These ideas are carried forth and developed further, viewing cerebral vascular amyloid deposition (cerebral amyloid angiopathy) [13, 14] as a characteristic of AD.

The review closes with directions for future research, including avenues to look at other dementing disorders as well as the contribution of concomitant cerebral vascular disease for the AD patient. Thus, while summarizing more than two decades of intensive clinical and research work, Reisberg and colleagues lay the groundwork for an additional two decades of clinical and research activity.

## REFERENCES

1. Reisberg B, Ferris S.H., de Leon M.J., Crook T. (1982) The Global Deterioration Scale for assessment of primary degenerative dementia. *Am. J. Psychiatry*, **139**: 1136–1139.
2. Reisberg B., London E., Ferris S.H., Borenstein J., Scheier L., de Leon M.J. (1983) The Brief Cognitive Rating Scale: language, motoric, and mood concomitants in primary degenerative dementia. *Psychopharmacol. Bull.*, **19**: 702–708.
3. Reisberg B. (1988) Functional assessment staging (FAST). *Psychopharmacol. Bull.*, **24**: 653–659.
4. Luc G., Bard J.M., Arveiler D., Evans A., Cambou J.P., Bringham A., Amouyel P., Schaffer P., Ruidavets J.B., Cambien F. (1994) Impact of apolipoprotein E polymorphism on lipoproteins and risk of myocardial infarction. The ECTIM Study. *Arteriosclerosis Thrombosis*, **14**: 1412–1419.
5. Namba Y., Tomonaga M., Kawasaki H., Otomo E., Ikeda K. (1991) Apolipoprotein E immunoreactivity in cerebral amyloid deposits and neurofibrillary tangles in Alzheimer's disease and kuru plaque amyloid in Creutzfeldt–Jakob disease. *Brain Res.*, **541**: 163–166.

6. De Deyn P.P., Rabheru K., Rasmussen A., Bocksbergen J.P., Dautzenberg P.L., Eriksson S., Lawlor B.A. (1999) A randomized trial of risperidone, placebo, and haloperidol for behavioural symptoms of dementia. *Neurology*, **53**: 946–955.
7. Katz I.R., Jeste D., Mintzer J.E., Clyde C., Napolitano J., Brecher M. (1999) Comparison of risperidone and placebo for psychosis and behavioural disturbances associated with dementia: a randomized, double-blind trial. *J. Clin. Psychiatry*, **60**: 107–115.
8. Bobinski M., Wegiel J., Wisniewski H.M., Tarnawski M., Reisberg B., Mlodzik B., de Leon M.J., Miller D.C. (1995) Atrophy of hippocampal formation subdivisions correlates with stage and duration of Alzheimer's disease. *Dementia*, **6**: 205–210.
9. Bobinski M., Wegiel J., Tarnawski M., Reisberg B., de Leon M.J., Miller D.C., Wisniewski H.M. (1997) Relationships between regional neuronal loss and neurofibrillary changes in the hippocampal formation and duration and severity of Alzheimer's disease. *J. Neuropathol. Exp. Neurol.*, **56**: 414–420.
10. Franssen E.H., Reisberg B., Kluger A., Sinaiko E., Boja C. (1991) Cognition-independent neurologic symptoms in normal aging and probable Alzheimer's disease. *Arch. Neurol.*, **48**: 148–154.
11. Franssen E.H., Kluger A., Torossian C.L., Reisberg B. (1993) The neurologic syndrome of severe Alzheimer's disease: relationship to functional decline. *Arch. Neurol.*, **50**: 1029–1039.
12. Franssen E.H., Reisberg B. (1997) Neurologic markers of the progression of Alzheimer disease. *Int. Psychogeriatrics*, **9**: 297–306.
13. Snowdon D.A., Greiner L.H., Mortimer J.A., Riley K.P., Greiner P.A., Markesbery W.R. (1997) Brain infarction and the clinical expression of Alzheimer's disease. The Nun Study. *JAMA*, **277**: 813–817.
14. Esiri M.M., Zsuzsanna N., Smith M.Z., Barnetson L., Smith A.D. (1999) Cerebrovascular disease and threshold for dementia in the early stages of Alzheimer's disease. *Lancet*, **354**: 193–214.

2.8
# Diagnosing Dementia: the Need for Improved Criteria

Gabriel Gold[1]

Reisberg *et al* report that the concept of dementia has entered its third millennium and that the term itself dates back to the first century AD. However, despite marked advances over the past century, the diagnosis of dementia and, particularly, of various dementia subtypes, remains a clinical challenge to this day. The Functional Assessment Staging (FAST) scale provides a detailed framework of the expected evolution of Alzheimer's disease (AD) and can support this diagnosis when the course is typical. Deviations from the FAST scheme can serve as a clue to a non-AD process.

[1] *Hôpital de Gériatrie, Route de Mon Idée, Thonex 1226, Switzerland*

Reisberg *et al* also provide convincing evidence that the FAST scale is superior to the Mini-Mental State Examination (MMSE) in measuring the longitudinal evolution of AD, particularly at advanced stages. This has important implications for drug trials that measure the impact of treatment on symptom or disease progression.

Another crucial point is the identification of early disease and of individuals at risk for the development of dementia. Ideally, clinical criteria for dementia should apply universally to all subtypes and should be able to identify initial stages as well as established cases. However, existing criteria for dementia do not always agree. In a study of 1879 elderly subjects, the proportion of subjects with dementia varied from 3.1% with ICD-10 criteria to 29.1% with DSM-III criteria [1]. Generally accepted definitions of dementia are strongly based on the clinical presentation of AD and must include memory deficits. This requirement may not be appropriate for other types of dementia, including frontotemporal dementias, where behavioural disorders and marked impairment in other cognitive domains, such as executive functions and language, may precede memory impairment. Severity requirements are also an issue: this has led Vladimir Hachinski to suggest that the term "vascular dementia" (VD) should be replaced by "vascular cognitive impairment", to stress early identification of affected patients across the whole spectrum of cognitive performance [2].

Differentiating VD from AD is a particularly challenging endeavour. Furthermore, both types of dementia often coexist, producing a mixed dementia (MD). As stated by Reisberg *et al*, "the characteristic presentation of AD as outlined with the FAST procedure is very different from the acute dementia which may result from stroke". However, the sensitivity and specificity of FAST for the detection of VD and MD are unknown. Although the clinical diagnosis of AD is based on criteria which have gained general acceptance and have been validated in clinicopathologic studies, this is not the case for VD, where many different criteria are still in use today. This points to the lack of a single generally accepted effective diagnostic methodology for VD. Several studies have demonstrated significant differences between VD criteria [3, 4]. Although most are effective in excluding AD, they generally suffer from low sensitivity and behave differently with regards to MD [4].

Clinicopathologic correlations represent a key method for the validation of clinical criteria. This raises the issue of a gold standard. The neuropathological diagnosis of AD is based on accepted criteria applied to dementia cases. Neuropathological severity scales have also been developed and validated in clinical studies [5–7]. Unfortunately, there is a lack of consensus on neuropathologic criteria for other dementias and particularly VD or MD. VD can result from several pathophysiological mechanisms, leading to multiple forms of the disease, such as multiple infarcts secondary to large vessel atherosclerosis or cardioembolism, a single strategic infarct, lacunae and white matter changes secondary to small vessel disease, hypoperfusion and haemorrhage. It is unlikely that a single set of clinical criteria can apply equally to all VD subtypes. Criteria for frontotemporal dementia and for Lewy body disease also need to be further assessed and validated.

A group of particular interest comprises individuals who present with mild cognitive impairment (MCI). It has been suggested that 6–15% of MCI cases progress to dementia each year [8, 9]. Validated criteria for MCI would allow appropriate targeting of prevention and early intervention trials.

Further studies, including neuropsychological and functional evaluations as well as neuroimaging and clinicopathological correlations, are needed to develop and validate better performing criteria, which could lead to a broader consensus on the clinical diagnosis of dementia and its various subtypes and could help identify individuals at risk for the development of dementia.

## REFERENCES

1. Erkinjuntti T., Ostbye T., Steenhuis R., Hachinski V. (1997) The effect of different diagnostic criteria on the prevalence of dementia. *N. Engl. J. Med.*, **337**: 1667–1674.
2. Hachinski V. (1994) Vascular dementia: a radical redefinition. *Dementia*, **5**: 130–132.
3. Verhey F.R., Lodder J., Rozendaal N., Jolles J. (1996) Comparison of seven sets of criteria used for the diagnosis of vascular dementia. *Neuroepidemiology*, **15**: 166–172.
4. Gold G., Giannakopoulos P., Montes-Paixao Junior C., Herrmann F.R., Mulligan R., Michel J.P., Bouras C. (1997) Sensitivity and specificity of newly proposed clinical criteria for possible vascular dementia. *Neurology*, **49**: 690–694.
5. Braak H., Braak E. (1991) Neuropathological staging of Alzheimer-related changes. *Acta Neuropathol.*, **82**: 239–259.
6. Gertz H.J., Xuereb J.H., Huppert F.A., Brayne C., McGee M.A., Paykel E., Harrington C., Mukaetova-Ladinska E., Arendt T., Wischik C.M. (1998) Examination of the validity of the hierarchical model of neuropathological staging in normal aging and Alzheimer's disease. *Acta Neuropathol.*, **95**: 154–158.
7. Gold G., Bouras C., Kövari E., Canuto A., Gonzales Glaria B., Malky A., Hof P.R., Michel J.P., Giannakopoulos P. (2000) Clinical validity of Braak Neuropathological Staging in the oldest old. *Acta Neuropathol.*, **99**: 579–582.
8. Wolf H., Grunwald M., Ecke G.M., Zedlick D., Bettin S., Dannenberg C., Dietrich J., Eschrich K., Arendt T., Gertz H.J. (1998) The prognosis of mild cognitive impairment in the elderly. *J. Neural Transm.*, **12** (Suppl.): 175–181.
9. Petersen R.C., Smith G.E., Waring S.C., Ivnik R.J., Tangalos E.G., Kokmen E. (1999) Mild cognitive impairment: clinical characterization and outcome. *Arch. Neurol.*, **56**: 303–308.

2.9
## Pitfalls in Diagnosing Alzheimer's Disease

Iwona Kloszewska[1]

The dementia syndrome, which, as Reisberg *et al* remind us, has been known for years, has gained much importance recently for epidemiological reasons. While the number of demented subjects is steadily growing, knowledge of aetiology and pathogenesis is still not sufficient to help the sufferers, and neither medical nor social resources can meet the needs of new cases and their families.

In the last decade, however, the state of knowledge has changed significantly. The dogma stating that 50% of dementia is caused by Alzheimer's disease (AD), 20% by vascular changes and 20% by the coexistence of the two, has fallen down. Pick's disease, which had been forgotten for some time, and other fronto-temporal dementias seem to be responsible for about 7% [1], and diffuse Lewy body disease for probably no less than 15% of all dementia cases [2]. Underdiagnosing AD in clinical practice has quite unexpectedly turned into the phenomenon of overdiagnosing this type of dementia. Clinical characteristics of AD have been described in great detail; careful studies on other degenerative dementias are urgently needed.

In clinical diagnosis of dementia, two steps are obligatory: first, dementia as a syndrome has to be identified, then its specific origin has to be determined. Although the definition of dementia found in the DSM-IV is quite satisfactory, still the question which remains open is: what are the boundaries between dementia and delirium when the two overlap? The more severe the dementia is, the more difficult clinical recognition of delirium becomes. DSM-IV states only that "delirium may be superimposed on a dementia". It is difficult to judge the level of consciousness in a moderately severe or severe dementia, as the contact with the patient or his ability to maintain attention are disturbed by the dementing process itself. Thus additional symptoms, such as visual hallucinations, transient delusions, psychomotor, emotional and sleep pattern disturbances, should be considered in the process of diagnosing the delirium, besides the disturbance of consciousness.

Although the presence and pattern of psychiatric symptoms accompanying cognitive impairment in dementia are not specific, the differences in frequency of hallucinations, depression, delusions and delusional misidentifications between AD and diffuse Lewy body disease are useful in discriminating the two processes [3].

Without the slightest doubt, Reisberg's Functional Assessment Staging (FAST) is an invaluable help in studying and understanding the

[1] *First Department of Psychiatry, Medical University of Lodz, Czechoslowacka 8/10, 92–216 Lodz, Poland*

clinical specificity of AD. Moreover, the use of both FAST and the Global Deterioration Scale in everyday practice lessens the likelihood of AD misdiagnosis. At the same time, the Mini-Mental State Examination (MMSE) has found a solid place in clinical practice and research on dementia, although it neither can nor pretends to monopolize the evaluation of dementia. One should keep in mind that the MMSE cannot be used to diagnose dementia by itself, without considering the clinical data. It is useful in assessment of severity of cognitive dysfunction in dementia of various origins, while the FAST outlines the course of AD specifically. These two measures are complementary and one cannot replace the other.

Retrogenesis is an intellectually attractive concept, which helps to understand the complicated phenomenology of AD. Obviously, the clinical symptoms only can be accounted for by the retrogenesis. β-amyloid and neurofibrillary tangles are the basic pathology of AD, which do not seem to fit into the retrogenic model. Degenerative dementias, other than AD, when their symptomatology attains the severe stage, are clinically not distinguishable one from another and from AD. Thus, in differential diagnosis of the advanced stages of dementia, the dynamics of the disease and its previous characteristics have to be taken into account.

## REFERENCES

1. Wilhelmsen K.C. (1998) Chromosome 17-linked dementias. *Cell. Mol. Life Sci.*, **54**: 920–924.
2. Luis C.A., Mittenberg W., Gass C.S., Duara R. (1999) Diffuse Lewy body disease: clinical, pathological, and neuropsychological review. *Neuropsychol. Rev.*, **9**: 137–150.
3. Ballard C., Holmes C., McKeith I., Neill D., O'Brien J., Cairns N., Lantos P., Perry E., Ince P., Perry R. (1999) Psychiatric morbidity in dementia with Lewy bodies: a prospective clinical and neuropathological comparative study with Alzheimer's disease. *Am. J. Psychiatry*, **156**: 1039–1045.

2.10

### Evaluating the Performance of Measures to Assess Dementia

David R. Gifford[1]

In order to deliver appropriate care to patients with dementia, clinicians need to be able to recognize patients as having a dementia syndrome and

[1] *Center for Gerontology and Health Care Research, Brown University, Box G-B 222, Providence, RI 02912, USA*

then determine the specific cause of dementia. However, nearly three-quarters of patients with moderate to severe dementia are unrecognized by primary care clinicians as having cognitive impairment [1]. Even when recognized, the appropriate evaluation is often lacking [1]. Clinicians also need to be able to accurately assess disease severity in order to select appropriate treatments, therapies and services, as well as to monitor the effectiveness of these interventions. Disease severity can be divided into three domains: cognitive function, functional ability and behaviour problems. There are numerous measures used to assess patients with dementia, but no single test has emerged as the established standard [2,3]. Reisberg and colleagues discuss one such measure of disease severity, the Functional Assessment Staging (FAST). Their discussion raises the issue of how dementia measures are evaluated.

Many dementia measures that initially show promise, are later found to be inaccurate, performing poorly in mild dementia and varying in accuracy depending on the patient's characteristics, such as age and educational level [4]. One reason for this discrepancy in performance is that initial evaluations often do not adhere to established methodological standards [4,5].

For any of these measures to be effective and helpful, they need to be simple to administer and accurate (i.e. reliable and valid) [5–7]. Busy clinicians will not use an instrument that takes too long or is too complicated to administer or interpret. Reliability refers to how reproducible or repeatable the test results are, while validity refers to the degree to which the measure correctly assesses what it purports to measure. There are three types of reliability—inter-rater reliability, intra-rater reliability and internal consistency, and three types of validity—content validity, construct validity and criterion validity [4]. All of these should be evaluated and reported for a diagnostic test [6,7], but also apply to dementia measures [4,5]. The remainder of this paper will briefly discuss these types of reliability and validity.

*Inter-rater and intra-rater reliability* measure the agreement in test results when performed by two or more individuals (inter-rater) or by the same individual two or more times (intra-rater). Test–retest reliability is a form of intra-rater reliability. If the test's inter-rater or intra-rater agreement is poor, then differences in test scores may reflect differences in reliability rather than true differences in the patients' status. Reliability is best measured by calculating a kappa value, which indicates the degree of agreement between ratings after correcting for chance agreement. Reliability can also be quantitated as a correlation coefficient. However, high correlation coefficients can be misleading, since responses can be correlated but disagree [4].

*Internal consistency* evaluates the extent to which all the items on a scale or questionnaire that make up a composite score reflect the same underlying construct. For example, questions on a cognitive function measure should evaluate different domains of cognition (e.g. memory, calculations, and visual-spatial function) and correlate with the composite score. Internal consistency is often assessed by calculating the Cronbach's coefficient alpha [4].

*Content validity* (often referred to as "face validity") represents the extent to which a test thoroughly and appropriately assesses the domain of interest. Experts reviewing the test question to see if they "look like" they measure what the test is designed to measure usually assess content validity. For example, a measure of dementia behaviours should have questions that evaluate behaviours (e.g. wandering), not cognitive function (e.g. memory) or functional ability (e.g. dressing).

*Construct validity* evaluates how well the new measure correlates with other measures assessing the same domain of interest (convergent validity) and does not correlate with measures of dissimilar characteristics (discriminate validity) [6]. When a new test relates well to other measures as hypothesized, construct validity is supported.

*Criterion validity* has two types: predictive and concurrent [4]. Predictive validity evaluates whether or not a new test predicts future performance. Concurrent validity evaluates whether or not a new test agrees with a "gold standard" measure administered concurrently. Concurrent validity is usually measured by calculating the sensitivity, specificity and the area under the receiver operator characteristic (ROC) curve. Sensitivity is the proportion of patients with the condition of interest (measured by the "gold standard") that have a positive test. Specificity is the proportion of patients without the condition (measured by the "gold standard") who have a negative test. In general, there is an inverse relationship between sensitivity and specificity. As one changes the cut-off score of a test to maximize sensitivity, the specificity decreases and vice versa. A ROC curve illustrates this trade-off between sensitivity and specificity. A ROC curve plots the true positive rate (i.e. sensitivity) on the vertical axis against the false-positive rate (i.e. specificity) on the horizontal axis for different cut-offs.

When evaluating the validity of a new test, the test's indices (e.g. sensitivity and specificity) may be imprecise due to small sample sizes [4,6]. Thus, the 95% confidence interval or standard error around the test's indices provides an estimate of the precision of these values and therefore should be reported [6]. In addition, attention needs to be paid to the patient sample used in the evaluation, since the sampling strategy can have profound impact on the results of an evaluation. For example, dementia measures are often evaluated by comparing patients with Alzheimer's disease with normal controls. However, most dementia measures are not used to distinguish normal individuals from dementia (except for measures to distinguish very mild dementia from normal aging). Rather, dementia measures need to discriminate between different types of dementia, different levels of disease severity, or changes in disease severity over time. Thus, when assessing dementia measures, they should be evaluated using adequate populations of patients with different forms of dementia and adequate sample sizes of patients with different degrees of disease severity.

It is both rare and difficult for a single evaluation of a new test or measure to evaluate and report each of these measures of reliability and valididity [6]. Yet, this information is necessary for clinicians when deciding which of the numerous measures available to select to use in their practice [6,7]. In their review, Reisberg and colleagues nicely summarize the growing evidence supporting the validity of FAST.

## REFERENCES

1. Callahan C.M., Henrie H.C., Tierney W.M. (1995) Documentation and evaluation of cognitive impairment in elderly primary care patients. *Ann. Intern. Med.*, **122**: 422–429.
2. Cummings J.L., Booss J., Dickinson B.D., Hazlewood M.G., Jarvik L.F., Matuszewski K.A., Mohs R.C. (1997) *Dementia Identification and Assessment: Guidelines for Primary Care Practitioners*, US Department of Veterans Affairs, Washington, DC, and University Health System Consortium, Oakbrook, IL.
3. Costa P.T. Jr, Williams T.F., Somerfield M. (1996) *Recognition and Initial Assessment of Alzheimer's Disease and Related Dementias*. Clinical Practice Guideline No. 19, US Department of Health and Human Services, Rockville, MD.
4. McDowell J., Newell C. (Eds) (1996) *Measuring Health: A Guide to Rating Scales and Questionnaires*, Oxford University Press, New York.
5. Gifford D.R., Cummings J.L. (1999) Evaluating screening tests for dementia: the methodologic standards used to evaluate their performance. *Neurology*, **52**: 224–227.
6. Reid M.C., Lachs M.S., Feinstein A.R. (1995) Use of methodological standards in diagnostic test research. *JAMA*, **274**: 645–651.
7. Jaeschke R., Guyatt G.H., Sackett D.L., for the Evidence-based Medicine Working Group (1994) Users' guides to the medical literature. III: How to use an article about a diagnostic test. A. Are the results of a study valid? *JAMA*, **271**: 389–391.

2.11
**Dementia as a Diagnostic Entity**
Sasanto Wibisono[1]

One classical aspect that has been used to characterize dementia aside from the various cognitive deficits is the presumption of existing structural brain defect. The practical clinical consequence is its irreversibility. Even though

[1] *Department of Psychiatry, University of Indonesia, Salemba 6, Jakarta 10430, Indonesia*

the biological criterion has been dropped, the irreversibility of the demented condition is still a relevant clinical characteristic that is worth considering.

Although some dementia cases will show improvement after treatment or supportive effort, in fact, it is assumed to be only a partial improvement caused by reorganization of the remaining functioning part of the brain. The process may, but not necessarily, be progressive and deteriorating: as mentioned in Prof. Reisberg's review, the term 'progressive and deteriorating' may be unsuitable in some cases. However, the temporary nature and possibility of complete recovery of the cognitive deficits should negate the diagnostic consideration of dementia (e.g. temporary cognitive deficits found in conditions such as drug intoxication, depression, anxiety, schizophrenia, etc.).

As also required by the DSM-IV, dementia as a diagnostic entity should always be followed by the identification of another clinical condition, directly or indirectly causing the dementia syndrome (Prof. Reisberg's "once the occurrence of dementia has been established, the clinician must determine the specific origin of the dementia, i.e. the specific dementing diagnostic entity").

Whatever the points of view that may be considered, dementia is a syndrome requiring a complex differential diagnosis. It seems that the clinical differentiation between "dementia as a symptom" and "dementia as a diagnostic entity" will always be a problem. It would be more reasonable not to use the term "dementia" for the description of a symptom, but instead, to use the term exclusively for a diagnostic entity. We can use descriptive terms to indicate symptoms of cognitive deficits.

In most cases in clinical practice, a thorough clinical history and examination will be able to differentiate the various types of "dementia" as a major clinical problem, as well as identifying a "secondary" and "temporary functional" cognitive deficit (e.g. in depression, schizophrenia, etc.). However, this should not be the end of the story. A depressed person, or a schizophrenic, may suffer from "pseudo-dementia" caused by functional disorganization which is temporary in nature. On the other hand, there is the possibility that the same person also suffers from a dementing disease, comorbid to the depression, schizophrenia or other condition, provided it can be proven.

It is undeniable that dementia (including Alzheimer's disease, AD) may coexist with other conditions such as schizophrenia, mood disorders (depression in particular), delirium, drug intoxication, etc. The comorbid condition may interfere with the symptomatic clinical manifestation of AD or vice versa, and obscure the diagnostic accuracy. For practically clinical reasons, we follow the conventional principle to hold the hierarchically (higher clinical manifestation as the primary diagnosis, provided that the clinical history and other relevant findings support it. The description of the DSM-IV is clinically suitable for various types of dementia, but unfortunately it would not allow a separate (comorbid) diagnosis (e.g. major depressive disorder, schizophrenia), denying the clinical possibility.

Concerning AD, exhaustive and expensive additional examination is available for diagnosis and differential diagnosis. Although diagnostic reliability is at present considered quite good, many of the final definite conclusions are still in the *postmortem* study. The Functional Assessment Staging procedure (FAST) [1] is indeed an important practical clinical aid in the diagnosis and management of AD.

There are currently no biological markers available for presymptomatic detection and diagnosis of AD, and diagnostic accuracy heavily relies on clinical judgement and clinician's experience. The DSM-IV criteria have some limitations [2], concerning their practical applicability. The clinician needs to know the course of the illness precisely and also the patient's functional ability in daily activities. In this respect, the FAST could be of great help in attaining clinical conclusions when applying the DSM-IV criteria (e.g. apraxia will be reflected by inability to prepare breakfast).

Aside from the extensive studies reviewed by Reisberg *et al* that supported the validity of FAST, there are other clinical advantages compared to the Mini-Mental State Examination (MMSE), such as: (a) MMSE evaluation relies on a direct information, subject to education, intelligence and literacy of the patient, whereas the FAST covers an assessment of a longer period of time, assuring higher objectivity; (b) the FAST is applicable for the assessment of advanced stages of AD, even when verbal communication has been lost. The practical, clinical shortcomings are that the reliance on second-hand information may produce a bias, and that cultural influence may lower the objectivity of the informed data. Conjoining FAST with the Clinical Dementia Rating Scale may minimize the problem.

## REFERENCES

1.  Reisberg B. (1988) Functional Assessment Staging (FAST). *Psychopharmacol. Bull.*, **24**: 653–659.
2.  Gauthier S. (1996) *Clinical Diagnosis and Management of Alzheimer Disease*, Dunitz, London.

# 3

# Neuropsychological and Instrumental Diagnosis of Dementia: A Review

## Ove Almkvist

*Division of Geriatric Medicine B84, Huddinge University Hospital, 14186 Huddinge, Sweden*

## INTRODUCTION

The present review summarizes the state of the art concerning the diagnosis of dementia syndromes using neuropsychological and instrumental methods. The paper is focused on the three most common dementia syndromes, namely Alzheimer's disease (AD), vascular dementia (VD) and frontotemporal dementia (FTD) [1]. The typical neuropsychological and instrumental findings in these syndromes are described, but first the principles of a neuropsychological and instrumental assessment are introduced.

There is no general pattern of neuropsychological or instrumental findings that is valid for all dementia syndromes. On the contrary, the characteristics of dementia appear to be disease-related and specific for the disease course, i.e. stage-related. The pattern of specific disease- and stage-related characteristics makes sense if the time course and the brain distribution of neuropathology is considered and related to behaviour.

## THE PRINCIPLES OF NEUROPSYCHOLOGICAL EVALUATION

The neuropsychological examination is one part of a comprehensive protocol for examination of suspected dementia. In this protocol the subject and a close informant are questioned about present symptoms and medical history. In addition, the patient is examined for somatic, neurological and

*Dementia, Second Edition.* Edited by Mario Maj and Norman Sartorius.
© 2002 John Wiley & Sons Ltd.

psychiatric symptoms. Laboratory analyses of blood, urine and often cerebrospinal fluid are made in order to exclude various systemic diseases. Heart and vessels are examined. Electroencephalogram is taken. Neuroimaging of the brain is performed using magnetic resonance imaging (MRI) or other methods. Finally, a careful assessment of functional status is made.

The main idea of functional diagnosis of all kinds of dementia is the difference principle, which states that it is necessary to examine the possible existence of a difference between pre-morbid and present level of functioning. The difference may concern cognition, personality, behavioural manifestations or activities of daily living (ADLs). The size of the difference and the time course of the change are also important. Finally, the pattern of changes vs. preserved functioning across various cognitive domains, personality characteristics and behaviour has to be carefully outlined.

## Pre-morbid Level of Functioning

The pre-morbid functioning may be assumed as normal when there is no relevant knowledge in the individual patient. It may also be predicted on the basis of demographic data such as age, level of education, profession, interests, history of intellectual or professional development. Such formulae of prediction can be found in the literature (see e.g. [2,3]). In addition, pre-morbid functioning may be assessed using specific tests such as the New Adult Reading Test (NART, [4]) or other tests based, for instance, on reading or lexical decisions of word/non-word (see e.g. [5]). Furthermore, pre-morbid functioning may be assessed on the basis of test profiles including functions that are both sensitive and relatively insensitive to change that occurs in dementia. Cognitive abilities that are acquired early in life, over-learned, and not limited by time allotted but rather by knowledge are less sensitive to change compared to those abilities that are acquired recently, less well learned, and dependent on speed of performance. Vocabulary [6] is an example of a verbal ability that is relatively insensitive to change, while interpretation of pictures depicting well-known scenes (Picture Completion in WAIS-R [6]) or objects may be a non-verbal example of the same kind. Finally, it has to be pointed out that the best measure of pre-morbid functioning is an assessment made before onset of the disease. This may be available for men tested prior to their military service or for anyone tested for educational or job counselling as a youngster.

The ideal situation when evaluating a patient is to know both his pre-morbid and present functioning. However, often this knowledge is lacking or uncertain. Then, the patient has to be compared with other persons as represented by norms based on population studies. Usually test manuals provide these norms. They may have a high quality when developed from population studies in which the criteria for defining the population are expressed in detail. It has to be concluded, however, that these details are often missing. It is not always clear whether individuals with disorders affecting brain function, or with latent disease (e.g. incident dementia), or carrying risk factors for brain dysfunction (e.g. hypertension, hypotension, diabetes, heart problems, endocrinological disturbance, psychiatric syndromes, etc.) are excluded or not. Of course, sensory and motor difficulties also have to be considered. With few exclusions made, the population will cover a large proportion of all individuals, which will result in relatively low values of mean performance and high values of distribution spread. On the other hand, with many exclusions made, the population will cover a small proportion of all individuals, which will result in relatively high values of mean performance and low values of distribution spread. Thus, the concept of normality, including as many individuals as possible or cleaning the population, will have profound consequences on the norms used and the evaluation of the individual patient. An illustration of this line of reasoning can be found in recent research on cognitive function in elderly individuals [7].

## Current Functioning

The current functioning has to be assessed by focusing on those functions in which early changes will appear, which have a differential diagnostic value. It is also important to adapt the level of difficulty to the patient's stage of dementia, because few instruments are adapted to the whole range of dementia development, from very early dementia, across mild and moderate dementia, to severe dementia. To fulfil this purpose, both cognitive functioning and personality have to be evaluated, and various aspects of memory (episodic and semantic, primary, procedural) have to be assessed.

## Methods of Assessment

### Neuropsychological Tests

Neuropsychological tests are described comprehensively elsewhere. For details of test descriptions, the interested reader is recommended to consult textbooks (e.g. [8]). Below, a short description of some standard tests is provided.

The most well-known neuropsychological test batteries for global cognition are the original and the revised version of Wechsler Adult Intelligence

Scale (WAIS [9]; WAIS-R [6]). The WAIS and WAIS-R have been translated to many European and other languages. The WAIS batteries assess verbal function by means of six tests (Information, Digit Span, Comprehension, Arithmetic, Vocabulary, Similarities) and performance by means of five tests (Picture Completion, Picture Arrangement, Block Design, Object Assembly, Digit Symbol). Although the WAIS batteries include 11 tests, these tests do measure only two or three cognitive functions, when the 11 summary scores are entered into a factor analysis [10–12]. The two-factor solution corresponds to Wechsler's categorization of verbal and performance subtests, while the three-factor solution suggests a verbal comprehension factor (including four verbal subtests), a perceptual organization factor (including four performance subtests), and a freedom-of-distraction factor (including Digit Span, Arithmetic, and Digit Symbol). These factor solutions seem to hold both for the original normal standardization sample and for neurologically impaired samples. The understanding of what is measured in the Wechsler batteries may be still more complex, if separate item scores are analysed [10]. For instance, it has recently been demonstrated that the 14 separate items in the Similarities test may be understood not as one single measure of verbal abstraction, but rather as two independent measures of search in semantic memory [13].

The Wechsler batteries are not designed for evaluation of dementia, since they do not cover all the changes that occur in dementia syndromes. Therefore, additional tests have to be added in order to get a comprehensive evaluation of dementia. Important cognitive domains not covered by standard batteries are executive functioning, naming, verbal fluency, reasoning, copying, tracking, perceptual abilities, motor skills, and procedural memory. To fulfil the purpose to assess these cognitive domains, specific tests are added at most clinical specialist centres. At some centres, tasks or principles from experimental cognitive psychology have been added to clinical assessment. For instance, the memory-scanning paradigm [14], the phonological loop idea [15] or examination of priming memory [16] have been used.

The original and the revised version of Wechsler Memory Scale (WMS [17]; WMS-R [18]) and the Benton Visual Retention test [19] are examples of often performed memory tests. The WMS included seven subtests (Personal and Current Information, Orientation, Mental Control, Logical Memory, Digit Span, Visual Reproduction, Associative Learning), which could be evaluated separately or in terms of a summary score. Among the drawbacks of the WMS were the overrepresentation of verbal tests, the disparate level of difficulty across subtests, the poor internal consistency, and the questionable validity in terms of factor structure. In factor analyses of subtest scores, two factors have emerged, a general memory and an attention/concentration factor, as well as associations with factors of intelligence [20]. As a response to the criticism of WMS, a revised version was developed, which was more oriented to modern concepts of memory, such as the distinction between short- and long-term memory and between verbal and figurative memory. The WMS-R includes eight subtests, which fall into two factors according to factor analyses with or without WAIS tests [18].

Although the WMS batteries are widely used for memory assessment, they are lacking the level of task difficulty that is required when assessing individuals in the borderline between dementia and healthy aging. Therefore, other tests may be added to meet the requirements of a comprehensive memory examination. Among the most common additional tests are the Rey Auditory Verbal Learning test [8] and the California Verbal Learning test [21] for the evaluation of verbal episodic memory and the Rey–Osterreith Retention test [8] for the assessment of visuospatial episodic memory. The common denominator of these tests is that the material to be remembered is too large to be kept in mind and that there is a retention period during which the subject is kept active in other activities besides memorizing, i.e. the primary memory is washed out and only material transformed to a more resistant store can be used for memorizing. For a more detailed description of the various memory processes, the reader is referred to modern textbooks in cognitive psychology (see e.g. [22]).

To assess executive functions, such as goal formulation, planning, carrying out goal-directed plans and evaluation of effective performance, there are no standard tests within neuropsychology, but a number of possible tests, including maze tests for planning, and Tinkertoy-like tests for purposive behaviour [8].

Word finding or naming performance may be assessed by means of the Boston Naming Test [23]. Another aspect of verbal abilities is verbal fluency, which is known to deteriorate during dementia [24], and may be assessed by the so-called FAS verbal fluency, referring to the ability to say as many words as possible initiated by letters F, A or S [8]. A related test is the category fluency test [8], in which the instruction is given: "Say the names of as many vegetables as possible in one minute".

The most common test for assessing copying performance is the Rey–Osterreith copy Test [8]. Another similar tool is the Cube copy test.

A brief overview of the most common neuropsychological tests used for dementia evaluation is presented in Table 3.1.

The main drawback associated with a comprehensive neuropsychological examination is its cost in terms of time and manpower. Therefore, short test batteries have been developed that can be used in epidemiological studies, clinical trials and at clinical settings, such as the battery of the Consortium to Establish a Registry of Alzheimer's Disease (CERAD [25,26]) and the Alzheimer's Disease Assessment Scale (ADAS-Cog [27]). These batteries have become almost a standard for the evaluation of cognitive deterioration. Another

TABLE 3.1  Some common tests for assessing cognitive functions in dementia

| Cognitive function | Test | Reference |
|---|---|---|
| Global cognition | WAIS-R or WAIS: FSIQ | Wechsler [6,9] |
| Verbal ability | Boston Naming | Kaplan et al [23] |
| | FAS fluency | Lezak [8] |
| Semantic memory | Information | Wechsler [6] |
| | Similarities | Wechsler [6] |
| | Vocabulary | Wechsler [6] |
| Visuospatial ability | Block Design | Wechsler [6] |
| | Rey–Osterreith Copying | Lezak [8] |
| Short-term memory, verbal | Digit Span | Wechsler [6] |
| Short-term memory, spatial | Corsi Span | Lezak [8] |
| Episodic memory, verbal | Rey Auditory Verbal Learning | Lezak [8] |
| | California Verbal Learning | Delis et al [21] |
| Episodic memory, spatial | Rey–Osterreith Retention | Lezak [8] |
| | Benton Visual Retention | Benton [19] |
| Attention | Digit Symbol | Wechsler [6] |
| | Trail Making | Lezak [8] |
| Executive | Mazes | Lezak [8] |
| | Tower of Hanoi | Lezak [8] |

WAIS, Wechsler Adult Intelligence Scale; WAIS-R, Wechsler Adult Intelligence Scale—Revised; FSIQ, Full Scale Intelligence Quotient

way to minimize costs is to use a computerized test battery, as exemplified by the Cambridge Neuropsychological Automated Battery (CANTAB [28]).

For severely demented patients, specific instruments are needed, because standard neuropsychological tests are not applicable. An example of a test battery for severely demented patients is the Severe Impairment Battery (SIB [29]), in which very simple tasks are utilized. The following tasks are examples from the SIB: orienting response to sudden stimuli, eye contact when greeting each other, answer by proper name when asked.

## Observation of Patient's Behaviour

Observation of behaviour during communication or testing may be used to further characterize the patient. This observation can be concerned with affective reactions (e.g. apathy, elated mood, panic, sadness), speech and communication peculiarities (e.g. anomia, articulation difficulties, confabulations, inadequate turn-taking behaviour, mutism, neologisms), as well as test behaviour (e.g. agnosia, bradykinesia, closing-in errors, degree of orderliness, distraction, fragmentation, intrusions, neglect, rotation errors,

TABLE 3.2  Stages of decline in dementia

| Stage | MMSE | CDR | GDS | ADAS-Cog | Typical features |
|---|---|---|---|---|---|
| None | 30 | 0 | 1 | 0 | No symptoms |
| MCI | 24–30 | 0.5 | 2 | 0–12 | Memory symptoms |
| Mild | 21–23 | 1 | 3 | 13–20 | Deficits in memory and cognition; depression |
| Marked | 18–20 | 1 | 4 | 21–28 | Clear cognitive deficits; compensatory coping |
| Moderate | 15–17 | 2 | 5 | 29–36 | Some assistance needed; psychiatric symptoms |
| Severe | 12–16 | 2 | 6 | 37–44 | Help with ADL needed; psychotic symptoms; aggressiveness |
| Grave | 0–11 | 3 | 7 | 45+ | Institutional care needed |

MMSE, Mini-Mental State Examination; CDR, Clinical Dementia Rating Scale; GDS, Global Deterioration Scale; ADAS-Cog, Alzheimer's Disease Assessment Scale; MCI, mild cognitive impairment

trial-and-error behaviour, utilization behaviour). No form of observation has met general acceptance; therefore the practitioner has to rely on clinical experience or textbooks in neuropsychology [8].

## Scales for Dementia Assessment

The most frequently used scales for assessment of dementia are the Clinical Dementia Rating Scale (CDR [30,31]), the Global Deterioration Scale (GDS [32]) and the Mini-Mental State Examination (MMSE [33]). These scales describe the development of dementia in terms of global functioning, from healthy ageing across mild cognitive changes to advanced dementia, in a number of stages or levels, as shown in Table 3.2.

To assess psychiatric symptoms, there are several scales. The Comprehensive Psychopathological Rating Scale (CPRS [34]), the Neuropsychiatric Inventory (NPI [35]) and the behavioural part of the Alzheimer's Disease Assessment Scale (ADAS-Behave [36]) are some of the most utilized.

## Instrumental Methods

ADLs incorporate self-care (e.g. toileting, dressing, eating, grooming, ambulating and bathing), whereas instrumental activities of daily living (IADLs) incorporate more complex activities, such as shopping, food preparation, housekeeping, use of private transportation, handling of apparatuses, and managing personal economy. There are a large number of instruments to be used for ADLs and IADLs, as reviewed by Nygård *et al* [37]. The primary advantage of these tools is their ecological validity as compared to neuropsychological methods. Some of them are briefly presented below.

The most commonly used ADL/IADL instrument is the Lawton and Brody scale [38], which is composed of two parts, assessing independence in physical self-maintenance (six tasks) and instrumental activities (eight tasks) by a five-point ordinal scale. The scale can be based on patient's self-reports or on information provided by family caregivers, which makes its application easy and at the same time open to inaccuracy because of the indirect method of observation.

The hierarchical index of Katz *et al* [39] is probably the most well-known instrument for assessing dependence in personal ADLs (bathing, dressing, toileting, transferring, continence and feeding). Each activity is graded in terms of dependence on a seven-point ordinal scale. The tool may be well adapted for late stages of dementia, but is less useful for mild dementia.

Recently, the Assessment of Motor and Process Skills (AMPS [40]) was developed to be an instrument for direct observation of performance with good scaling properties that could be used also in mild dementia. To use this instrument, specific training is required, which represents its main drawback. However, promising data have been gained by using it in clinical trials as well as in clinical settings [37,41].

## Evaluation of Results

Usually results from neuropsychological testing are reported verbally and/ or graphically in domains of cognition such as global cognition (e.g. the Full Scale Intelligence Quotient of the WAIS-R battery (FSIQ [6])), verbal abilities, visuospatial functioning, attention, memory, sensory and motor performance. The results are transformed to standard scores using test manuals and departing from the assumption that test scores are normally distributed in the population. The interested reader is referred to textbooks of neuropsychological assessment for details (see e.g. [8]).

The interpretation of neuropsychological test results has to consider the size of change (present performance in relation to assumed or assessed premorbid performance), the pattern of performance across cognitive domains, and the pattern of change across time. A very important aspect is whether follow-up data are available; if so, the interpretation of a neuropsychological examination is more powerful. Finally, it has to be pointed out that neuropsychological tests are among the most powerful methods in an examination of suspected dementia, because of the rigorous standardization of test presentation, scoring and interpretation. The data on reliability and validity are to be found in manuals and textbooks of neuropsychology [8].

## NEUROPSYCHOLOGICAL AND INSTRUMENTAL CHARACTERISTICS OF ALZHEIMER'S DISEASE (AD)

The pattern of neuropathological findings in AD brains includes neurofibrillary tangles (NFTs), senile plaques (SPs), and a number of other changes [42]. Both NFTs and SPs are distributed in the brain in a specific topographic manner. For instance, NFTs begin to appear in the medial temporal lobes in the preclinical period of AD, spread to posterior association areas during the early clinical period of the disease, and later also to frontal areas of the brain, although primary projection areas are almost spared from pathology during the course of the disease [43]. This pattern is interesting to consider in relation to the corresponding neuropsychological findings.

### Neuropsychological Characteristics

Detection of AD may be accomplished by using a few neuropsychological tests tapping episodic memory, semantic memory (including verbal fluency and confrontation naming), visuospatial functioning, and psychomotor speed [25,44–49]. A summary of the cognitive findings in AD is presented in Table 3.3.

The sensitivity of episodic memory for early AD can be somewhat higher if processes of memory such as encoding, consolidation and retrieval are considered. There is a general consensus that encoding and delayed retrieval are efficient measures of episodic memory performance.

Although AD is said to be characterized by a continuous decline in global cognitive functioning, it is worth noticing that not all cognitive functions are affected. Some abilities seem to be preserved in early AD and, interestingly enough, some functions seem to be preserved even in advanced dementia. Examples of relatively preserved functions in early AD are primary memory, procedural memory and perceptual functions, as well as motor and sensory functions. The pattern of affected and preserved functions, as well as the course of change in these functions, may be understood in terms of neuropathology in AD and of brain–behaviour relationships in general.

In cognitive psychology, there is a distinction between various memory systems (see [50] for a review), which is based both on results from experimental manipulation of memory performance and on brain–behaviour relationships as shown in lesion studies and brain activation studies. First,

TABLE 3.3  Neuropsychological features of Alzheimer's disease across stages of dementia

*Preclinical period*
  Impairment of verbal and spatial episodic memory
  No other cognitive dysfunction, or very mild impairment

*Mild stage of dementia*
  Severe impairment of verbal and spatial episodic memory
  Impairment of semantic memory
  Impairment of visuospatial functioning
  Impairment of complex attention, but intact vigilance
  Impaired executive functions
  Intact primary and procedural memory
  Intact sensory-motor skills
  Intact personality, but affected adaption to environmental demands

*Advanced stage of dementia*
  Severe cognitive and personality changes as well as ADL dysfunction
  Changes of sensory-motor function

ADL, activities of daily living

there is a separation of memory traces that represent knowledge and information preserved across time. This knowledge or information may be concerned with motor skills or mental procedures (procedural memory), factual knowledge about the world (semantic memory), or context-related information, i.e. associated with a specific person, time and spatial location (episodic memory). There is also a memory system relating objects to sensory qualities (perceptual representation system). In contrast, there are memory traces representing small amounts of information, which are in mind for a short period of time (short-term memory) or operated upon in real time (working memory).

Schematically, the episodic memory is changed dramatically in early AD, which can be related to the early neuropathological changes within the medial temporal lobe, particularly in the transentorhinal cortex [43]. This pattern of brain–behaviour relationship is supported by recent brain activation studies showing that the activity in areas related to hippocampus are changed in early AD compared to aged-matched healthy individuals [51].

In contrast, it has been shown repeatedly that short-term memory is preserved in early dementia of the AD type [45,47,52]. Implicit memory as exemplified by priming effects, i.e. the unconscious facilitation of performance following prior exposure to target items or related items, is also relatively unaffected in early AD both according to behavioural studies [16] and brain activation studies [53].

The linguistic changes in AD are manifold and vary according to the level of decline. Among the possible language symptoms are anomia, reduced verbal fluency, semantic vagueness [54], generalized speech [55], and confabulation [56].

A study of confabulation in AD patients revealed that the total number of confabulations was highly correlated to the level of cognitive deterioration, as shown by the MMSE score, and to autobiographical memory [57]. Interestingly, confabulations were not related to free recall of a recently presented word list (episodic memory), which demonstrated a dissociation between autobiographical and item memory. Furthermore, confabulations could be described as four different categories varying in semantic remoteness to the target.

Several studies have reported evidence of subgroups of AD in terms of three profiles of neuropsychological characteristics, one showing a generalized impairment in both verbal and visuospatial function, a second with a predominantly verbal impairment, and a third with a predominantly visuospatial impairment [58,59]. The probable reason for these different profiles is the fact that individuals differ in pre-morbid profiles of cognitive function.

## Instrumental Characteristics

The first changes are noted in complex activities, for example at work [60] or in social activities [61]. Much later, when cognitive deterioration has progressed into moderate dementia, there is a change of the ability to perform self-care activities [36]. Not only is the distinction between IADLs and ADLs interesting to observe, but so too is the ability to perform various activities within IADLs and ADLs. As an example, the ability to use cutlery vs. using a comb may vary in a progression-related manner: typically the former is most often preserved longer during disease progression than is the latter [62]. However, studies usually demonstrate only a weak to moderate strength of relationship between ADLs/IADLs and cognition [37].

## Relationship between Neuropsychology and Markers of Neuropathology

Empirical studies on the relationship between neuropsychological measures and the number of NFTs have met limited success, showing a common variance ranging from 6% [63] to 60% [64]. The corresponding data on cognition and SPs are around 15% [63,64]. These findings are reflected in the relatively high correlation between global cognition and NFTs and the poor correlation between global cognition and SPs [65,66].

## Neuroimaging Findings

In early AD, the typical neuroimaging finding is a bilateral hypometabolism in temporoparietal association areas with a relative preservation of primary sensory and motor cortices, basal ganglia and cerebellum, as demonstrated by positron emission tomography (PET) using glucose as a marker [67,68] and single photon emission tomography (SPECT) [68,69]. Already in the pre-clinical period of AD, when a clinical diagnosis is not possible, a change in the pattern of blood flow can be visualized by SPECT [70,71].

Using morphological methods such as MRI, a very good predictive power has been reported for specific measures, i.e. hippocampal atrophy or other measures of the temporal lobes, in relation to development of AD in pre-clinical cases (see e.g. [72–74]). Also measures of general brain atrophy are associated with dementia [75].

## Differential Diagnosis

The most common clinical diagnostic issue is related to depression. To handle this issue, several differentiating neuropsychological and clinical characteristics have been suggested (Table 3.4).

TABLE 3.4 Differentiating neuropsychological and clinical characteristics in Alzheimer's disease (AD) and major depression (MD)

| Characteristic | Typical for AD | Typical for MD |
|---|---|---|
| Mood pattern | Enduring | Episodic |
| Mood easily influenced | Yes | No |
| Delusions | Mood-independent | Mood-congruent |
| Awareness of forgetfulness | No | Yes |
| Recognition memory | Impaired | Intact |
| Memory prompting | Unhelpful | Helpful |
| Non-incidental memory | Impaired | Intact |
| Procedural memory | Intact | Impaired |
| SPECT pattern | Parietal hypoperfusion | Frontal hypoperfusion |
| EEG activity | Abnormal | Normal |

SPECT, single photon emission tomography; EEG, electroencephalogram

# NEUROPSYCHOLOGICAL AND INSTRUMENTAL CHARACTERISTICS OF VASCULAR DEMENTIA (VD)

VD may be the consequence of a large brain infarction resulting from the occlusion of a major cerebral artery, which may occur suddenly and be followed by gross changes in behaviour (e.g. aphasia, apraxia, agnosia) as well as impairment of sensory and motor performance. The type of impairment may vary due to the specific vessel affected. In other cases VD may be due to multiple minor infarctions or haemorrhages, mainly in subcortical areas, affecting a variety of cognitive functions involving mental tempo, attention, memory and mood, and possibly producing gait disturbance, urinary incontinence and pyramidal signs. Third, VD can be caused by thickening of blood vessel walls associated with cerebral amyloid angiopathy, hyalinosis and sclerotic factors. These processes are found in small arteries and arterioles; consequently, this type of VD is a small-vessel disease. Long penetrating vessels supplying deep white matter and located in watershed areas are thought to be especially sensitive. Fourth, VD can be associated with general disturbance of brain perfusion resulting from heart arrest and hypotension. Fifth and last, VD can be associated with bleeding owing to subdural haematoma or subarachnoidal haemorrhage.

The clinical diagnosis of VD is most frequently based on DSM-IV [76], or the criteria suggested by the National Institute of Neurological Disorders and Stroke and the Association Internationale pour la Recherche et l'Enseignement en Neurosciences (NINDS–AIREN [77]). These criteria state that the diagnosis of VD has to be connected with confirming neuroimaging observations in addition to a relevant time relation between cerebrovascular disease and dementia. When neuroimaging examination is lacking, it is possible to use a clinical evaluation of cerebrovascular factors. For instance, it has recently been confirmed that the Hachinski Ischemic Score (HIS [78]) has a high degree of validity when examined in relation to neuropathological data [79].

There are a number of reports showing differences between VD and other dementias in specific domains such as personality disturbance, executive dysfunction and motor performance, as well as biologically basic behaviours [80]. However, the conclusion from reviews and experimental studies is that differences between VD and AD are hard to detect, when groups of patients are compared [45,81–83]. This probably reflects the fact that unselected groups of VD are usually examined, and it does not exclude the possibility that specific subgroups of VD may demonstrate distinctive features of behaviour and neuropsychological test results.

In connection with VD, white-matter changes (WMC) have to be mentioned, because they occur frequently. There are a number of studies

TABLE 3.5   Neuropsychological features of vascular dementia

Possible selective deficits in verbal and spatial functions due to distribution of
  lesions
Possible selective deficits in verbal and spatial episodic memory
Frequent changes in sensory-motor performance, general or asymmetric
Personality changes, e.g. emotional incontinence
Impaired executive function due to frontal involvement
General slowness in speeded performance, mentally or in motor skills
Fluctuations of performance
Pattern of decline may not be continuous, but stepwise or stable

showing slowing of mental processes and motor skills as the general effect linked to WMC [84–88]. No clear localization effect has been documented, but there is a mass effect of WMC [85].

The specific linguistic changes in VD are often concerned with basic language processes due to circumscribed selective brain infarction, whereas AD is concerned with ideational impoverishment due to the brain affection of temporal association areas. As an example of specific linguistic disturbance in VD, confabulation may be mentioned, which has been reported as a typical phenomenon linked to a disturbance in the understanding of basic time and space concepts caused by a right hemispheric posterior infarction [57].

In individual patients, characteristic features may exist involving, for instance, sensory–motor abnormalities, which can be asymmetric or general, and this type of findings is almost non-existent in early AD or FTD. The possible characteristic features of VD are summarized in Table 3.5.

In VD, the typical findings in brain imaging examinations are brain infarctions and an increased amount of white matter hyperintensities (WMH). The brain infarctions are visualized as areas with high intensities on $T_2$-weighted images and low signal intensities on $T_1$-weighted images, whereas WMH are seen as high signal intensities on $T_2$-weighted images [89].

## NEUROPSYCHOLOGICAL AND INSTRUMENTAL CHARACTERISTICS OF FRONTOTEMPORAL DEMENTIA (FTD)

The predominant location of brain pathology in FTD is the premotor frontal lobes and the anterior part of the temporal lobes [90,91]. Sometimes, the pathology is more pronounced in one hemisphere than in the other.

Nowadays, the diagnosis is based on the clinical criteria suggested by the Lund and Manchester groups [90]. The clinical picture of FTD is defined by

TABLE 3.6  Neuropsychological features of frontotemporal dementia

Early changes of personality
Impaired executive functions
Relatively intact verbal and spatial functions
Relatively intact verbal and spatial memory
Intact sensory-motor skills

profound alteration of personality and social conduct, loss of drive, blunted emotions, lost insight, stereotypic behaviours, reduced speech, cognitive changes due to impairment of mental control [91,92]. In addition to the prototypical FTD, the clinical diagnosis also covers progressive non-fluent aphasia [93] and semantic dementia [94].

The typical neuropsychological findings in FTD are concerned with personality or behavioural changes as the most conspicuous features, in addition to specific cognitive changes related to quality rather than type of performance [95–100]. There are also areas of no change, which can be illustrated by preserved sensory and motor functions. The main characteristics of early FTD are presented in Table 3.6.

The specific cognitive and behavioural features of FTD can vary due to the specific brain area that is affected by the disease as well as the extent of lesion [101]. Recently, it has been demonstrated that the first symptom in FTD was related to the predominance of atrophy, being right, left or bilateral, as observed by blinded ratings of neuroimaging examinations using SPECT [102]: predominant left atrophy was related to deviant language, whereas predominant right atrophy was related to disinhibition, and bilateral atrophy to executive problems. Some symptoms that are frequent in FTD did not occur as a first symptom (e.g. hyperorality, compulsions) and some symptoms had no specific relation to brain atrophy. Failing memory never occurred as the first symptom in FTD, while it was the most prominent first symptom in early AD [102].

The specific linguistic changes in FTD have not been described in detail except for test results showing reduced verbal fluency [98]. However, recent research on FTD patients [103,104] has demonstrated that FTD patients produce confabulations of two types. In one type of confabulation, the patient substituted the present situation by an old and well-known situation related to his own previous life history. In a second type, the patient substituted the present situation by using irrelevant concepts or words [104]. FTD patients with predominant left hemispheric atrophy demonstrated relatively more stereotypic and less specified utterances compared to FTD patients with predominant right hemispheric atrophy [103].

## SUMMARY

### Consistent Evidence

There is consistent evidence that neuropsychological, instrumental and behavioural characteristics of dementia syndromes are specific for the disease and degree of deterioration, that is, features are both disease-related and stage-related.

The onset of AD is related to impairment of episodic memory without any other clear cognitive symptoms, whereas the early clinical stage of AD is characterized by multiple cognitive deficits, mainly involving episodic and semantic memory, verbal functions (e.g. anomia) visuospatial functions, executive function and attention. These changes may be compensated for or supported in order to handle ADL. In the advanced stage of AD, primary memory and implicit memory related to sensory and motor performance will be clearly affected in addition to perception. During this stage, the individual requires support and help with ADL.

In VD, the onset is connected with sudden or progressive changes of cerebrovascular supply, which can imply slowing of both motor and mental activities, which is typical during the early clinical stage. In advanced VD, other cognitive deficits add on. The progression follows a stepwise or monotonic fashion. Frequently, VD is associated with asymmetric sensory and/or motor impairments, which is specific for this syndrome.

The onset of FTD is marked by abnormal affective function and behaviour together with a relatively intact cognitive function. However, cognitive functioning may be disturbed secondarily due to abnormal personality characteristics that influence motivation and strategy utilization. In advanced stages of FTD, there is also a clear cognitive dysfunction in addition to grossly abnormal personality and behaviour. Progression is typically continuous.

### Incomplete Evidence

The main difficulty with dementia studies is bound to the fact that the dementia diseases are progressive and there are still only very rough indicators of their time course. Second, the behavioural features and symptoms of dementia disorders are dependent on the specific pre-morbid abilities of the individual, and there is no simple way to take into account the pre-morbid abilities when evaluating the present status of cognitive function. Third, the time course of change in cognition, personality and behaviour has to be analysed in more detail, particularly in relation to healthy ageing. Fourth, the characteristics of healthy ageing have to be described.

## Areas Still Open to Research

At the general level, knowledge of the brain–behaviour relationship in healthy individuals and patients with various dementia diseases is far from complete. Future research has to study in detail the networks of brain activity that are responsible for the tasks that are critically involved in various dementia diseases, for instance, episodic memory in early AD, cognitive slowing in VD and abnormal behaviour in FTD.

More specifically, there is a need to clarify the relationship between neuropsychological measures and neurochemical as well as neuropathological markers of disease in AD, VD and FTD.

## ACKNOWLEDGEMENT

Financial support to write this review was provided by Alzheimerfonden, Gamla Tjänarinnor, and the Swedish Medical Research Council, which is gratefully acknowledged.

## REFERENCES

1. Cummings J.L., Benson D.F. (1992)   *Dementia: a Clinical Approach*, 2nd edn, Butterworth-Heineman, Boston.
2. Crawford J.R., Stewart L.E., Cochrane R.H., Foulds J.A., Besson J.A., Parker D.M. (1989)   Estimating premorbid IQ from demographic variables: regression equations derived from a UK sample. *Br. J. Clin. Psychol.*, **28**: 275–278.
3. Paolo A.M., Ryan J.J., Troster A.I. (1997)   Estimating premorbid WAIS-R intelligence in the elderly: an extension and cross validation of new regression equations. *J. Clin. Psychol.*, **53**: 647–656.
4. Nelson N.E., McKenna P. (1975)   The use of current reading ability in the assessment of dementia. *Br. J. Soc. Clin. Psychol.*, **14**: 259–267.
5. Baddeley A., Emslie H., Nimmo-Smith I. (1993)   The Spot-the-Word test: a robust estimate of verbal intelligence based on lexical decision. *Br. J. Clin. Psychol.*, **32**: 55–65.
6. Wechsler D. (1981)   *Wechsler Adult Intelligence Scale-Revised: Manual*, Psychological Corporation, New York.
7. Wilson R.S., Beckett L.A., Bennet D.A., Albert M.S., Evans D.A. (1999)   Change in cognitive function in older persons from a community population. *Arch. Neurol.*, **56**: 1274–1279.
8. Lezak M. (1995)   *Neuropsychological Assessment*, 3rd edn, Oxford University Press, New York.

9. Wechsler D. (1955) *Wechsler Adult Intelligence Scale: Manual*, Psychological Corporation, New York.
10. Beck N.C., Tucker D., Frank R., Parker J., Lake R., Thomas S., Lichty W., Horowitz B., Merritt F. (1989) The latent factor structure of the WAIS-R: a factor analysis of individual item responses. *J. Clin. Psychol.*, **45**: 281–293.
11. Burgess A., Flint J., Adshead H. (1992) Factor structure of the Wechsler Adult Intelligence Scale—Revised (WAIS-R): a clinical sample. *Br. J. Clin. Psychol.*, **31**: 336–338.
12. Enns R.A., Reddon J.R. (1998) The factor structure of the Wechsler Adult Intelligence Scale—Revised: one or two but not three factors. *J. Clin. Psychol.*, **54**: 447–459.
13. Fernaeus S.E., Bronge L., Östberg P., Julin P., Winblad B., Wahlund L.O., Almkvist O. Lexical access and conceptual elaboration are related to different types of brain lesions (in preparation).
14. Kerr B., Vitiello M.V., Calogero M., Wilkie F., Prinz P.N. (1998) Memory-scanning task performance in Alzheimer's disease. *Aging*, **10**: 401–410.
15. Collette F., Van der Linden M., Bechet S., Salmon E. (1999) Phonological loop and central executive functioning in Alzheimer's disease. *Neuropsychologia*, **37**: 905–918.
16. Fleishman D.A., Gabrieli J.D., Gilley D.W., Hauser J.D., Lange K.L., Dwornik L.M., Bennett D.A., Wilson R.S. (1999) Word-stem completion priming in healthy aging and Alzheimer's disease: the effects of age, cognitive status, and encoding. *Neuropsychology*, **13**: 22–30.
17. Wechsler D. (1945) A standardized memory scale for clinical use. *J. Psychol.*, **19**: 87–95.
18. Wechsler D. (1981) *Wechsler Memory Scale-Revised: Manual*, Psychological Corporation, New York.
19. Benton A.L. (1974) *The Revised Visual Retention Test*, 4th edn, Psychological Corporation, New York.
20. Larrabee G.J., Kane R.L., Schuck J.R. (1983) Factor analysis of the WAIS and Wechsler Memory Scale: an analysis of the construct validity of the Wechsler Memory Scale. *J. Clin. Neuropsychol.*, **5**: 159–168.
21. Delis D.C., Freeland J., Kramer J.H., Kaplan E. (1988) Integrating clinical assessment with cognitive neuroscience: construct validation of the California Verbal Learning Test. *J. Consult. Clin. Psychol.*, **56**: 123–130.
22. Anderson J.R. (1995) *Cognitive Psychology and its Implications* (4th edn), Freeman, New York.
23. Kaplan E.F., Goodglass H., Weintraub S. (1978) *The Boston Naming Test*, Kaplan and Goodglass, Boston.
24. Monsch A.U., Bondi M.W., Butters N., Paulsen J.S., Salmon D.P., Katzman R., Swenson M.R. (1994) A comparison of category and letter fluency in Alzheimer's disease and Huntington's disease. *Neuropsychology*, **8**: 25–30.
25. Welsh K.A., Butters N., Hughes J.P., Mohs R.C., Heyman A. (1992) Detection and staging of dementia in Alzheimer's disease: use of neuropsychological measures developed for the Consortium to establish a Registry for Alzheimer's Disease (CERAD). *Arch. Neurol.*, **49**: 448–452.
26. Welsh K.A., Butters N., Mohs R.C., Beekly D., Edland S., Fillenbaum G., Heyman A. (1994) Consortium to Establish a Registry for Alzheimer's Disease (CERAD). Part V. A normative study of the neuropsychological battery. *Neurology*, **44**: 609–614.

27. Rosen W.G., Mohs R.C., Davis K.L. (1984) A new rating scale for Alzheimer's disease. *Am. J. Psychiatry*, **141**: 1356–1364.
28. Robbins T.W., James M., Owen A.M., Sahakian B.J., McInnes L., Rabbitt P. (1994) Cambridge neuropsychological automated battery (CANTAB): a factor analytic study of a large sample of normal elderly volunteers. *Dementia*, **5**: 266–281.
29. Saxton J., McGonigle K.L., Swihart A.A., Boller F. (1993) *The Severe Impairment Battery*, Thames Valley Test Company, Bury St. Edmunds.
30. Hughes C.P., Berg L., Danziger W.L., Coben L.A., Martin R.L. (1982) A new clinical scale for the staging of dementia. *Br. J. Psychiatry*, **140**: 566–572.
31. Morris J.C. (1993) The Clinical Dementia Rating (CDR): current version and scoring rules. *Neurology*, **43**: 2412–2414.
32. Reisberg B., Ferris S., deLeon M.J., Crook T. (1982) The Global Deterioration Scale for assessment of primary degenerative dementia. *Am. J. Psychiatry*, **139**: 1136–1139.
33. Folstein M.F., Folstein S.E., McHugh P.R. (1975) "Mini-Mental State": a practical method for grading the cognitive status of the patient for the clinician. *J. Psychiatr. Res.*, **12**: 189–198.
34. Åsberg M., Perris C., Schalling D., Sedvall G. (1978) The CPRS: development and application of a psychiatric rating scale. *Acta Psychiatr. Scand.*, **271** (Suppl.).
35. Cummings J.L., Mega M., Gray K., Rosenberg-Thompson S., Carusi D.A., Gornbein J. (1994) The Neuropsychiatric Inventory: comprehensive assessment of psychopathology in dementia. *Neurology*, **44**: 2308–2314.
36. Reisberg B., Auer S.R., Monteiro I.M. (1996) Behavioral pathology in Alzheimer's disease (Behave-AD) rating scale. *Int. Psychogeriatrics*, **8** (Suppl. 3): 301–308.
37. Nygård L., Amberla K., Bernspång B., Almkvist O., Winblad B. (1998) The relationship between cognition and instrumental daily activities in cases of mild Alzheimer's disease. *Am. J. Occup. Ther.*, **5**: 160–166.
38. Lawton M.P., Brody E.M. (1969) Assessment of older people: self-maintaining and instrumental activities of daily living. *Gerontologist*, **9**: 179–186.
39. Katz S., Ford A.B., Moskowitz R.W., Jackson B.A., Jaffee M.W. (1963) The index of ADL: a standardized measure of biological and psychosocial function. *JAMA*, **185**: 914–919.
40. Fisher A.G. (1997) *Assessment of Motor and Process Skills*, 2nd edn. *Test Manual*, Department of Occupational Therapy, Colorado State University, Three Star Press, Fort Collins.
41. Nygård L. (1998) Assessing ADL/IADL in persons with dementia. In *Health Economics of Dementia* (Eds A. Wimo, B. Jönsson, B. Winblad), pp. 371–378, Wiley, Chichester.
42. Hardy J., Higgins G. (1992) Alzheimer's disease: the amyloid cascade hypothesis. *Science*, **256**: 184–185.
43. Braak H., Braak E. (1995) Staging of Alzheimer's disease-related neurofibrillary changes. *Neurobiol. Aging*, **16**: 271–284.
44. Almkvist O. (1996) Neuropsychological features of early Alzheimer's disease: preclinical and clinical stages. *Acta Neurol. Scand.*, **165** (Suppl.): 21–29.
45. Almkvist O., Bäckman L., Basun H., Wahlund L.O. (1993) Patterns of neuropsychological performance in Alzheimer's disease and vascular dementia. *Cortex*, **29**: 661–673.
46. Herlitz A., Hill R.D., Fratiglioni L., Bäckman L. (1995) Episodic memory and visuospatial ability in detecting and staging of dementia in a community-based sample of very old adults. *J. Gerontol. Med. Sci.*, **50A**: M107–M113.

47. Small B.J., Herlitz A., Fratiglioni L., Almkvist O., Bäckman L. (1996)  Cognitive predictors of incident Alzheimer's disease: a prospective longitudinal study. *Neuropsychology*, **11**: 1–8.
48. Storandt M., Hill R. (1989)  Very mild senile dementia of the Alzheimer type: II. Psychometric test performance. *Arch. Neurol.*, **46**: 383–386.
49. Tierney M.C., Szalai J.P., Snow W.G., Fisher R.H., Nores A., Nadon G., Dunn E., St. George-Hyslop P.H. (1996)  Prediction of probable Alzheimer's disease in memory-impaired patients: a prospective longitudinal study. *Neurology*, **46**: 661–665.
50. Tulving E., Schacter D.L. (1990)  Priming and human memory systems. *Science*, **247**: 301–305.
51. Bäckman L., Andersson J.L.R., Nyberg L., Winblad B., Nordberg A., Almkvist O. (1999)  Brain regions associated with episodic retrieval in normal aging and Alzheimer's disease. *Neurology*, **52**: 1861–1870.
52. Simon E., Leach L., Winocur G., Moscovitch M. (1995)  Intact primary memory in mild to moderate Alzheimer's disease: indices from the California Verbal Learning Test. *J. Clin. Exp. Neuropsychol.*, **16**: 414–422.
53. Bäckman L., Almkvist O., Nyberg L., Andersson J. (2000)  Functional changes in brain activity during priming in Alzheimer's disease. *J. Cogn. Neurosci.*, **12**: 134–141.
54. Chan A.S., Butters N., Salmon D. (1997)  The deterioration of semantic networks in patients with Alzheimer's disease: a cross-sectional study. *Neuropsychologia*, **35**: 241–248.
55. Orange J.B., Lubinski B., Higginbotham D.J. (1996)  Conversational repair by individuals with dementia of the Alzheimer type. *J. Speech Hearing Res.*, **39**: 881–895.
56. Tallberg I.M., Almkvist O. (2001)  Confabulation and memory in patients with Alzheimer's disease. *J. Clin. Exp. Neuropsychol.*, **23**: 172–184.
57. Tallberg I.M.  Deictic disturbances after right hemisphere stroke. Submitted for publication.
58. Fisher N.J., Rourke B.P., Bieliauskas L.A. (1999)  Neuropsychological subgroups of patients with Alzheimer's disease: an examination of the first 10 years of CERAD data. *J. Clin. Exp. Neuropsychol.*, **21**: 488–518.
59. Martin A., Brouwers P., Lalonde F., Cox C., Teleska P., Fedio P., Foster N.L., Chase T.N. (1986)  Towards a behavioural typology of Alzheimer's patients. *J. Clin. Exp. Neuropsychol.*, **8**: 594–610.
60. Robinson P., Ekman S.L., Meleis A., Winblad B., Wahlund L.O. (1997)  Suffering silence: the experience of early memory loss. *Health Care in Later Life*, **2**: 107–120.
61. DeJong R., Osterlund O.W., Roy G.W. (1989)  Measurement of quality-of-life changes in patients with Alzheimer's disease. *Clin. Ther.*, **11**: 545–554.
62. Borell L., Rönnberg L., Sandman P.O. (1996)  The ability to use familiar objects among patients with Alzheimer's disease. *Occup. Ther. J. Res.*, **15**: 111–121.
63. Kanne S.M., Balota D.A., Storandt M., McKeel D.W., Jr, Morris J.C. (1998)  Relating anatomy to function in Alzheimer's disease: neuropsychological profiles predict regional neuropathology 5 years later. *Neurology*, **50**: 979–985.
64. Gomez-Isla T., Hollister R., West H., Mui S., Growdon J.H., Petersen R.C., Parisi J.E., Hyman B.T. (1997)  Neuronal loss correlates with but exceeds neurofibrillary tangles in Alzheimer's disease. *Ann. Neurol.*, **41**: 17–24.

65. Arriagada P.V., Marzloff K., Hyman B.T. (1992)   Distribution of Alzheimer-type pathologic changes in nondemented elderly individuals matches the pattern of Alzheimer's disease. *Neurology*, **42**: 1681–1688.
66. Wilcock G.K., Esiri M.M. (1982)   Plaques, tangles, and dementia: a quantitative study. *J. Neurosci.*, **56**: 343–356.
67. Herholz K., Nordberg A., Salmon E., Perani D., Kessler J., Mielke R., Halber M., Jelic V., Almkvist O., Collette F. *et al* (1999)   Impairment of neocortical metabolism predicts progression in Alzheimer's disease. *Dement. Geriatr. Cogn. Disord.*, **10**: 494–504.
68. Wahlund L.O., Basun H., Almkvist O., Julin P., Viitanen M., Axelman K., Shigeta M., Jelic V., Nordberg A., Lannfelt L. (1999)   A follow-up study of a family with the Swedish Alzheimer mutation. *Dement. Geriatr. Cogn. Disord.*, **10**: 526–533.
69. Jagust W.J. (1994)   Functional imaging in dementia: an overview. *J. Clin. Psychiatry*, **55** (Suppl.): 5–11.
70. Johnson K.A., Jones K., Holman B.L., Becker J.A., Spiers P.A., Satlin A., Albert M.S. (1998)   Preclinical prediction of Alzheimer's disease using SPECT. *Neurology*, **50**: 1563–1571.
71. Julin P., Almkvist O., Basun H., Lannfelt L., Svensson L., Winblad B., Wahlund L.O. (1998)   Brain volumes and regional cerebral blood flow in carriers of the Swedish Alzheimer amyloid mutation. *Alz. Dis. Assoc. Disord.*, **12**: 49–53.
72. DeLeon M.J., George A.E., Golomb J., Tarshish C., Convit A., Kluger A., DeSanti S., McRae T., Ferris S.H., Reisberg B. *et al* (1997)   Frequency of hippocampal atrophy in normal aging and Alzheimer's disease. *Neurobiol. Aging*, **19**: 1–11.
73. Jack C.R., Jr., Petersen R.C., Xu Y.C., O'Brien P.C., Smith G.E., Ivnik R.J., Boeve P.F., Waring S.C., Tangalos E.G., Kokmen E. (1999)   Prediction of AD with MRI-based hippocampal volume in mild cognitive impairment. *Neurology*, **52**: 1397–1403.
74. Scheltens P., Leys D., Barkhof F., Huglo D., Weinstein H.C., Vermersch P., Kuiper M., Steinling M., Wolters E.C., Valk J. (1992)   Atrophy of the medial temporal lobes on MRI in probable Alzheimer's disease and normal ageing: diagnostic value and neuropsychological correlates. *J. Neurol. Neurosurg. Psychiatry*, **55**: 967–972.
75. Fox N.C., Scahill R.I., Crum W.R., Rossor M.N. (1999)   Correlation between rates of brain atrophy and cognitive decline in AD. *Neurology*, **52**: 1687–1689.
76. American Psychiatric Association (1994)   *Diagnostic and Statistical Manual of Mental Disorders*, 4th edn, *American Psychiatric Association*, Washington, DC.
77. Román G., Tatemichi T.K., Erkinjuntti T., Cummings J.L., Masdeu J.C., Garcia J.H., Amaducci L., Orgogoto J.M., Brun A., Hofman A. *et al* (1993)   Vascular dementia: diagnostic criteria for research studies. *Neurology*, **43**: 250–260.
78. Hachinski V.C., Iliff L.D., Zilkha E., DuBolay G.H., McAlister V.L., Marshall J., Ross-Russell R.W., Symon L. (1975)   Cerebral blood flow in dementia. *Arch. Neurol.*, **32**: 632–637.
79. Moroney J.T., Bagiella E., Desmond D.W., Hachinski V.C., Mölsä P.K., Gustafson L., Brun A., Fischer P., Erkinjuntti T., Rosen W. *et al* (1997)   Meta-analysis of the Hachinski Ischemic Score in pathologically verified dementias. *Neurology*, **49**: 1096–1105.
80. Mega M.S., Cummings J.L. (1994)   Frontal-subcortical circuits and neuropsychiatric disorders. *J. Neuropsychiatry Clin. Neurosci.*, **6**: 358–370.

81. Almkvist O. (1994) Neuropsychological deficits in vascular dementia in relation to Alzheimer's disease: reviewing evidence for functional similarity or divergence. *Dementia*, **5**: 203–209.
82. Almkvist O., Fratiglioni L., Aguero-Torres H., Viitanen M., Bäckman L. (1999) Cognitive support at episodic encoding and retrieval: similar patterns of utilization in community-based samples of Alzheimer's disease and vascular dementia patients. *J. Clin. Exp. Neuropsychol.*, **21**: 816–830.
83. Erkinjuntti T., Laaksonen R., Sulkava R., Syrjäläinen R., Palo J. (1986) Neuropsychological differentiation between normal aging, Alzheimer's disease, and vascular dementia. *Acta Neurol. Scand.*, **74**: 393–403.
84. Almkvist O., Wahlund L.O., Andersson-Lundman G., Basun H., Bäckman L. (1992) White-matter hyperintensity and neuropsychological functions in dementia and healthy aging. *Arch. Neurol.*, **49**: 626–632.
85. Boone K.B., Miller B.L., Lesser I.M., Mehringer C.M., Hill-Gutierrez E., Goldberg M.A., Berman N.G. (1992) Neuropsychological correlates of white-matter lesions in healthy elderly subjects: a threshold effect. *Arch. Neurol.*, **49**: 549–554.
86. Junque C., Puiol J., Vendrell P., Bruna O., Jódar M., Ribas C.J., Vinas J., Capdevila A., Marti-Vilalta J.L. (1990) Leuko-araiosis on magnetic resonance imaging and speed of mental processing. *Arch. Neurol.*, **47**: 151–156.
87. Tupler L.A., Coffey C.E., Logue P.E., Djang W.T., Fagan S.M. (1992) Neuropsychological importance of subcortical white matter hyperintensity. *Arch. Neurol.*, **49**: 1248–1252.
88. Ylikoski R., Ylikoski A., Erkinjuntti T., Sulkava R., Raininko R., Tilvis R. (1993) White matter changes in healthy elderly persons correlate with attention and speed of mental processing. *Arch. Neurol.*, **50**: 818–824.
89. Wahlund L.O. (1994) Brain imaging and vascular dementia. *Dementia*, **5**: 193–196.
90. The Lund and Manchester Groups (1994) Clinical and neuropathological criteria for frontotemporal dementia. *J. Neurol. Neurosurg. Psychiatry*, **57**: 416–418.
91. Neary D. (1999) Overview of frontotemporal dementias. *Dement. Geriatr. Cogn. Disord.*, 10 (Suppl. 1): 6–9.
92. Gustafson L. (1993) Clinical picture of frontal lobe degeneration of the non-Alzheimer type. *Dementia*, **4**: 143–148.
93. Mesulam M.M. (1982) Slowly progressive aphasia without dementia. *Ann. Neurol.*, **11**: 592–598.
94. Hodges J.R., Patterson K., Oxbury S., Funnell E. (1992) Semantic dementia: progressive fluent aphasia with temporal lobe atrophy. *Brain*, **115**: 1783–1806.
95. Elfgren C., Passant U., Risberg J. (1993) Neuropsychological findings in frontal lobe dementia. *Dementia*, **4**: 214–219.
96. Förstl H., Besthorn C., Hentschel F., Geiger-Kabisch X., Sattel H., Schreiter-Gasser U. (1996) Frontal lobe degeneration and Alzheimer's disease: a controlled study on clinical findings, volumetric brain changes and quantitative electroencephalographic data. *Dementia*, **7**: 27–34.
97. Lebert F., Pasquier F., Petit H. (1995) Personality traits and frontal lobe dementia. *Int. J. Geriatr. Psychiatry*, **10**: 1047–1049.
98. Lindau M., Almkvist O., Johansson S.E., Wahlund L.O. (1998) Neuropsychological characteristics of frontal lobe dementia in contrast to Alzheimer's disease. *Dement. Geriatr. Cogn. Disord.*, **9**: 205–213.
99. Miller B., Cummings J.L., Villanueva-Meyer J., Boone K., Mehringer C.M., Lesser I.M., Mena I. (1991) Frontal lobe degeneration: clinical, neuropsychological, and SPECT characteristics. *Neurology*, **41**: 1374–1382.

100. Neary D., Snowdon J.S., Northen B., Goulding P.J. (1988)  Dementia of frontal type. *J. Neurol. Neurosurg. Psychiatry*, **51**: 353–361.
101. Lindau M., Andersen C., Julin P., Blomberg M., Wahlund L.O., Almkvist O. Neuropsychological findings and volumetric brain measurements in fronto-temporal dementia and healthy controls. Submitted for publication.
102. Lindau M., Almkvist O., Kushi J., Boone K., Johansson S.E., Wahlund L.O., Cummings J.L., Miller B.L. (2000)  First symptoms—frontotemporal dementia versus Alzheimer's disease. *Dement. Geriatr. Cogn. Disord.*, **11**: 286–293.
103. Tallberg I.M., Persson H., Wångmar L., Wahlund L.O., Almkvist O. (2002) Semantic range and relevance of emotive utterances in frontotemporal degeneration. *Brain Lang.*, **82**: 146–158.
104. Tallberg I.M. (1999)  Projection of meaning in frontotemporal dementia. *Discourse Studies*, **1**: 455–477.

# Commentaries

3.1

## Improving Diagnosis of Dementia

Martin Rossor[1]

We have come a long way in the last 20 years in our ability to diagnose the different dementing disorders. Indeed, the term "dementia" is now as much a hindrance as a help. The term was developed to distinguish patients with multiple domains of cognitive impairment from those who had either a focal deficit or a confusional state. The former would lead to an intensive search for a focal lesion, such as a neoplasm, which might have therapeutic implications. The latter, i.e. patients with confusional states and marked impairment of attention, often had an underlying metabolic disorder, the recognition of which was essential. By contrast, patients presenting with multiple domains of cognitive impairment who did not fulfil the criteria for a confusional state or delirium were usually found to suffer from one of the degenerative disorders, such as Alzheimer's disease (AD). The diagnostic process usually stopped at the level of dementia.

In order to fulfil the criteria for dementia, there has to be impairment of memory plus at least one other domain of cognitive dysfunction, and this must be sufficiently severe to interfere with social or work. In order to fulfil the diagnostic criteria for AD, it is necessary also to fulfil the criteria for dementia. Clearly this is at a more advanced stage than one would ideally identify the disease. Thus, we are now employing terms such as "mild cognitive impairment" (MCI), which is known to include a number of patients who have early AD and indeed, on average, 15% per annum of MCI patients will progress to dementia [1]. The idea that such patients go on to develop AD only when they fulfil the dementia criteria is clearly conceptually incorrect.

Many of the earlier definitions imply that the cognitive impairment is global. Whilst this may be true in the end stage of the disease, it is certainly not so early on. A number of the dementia disorders have characteristic modes of onset reflecting the regional selectivity of the disease process.

[1] *Dementia Research Group, National Hospital for Neurology and Neurosurgery, Queen Square, London WC1N 3BG, UK*

Thus, early impairment of event or episodic memory characterizes AD, whereas impairment of language or frontal executive functions reflects those diseases preferentially affecting the frontotemporal cortices.

It is, of course, change within an individual that reflects the onset of the disease, and our ability to identify that change in the individual is critically important in the diagnostic process. It is one thing to be able to demonstrate changes at a group level, but entirely different to identify reliably change at an individual level. It is, however, the latter which is of greatest value in the diagnostic process. Almqvist points out the essential features to achieve this measurement of change in cognitive tests. We rarely have the luxury of premorbid assessment, and the National Adult Reading Test can provide some estimate of premorbid intellect. This serves well in patients with classical AD, but fails in some of the patients with frontotemporal degeneration. In particular, patients with a semantic dementia will often demonstrate an early surface dyslexia and an inability to perform adequately on tests of reading (lexical) skills. Neuropsychological tests which are able to measure change should avoid ceiling and floor effects, and thus early in the disease the best tests are those of graded difficulty which are normally distributed in the general population. Tests that are very difficult may be sensitive to the early stage of the disease, but also sensitive to a host of other confounding factors. Clearly a different set of tests are needed to measure change in those more severely affected.

The same criteria apply to imaging modalities, increasingly important in the differential diagnosis of the patient presenting with cognitive impairment. Again, one may be able to demonstrate differences at a group level, but abnormalities within the individual are of critical importance. Functional imaging may show changes early in the disease, but there is substantial overlap at the individual level. Again, the key feature is change, and an imaging modality that allows frequent imaging is advantageous. The ideal would be imaging modalities to affect the underlying molecular pathology of amyloid, tau, prion or synuclein deposition. There are advances being made in amyloid imaging, but not yet in clinical practice. Magnetic resonance spectroscopy shows some promise for looking at neuronal markers such as $N$-acetylaspartate and myo-inositol as a glial signal [2], but again, not in routine practice. Structural imaging can measure atrophy as a surrogate measure of tissue disintegration, and there are now techniques for positional registration of volume magnetic resonance (MR) images which can provide a very precise quantitation of tissue loss [3]. Whilst total brain volume, ventricular volume or hippocampal volume may be reduced in AD, there is an overlap between the disease and control groups. By contrast, the rate of change, i.e. the tissue loss over a 6-month or 1-year period, is significantly greater in the AD group than in controls [4].

The goal is to make a precise molecular pathological diagnosis. However, whilst one can now predict AD with some accuracy, it is a far greater challenge with the non-AD dementias. In particular, the clinical syndrome of frontotemporal dementia can be particularly problematic. The variable combination of frontal and temporal lobe features, with the prototypic syndromes of a frontal dysexecutive syndrome, primary progressive aphasia and semantic dementia [5], reflects the frontotemporal degeneration. However, there are a whole variety of underlying disease processes, which include a non-specific degeneration also referred to as dementia without histological features, classical Pick's disease with tau-positive ubiquitin-positive inclusions, the hereditary tauopathies, corticobasal degeneration and rarely AD and prion disease. Ubiquitin-positive tau-negative inclusions, similar to those seen in motor neurone disease, can also be associated with frontotemporal degeneration and, indeed, were found to be the underlying histopathology in the prototypic semantic dementia cases [6].

We have moved beyond using the dementia syndrome to separate focal lesions and confusional states from the degenerative dementias. We are now able to recognize a number of diseases by virtue of their topological selectivity; the challenge is now on for more precise molecular diagnoses, essential if we are to take therapeutic intervention further.

## REFERENCES

1. Petersen R.C., Smith G.E., Waring S.C., Ivnik R.J., Tangalos E.G., Kokmen E. (1999) Mild cognitive impairment: clinical characterization and outcome. *Arch. Neurol.*, **56**: 303–308.
2. Jack C.R., Petersen R.C., Xu Y.C., O'Brien P.C., Smith G.E., Ivnik R.J., Boeve B.F., Waring S.C., Tangalos E.G., Kokmen E. (1999) Prediction of AD with MRI-based hippocampal volume in mild cognitive impairment. *Neurology*, **52**: 1397–1403.
3. Fox N.C., Freeborough P.A. (1997) Brain atrophy progression measured from registered serial MRI: validation and application to Alzheimer's disease. *J. Magnetic Resonance Imaging*, **7**: 1069–1075.
4. Fox N.C., Freeborough P.A., Rossor M.N. (1996) Visualisation and quantification of atrophy in Alzheimer's disease. *Lancet*, **348**: 94–97.
5. Neary D., Snowden J.S., Gustafson L., Passant U., Stuss D., Black S., Freedman M., Kertesz A., Robert P. H., Albert M. *et al* (1998) Frontotemporal lobar degeneration: a consensus on clinical diagnostic criteria. *Neurology*, **51**: 1546–1554.
6. Rossor M.N., Revesz T., Lantos P.L., Warrington E.K. (2000) Semantic dementia with ubiquitin-positive tau-negative inclusion bodies. *Brain*, **123**: 267–276.

3.2
## The Contribution of Neuropsychology to the Assessment of Dementia Syndromes

Karen Ritchie[1]

Neuropsychological assessment involves the observation of an individual's behaviour in relation to a given stimulus, selected for its likelihood to provoke an abnormal response in the face of damage to specific neuroanatomical structures. The theoretical basis of neuropsychological assessment is derived, on the one hand, from cognitive psychology, which is concerned with the development of cognitive tests for the demonstration of theoretical models of normal cognitive functioning, and on the other hand, from behavioural neurology in the tradition of Luria, which aims at the classification of normal and pathological responses to cognitive stimuli with a view to screening central nervous system disorder. Ove Almkvist's review of neuropsychological assessment in dementia emphasizes the importance for diagnosis of considering both normal models of cognitive functioning, such as the dissociation of primary, episodic and procedural memory, and the features of pathological central nervous system functioning typical of these disorders, such as aphasia, hallucinations and personality disorder.

The author also reminds us that, despite the identification in recent years of a number of potential biological markers for these disorders, diagnosis still relies primarily on accurate behavioural observation. Much of the work conducted in relation to dementia follows Luria's process-achievement approach, which emphasizes the need for detailed analysis of neuropsychological data to uncover different cognitive processes responsible for patients' overall performance. This approach has also been used to differentiate diseases and clinical syndromes, for example, between frontotemporal degeneration, Lewy body dementia, Alzheimer's disease (AD) and Parkinson's disease dementia, between AD and cerebrovascular disease, and within some of these forms of dementia, in terms of clinical heterogeneity.

Neuropsychological assessment has played an important role in the differentiation of dementia subtypes in the past decade. While generic terms such as "organic brain disease" were freely applied up until the 1980s (when specific diagnostic algorithms for dementia appeared in disease classifications), the differentiation of homogeneous behavioural subgroups and their relationship to distinct underlying forms of brain pathology allows us now to differentiate a large number of dementia subtypes, such

[1] *Research Group on the Epidemiology of Central Nervous System Pathologies, Institut National de la Santè et de la Recherche Mèdicale (INSERM), Montpellier, France*

as Lewy body dementia, frontotemporal dementia, semantic dementia, vascular dementia, early and late onset AD. Within dementia syndromes it is, furthermore, now recognized that many of the differences in disease presentation once attributed to individual differences are a function of different patterns of degeneration, suggesting the existence of subtypes [1].

However, despite the proliferation of neuropsychological testing methods in the field of information processing research in dementia, surprisingly few of these fine-tuned methods are being carried over into clinical practice and routine diagnosis. Investigations carried out in a number of countries suggest that reliance is predominantly placed on older tests, notably the Wechsler intelligence and memory scales, due to the accumulation of normative and pathology-specific data [2]. While more recent, and in particular computer-generated, testing procedures are recognized as having considerable advantages over older tests, precedence is clearly given to paper-and-pencil techniques, which have been widely used. Given that neuropsychological testing even in a research context is generally conducted on small numbers of subjects, the trend is against innovation, due to lack of normative data, although meta-analytic techniques are now being applied to clinical neuropsychological studies to alleviate this situation.

Finally, interest in normal and pathological brain ageing has presented a new challenge to research in the dementias—that of differentiating pathological and ageing-related physiological change. The appearance of subclinical nosological entities, such as mild cognitive disorder, which may herald more serious disease, or even warrant therapeutic intervention in themselves, emphasizes the present interest in borderline states. The establishment of a normal range in heterogeneous elderly populations has been extremely difficult, due principally to the erroneous practice of using younger control groups to estimate rates of ageing-related cognitive decline. In so doing, cohort effects or generation differences have been confounded with neurodegenerative processes. As Almkvist's review points out, there has consequently been considerable interest in developing tests which permit estimation of premorbid young adult levels so that the present results achieved by an individual may be compared with his own optimal performance [3,4]. Focus may thus be turned on the individual rate of decline over time, which is theoretically closer to the essential notion of dementia than statistical differences in performance estimated from population means.

## REFERENCES

1. Leibovici D., Ritchie K. (1995) Heterogeneity in senile dementia and normal cognitive ageing. *Alzheimer's Res.*, **1**: 17–22.

2. Sullivan K., Bowden S. (1997)  Which tests do neuropsychologists use? *J. Clin. Psychol.*, **53**: 657–661.
3. Taylor K., Salmon D., Rice V.A., Bondi M., Hill L. (1996)  Longitudinal examination of American National Adult Reading Test (AMNART) performance in dementia of the Alzheimer type: validation and correction based on degree of cognitive decline. *J. Clin. Exp. Neuropsychol.*, **18**: 883–891.
4. Carswell L.M., Graves R., Snow W., Tierney M. (1997)  Postdicting verbal IQ of elderly individuals. *J. Clin. Exp. Neuropsychol.*, **19**: 914–921.

3.3
## Neuropsychological and Instrumental Diagnosis of Dementia: the Evidence
Philip Scheltens[1]

Ove Almkvist describes in his review typical neuropsychological and instrumental findings in several dementia syndromes. He concludes that there is some consistent evidence pointing to the specificity of these characteristics for the disease and the degree of dementia severity. Inconsistencies remain, mainly concerning the premorbid abilities of the patient and the lack of sufficient knowledge of the normal ageing process. However, how is the "evidence" given by the author defined?

When reviewing studies for "evidence" (or lack thereof), often used criteria are: (a) Were there appropriate comparison groups, at least one of which was free of the target disorder? (b) Was there an independent and blind comparison with an appropriate reference ("gold") standard? (c) Was the spectrum of patients and controls clearly described, so that generalizability of results to clinical practice can be assessed? (d) Were data provided to enable calculation of sensitivity, specificity and likelihood ratios (LR)?

Following these criteria, studies may then be subdivided according to the presence of class I evidence (prospective) vs. class II (retrospective), and as Ia or IIa (broad spectrum of patients and controls) vs. Ib or IIb (narrow spectrum of patients and controls). A prospective design decreases the likelihood of work-up bias (i.e. where the decision to perform the reference standard is influenced by the test result).

Recently, Tierney [1] reviewed the existing literature on neuropsychological measurements for diagnosing dementia, using these criteria for guidance. She found only two studies meeting Ia criteria [2,3] and six meeting Ib

[1] *Department of Neurology, Research Institute of Neurosciences, Vrije Universiteit, Amsterdam, The Netherlands*

criteria [4–9]. The study of Incalzi *et al* [2] was cross-sectional and prospective and included a broad range of elderly patients who were admitted to the same hospital in Italy for minor surgery (two control samples) or to the Neurology or Geriatrics wards (dementia sample). All participants were screened to determine whether they met DSM-III-R criteria for dementia. The dementia sample was further screened to select those who met the National Institute of Neurological and Communicative Disorders–Alzheimer's Disease and Related Disorders Association (NINCDS–ADRDA) criteria for Alzheimer's disease (AD). The investigators excluded very impaired patients, thereby including only patients with mild to moderate levels of the disease. The neuropsychological tests that accounted for discrimination among groups were five subtests of the Rey Auditory Verbal Learning Test (RAVLT) (forgetting, immediate and delayed recall, false positive recognition, and middle of the list serial position effect) and the Wechsler Adult Intelligence Scale—Revised (WAIS-R) Digit Span backwards. The sensitivity for AD was 81%, with a specificity of 90% (likelihood ratio 8.3). The study of Tierney *et al* [3] was prospective and longitudinal and conducted among patients referred because of concern about their memory loss. All subjects were screened to ensure they did not meet DSM-III-R criteria for dementia upon entry to study. Eligible subjects were first administered a battery of neuropsychological tests and then followed for 2 years. After 2 years, all subjects were given another diagnostic work-up for dementia (DSM-III-R) and AD (NINCDS–ADRDA). Logistic regression analyses revealed that two of the tests administered at baseline, RAVLT delayed recall and the Mental Control subtest of the Wechsler Memory Scale (WMS), showed classification accuracy as robust as the larger battery of tests. The likelihood ratio was 11.86, representing a large shift from pre- to post-test probability. The likelihood ratios in the Ib studies ranged from 2 to 12 depending on the test used.

The great majority of studies in this field lack the presence of people who are representative of the spectrum of patients who are seen in clinical practice. Normal high-functioning individuals, who comprised the comparison groups in most of the studies reviewed by Almkvist, are unlikely to be part of the spectrum of participants to whom the diagnostic tests will be applied in the clinical setting. Also, comparisons between normal controls and dementia cases are likely to produce much bigger differences than comparisons with non-demented people who may have cognitive, affective or medical problems.

Future studies should be designed to include a set of potentially useful tests in a single study. Examining the accuracy of only one test provides limited information, whereas inclusion of many potentially useful tests in a multivariate regression model allows for the examination of the combined effect of all the tests, as well as the individual contribution of each test. This information allows for the development of the shortest test battery with the highest accuracy rate in diagnosing AD and separating it from other dementias.

## REFERENCES

1. Tierney M. (in press) Mental status exam and neuropsychological test. In *Evidence Based Dementia* (Eds N. Qizilbash, L. Schneider, H. Chui, H. Brodaty, J. Kaye, T. Erkinjuntti), Blackwell Science, Oxford.
2. Incalzi R.A., Capparella O., Gemma A., Marra C., Carbonin P. (1995) Effects of aging and of Alzheimer's disease on verbal memory. *J. Clin. Exper. Neuropsychol.*, **17**: 580–589.
3. Tierney M.C., Szalai J.P., Snow W.G., Fisher R.H., Nores A., Nadon G., Dunn E., St. George-Hyslop P.H. (1996) Prediction of probable Alzheimer's disease in memory-impaired patients: a prospective longitudinal study. *Neurology*, **46**: 661–665.
4. Buschke H., Kuslansky G., Katz M., Stewart W., Sliwinski M., Lipton R. (1999) Screening for dementia with the Memory Impairment Screen. *Neurology*, **52**: 231–238.
5. Grut M., Fratiglioni L., Viitanen M., Winblad B. (1993) Accuracy of the Mini-Mental Status Examination as a screening test for dementia in a Swedish elderly population. *Acta Neurol. Scand.*, **87**: 312–317.
6. Heun P., Jennssen F. (1998) The validity of psychometric instruments for detection of dementia in the elderly population. *Int. J. Geriatr. Psychiatry*, **13**: 368–380.
7. Ritchie K., Fuhrer R. (1992) A comparative study of the performance of screening tests for senile dementia using receiver operating characteristics analysis. *J. Clin. Epidemiol.* **45**: 627–637.
8. Welsh K., Butters N., Hughes J., Mohs R., Heyman A. (1991) Detection of abnormal memory decline in mild cases of Alzheimer's disease using CERAD neuropsychological measures. *Arch. Neurol.*, **48**: 278–281.
9. Welsh K., Butters N., Hughes J., Mohs R., Heyman A. (1992) Detection and staging of dementia in Alzheimer's disease: use of the neuropsychological measures developed for the Consortium to Establish a Registry for Alzheimer's disease. *Arch. Neurol.*, **49**: 448–452.

3.4
## Some Clinical Aspects and Research Issues in the Neuropsychological Assessment of Dementia

Andreas U. Monsch[1]

Within neuropsychology, the assessment of dementia is probably one of the most interesting, fascinating and challenging endeavours. Health care sys-

[1] *Memory Clinic, Geriatric University Hospital, Kantonsspital, Hebelstrasse 10, 4031 Basel, Switzerland*

tems are required to accurately and efficiently diagnose patients suffering from dementia. This is especially important, since some drug treatment is now available and family members need to be assisted in and prepared for what is ahead of them. It seems obvious that the earlier the diagnosis can be made, the better the health care system is able to react and provide appropriate help.

The multidimensional assessment of dementia in general and of Alzheimer's disease (AD) in particular requires well trained personnel and an assessment procedure that will work accurately, efficiently and quickly. However, which neuropsychological instrument should be utilized for the neuropsychological assessment of dementia? What are the objectives that need to be met in everyday clinical practice? When one examines the available tools and common procedures, the situation seems rather problematic. Often results are judged solely from a clinical point of view; some normative data are available but are often far from really being useful for everyday clinical practice. The Mini-Mental State Examination (MMSE [1]) may serve as an example: the advantage is that this tool is probably the most widespread dementia instrument and therefore serves as a common language among clinicians and researchers. On the other hand, neuropsychological research has enabled us to diagnose patients in much earlier stages. The MMSE's cut-off score needs to be adjusted and the instrument may continue to serve as a staging instrument.

In Switzerland we have set forward an easy system for identifying and diagnosing patients in their earliest stages [2]. With respect to neuropsychology, the family physician first performs a screening procedure (first step), utilizing a combination of the Clock Drawing Test and the MMSE [3]. If a suspicion of dementia arises, the patient is referred to one of the 12 Memory Clinics currently in operation in Switzerland. The second step includes the quantitative and qualitative neuropsychological assessment of the patient's cognitive functions, which has the following objectives: (a) to aid in diagnosing patients at the earliest stage of dementia; (b) to contribute to the differential diagnostic process; (c) to document disease progression and therapy outcomes; (d) to identify relatively intact areas of cognition to serve as a basis for therapy. A specific challenge within this second step is the appropriate neuropsychological examination that will allow for a common language, quite similar to that achieved with the MMSE. In a collaborative effort, the German-speaking Memory Clinics in Europe decided to utilize the German translation of the Consortium to Establish a Registry for Alzheimer's Disease–Neuropsychological Assessment Battery (CERAD–NAB) [4] as a minimal common assessment tool. The CERAD–NAB consists of "verbal fluency, animals"; "Boston Naming Test, 15 items"; MMSE; "word list learning"; "constructional praxis"; "word list delayed recall"; "word list recognition"; and recall of items presented in constructional praxis (i.e. "visual memory") [5,6]. Based on the results, which have to be demographically adjusted, the neuropsychologist can then decide him- or herself which further testing is appropriate. The CERAD–NAB is a well-established and neuropathologically validated diagnostic battery [7], which offers clinicians and researchers a neuropsychological standard for diagnosing AD and other dementias. Furthermore, the data are internationally comparable and allow for the rapid evaluation of new treatment concepts, thus enhancing the pace of progress in treating the increasing number of older persons with neurodegenerative diseases. In Basel we have collected normative data for the German CERAD–NAB on 617 healthy elderly individuals. This assessment instrument, as well as a program to obtain gender-, age- and education-adjusted standard scores, is now available for professionals on the Internet (www.healthandage.com).

Another problematic situation can be found when results of neuropsychological assessments are to be correlated to neuropathology findings: the time points are often years apart. For this purpose, a series of instruments were developed that can be used even in severe dementia and therefore in close temporal proximity to death.

The identification of relative strengths and weaknesses of advanced dementia patients in specific areas of cognition could help to: (a) reveal aetiology-specific cognitive patterns of impairment, which allow determination of strategies to enhance communication and interactions with patients, and therefore improve the care of institutionalized individuals; and (b) produce detailed neuropsychological profiles in close temporal proximity to death. However, no German instrument is presently available to assess patients in advanced stages of dementia. We translated (culturally and literally) two American assessment instruments (Severe Cognitive Impairment Profile, SCIP [8]; and Severe Impairment Battery, SIB [9]) into German and examined 57 severely demented patients (42 females, 15 males; age $= 83 \pm 9$ years; MMSE $= 5.7 \pm 5.3$) (inclusion criterion: MMSE $\leqslant$ 15) with both instruments. The results revealed high inter-rater reliability (0.992–1.0) in both instruments. Thirteen of 14 patients with an MMSE score of zero still obtained measurable scores on the SCIP, and 10/14 obtained a score on the SIB. Therefore, both instruments showed that the floor-effect commonly encountered in these patients using the MMSE could be avoided.

# REFERENCES

1.  Folstein M.F., Folstein S.E., McHugh P.R. (1975) "Mini Mental State"—a practical method for grading the cognitive state of patients for the clinician. *J. Psychiatr. Res.*, **12**: 189–198.

2. Stähelin H.B., Monsch A.U., Spiegel R. (1997)   Early diagnosis of dementia via a two-step screening and diagnostic procedure. *Int. Psychogeriatrics*, **9** (Suppl. 1): 123–130.
3. Thalmann B., Spiegel R., Stähelin H.B., Ermini-Fünfschilling D., Bläsi S., Monsch A.U.   Dementia screening in general practice: combining the Mini-Mental Status Examination and the Clock Drawing Test (submitted for publication).
4. Morris J.C., Heyman A., Mohs R.C., Hughes J.P., van Belle G., Fillenbaum G., Mellits E.D., Clark C. and CERAD investigators (1989)   The Consortium to Establish a Registry for Alzheimer's Disease (CERAD). Part I. Clinical and neuropsychological assessment of Alzheimer's disease. *Neurology*, **39**: 1159–1165.
5. Welsh K., Butters N., Hughes J., Mohs R., Heyman A. (1991)   Detection of abnormal memory decline in mild cases of Alzheimer's disease using CERAD neuropsychological measures. *Arch. Neurol.*, **48**: 278–281.
6. Welsh K.A., Butters N., Mohs R.C., Beekly D., Edland S., Fillenbaum G., Heyman A. (1994)   The Consortium to Establish a Registry for Alzheimer's Disease (CERAD). Part V. A normative study of the neuropsychological battery. *Neurology*, **44**: 609–614.
7. Mirra S.S., Heyman A., McKeel D., Sumi S.M., Crain B.J., Brownlee L.M., Vogel F.S., Hughes J.P., van Belle G., Berg L. and CERAD investigators (1991)   The Consortium to Establish a Registry for Alzheimer's Disease (CERAD). Part II. Standardization of the neuropathologic assessment of Alzheimer's disease. *Neurology*, **41**: 479–486.
8. Peavy G.M., Salmon D.P., Rice V.A., Galasko D., Samuel W., Taylor K.I., Ernesto C., Butters N., Thal L. (1996)   Neuropsychological assessment of severely demented elderly: the severe cognitive impairment profile. *Arch. Neurol.*, **53**: 367–372.
9. Saxton J., McGonigle K.L., Swihart A.A., Boller F. (1993)   *The Severe Impairment Battery*, Thames Valley Test Company, Bury St. Edmunds.

3.5
# The Role of Cognitive and Functional Evaluation in the Care of Patients with Dementia

Richard C. Mohs[1]

By definition, all patients with dementia have both cognitive and functional impairment. Assessment in both domains is a key component of any dementia evaluation, and Prof. Almkvist has provided an excellent overview of the current state of the art in this area. The review highlights several issues of great importance for understanding the use of these assessments, both in clinical practice and in research designed to elucidate pathophysiologic mechanisms of disease. This discussion will amplify Prof. Almkvist's review in three areas: strengths and limitations of neuropsychological

[1] *Department of Psychiatry, Mount Sinai School of Medicine, VA Medical Center, 130 West Kingsbridge Road, Bronx, NY 10468, USA*

tests in differential diagnosis, the importance of longitudinal data in neuro-degenerative disease, and the relationship of clinical change to pathophysiology.

*Strengths and limitations of neuropsychological tests.* There is ample evidence that many elderly persons with dementia remain undiagnosed and untreated. Community-based epidemiologic studies [1] indicate that a very high proportion of all elderly persons living at home meet currently accepted criteria for dementia, but many of them have never received that diagnosis and have never been treated. Clinic-based epidemiologic studies conducted in geriatric medicine practices [2] also find that a high proportion of patients meet criteria for dementia, but relatively few have received the diagnosis or been treated. Of the many factors contributing to this low recognition of the dementia syndrome, one that could be rectified fairly easily is the limited use of neuropsychological and functional screening instruments to identify patients who may have impairments. Recent clinical guidelines [3] have described how such screens can be incorporated into clinical practices that, because of the age of their patients, are likely to have many cases of dementia. Greater familiarity with and use of cognitive and functional assessment would improve the recognition and treatment of dementia patients in clinical practice.

Scores on cognitive and functional tests must always be viewed in light of other clinical data, and Prof. Almkvist describes very clearly some of the factors that must be taken into account in interpreting test scores. Premorbid capacity varies widely, and the same score on a cognitive test may mean different things, depending upon the patient's background, previous level of functioning and current medical condition. Norms can help but, as Prof. Almkvist describes, they are limited by the characteristics of the population from which they were drawn.

Differentiating cases of dementia by etiology is even more difficult and fraught with ambiguity than is the identification of dementia. The tables provided in the review give useful information about the features clinicians should consider in differentiating among dementias, but hard data on diagnostic accuracy are generally lacking.

*Importance of longitudinal data.* Alzheimer's disease (AD) and the other dementias of aging are progressive, degenerative conditions leading ultimately to death. Measuring change is often as important as measuring absolute level of functioning. In addition to the clinical progression described in Prof. Almqvist's review, a number of studies have investigated the rate of change on semi-quantitative measures of cognitive and functional status administered over time to patients with AD. The Mini-Mental State Examination (MMSE) has been used in a number of longitudinal studies and, typically, AD patients' scores decline by about 2–3 points per year [4]. Extensive data are also available on the rate of change for patients tested over time with the Alzheimer's Disease Assessment Scale (ADAS) [5]. Of some interest is the fact that on both these and other measures the rate of decline is slower for patients with very mild disease than it is for patients with more advanced dementia [5]. The fact that cognitive change is very gradual at the onset of AD may contribute to the difficulty in identifying cognitive decline early in the course of disease.

Longitudinal studies of functional decline have also been published, and Almqvist describes the sequence in which patients with dementia typically lose the ability to perform basic and instrumental activities of daily living (ADLs). Because the ability to perform instrumental activities is impaired early in the course of dementia, there have been efforts recently to develop more sensitive and universally applicable inventories to assess instrumental ADL performance [6]. Decline in ADL performance over time is highly correlated with the loss of cognitive function [7], while the relationship of function to psychiatric symptoms such as psychosis and agitation is more modest [7].

*Relationship of clinical change to pathophysiology.*   One key to understanding the pathophysiology of AD is to determine which of the many patho-physiologic changes found in AD patients are closely related to changes in clinical state. Almqvist briefly describes some of the studies looking for correlations between cognitive and biologic measures. These relationships may be complex, however, since the pathologic events driving clinical change may vary with stage of disease. Autopsy studies indicate that the most pronounced difference between non-demented persons and those with very mild AD is an increase in neocortical plaques [8] and amyloid-β 1–42 [9]. An increase in tangles [10] and a loss of cholinergic markers [11] is more pronounced in comparisons of mild vs. moderate and moderate vs. severe AD. Simple correlations across the entire spectrum of dementia severity may not reveal these relationships that are specific to certain periods during disease progression. Additional analyses of the type described by Almkvist will further our understanding of these important relationships and will help guide the development and evaluation of new treatments.

# REFERENCES

1.   Evans D.A., Scherr P.A., Cook N.R., Albert M.S., Funkenstein H.H., Smith L.A., Hebert L.E., Wetle T.T., Branch L.G., Chown M. *et al* (1990)   Estimated prevalence of Alzheimer's disease in the United States. *Milbank Quarterly*, **68**: 267–289.

2. Callahan C.M., Hendrie H.C., Tierney W.M. (1995)   Documentation and evaluation of cognitive impairment in elderly primary care patients. *Ann. Intern.
   Med.*, **122**: 422–429.
3. Small G.W., Rabins P.V., Barry P.P., Buckholtz N.S., DeKosky S.T., Ferris S.H.,
   Finkel S.I., Gwyther L.P., Khachaturian Z.S., Lebowitz B.D. *et al* (1997)   Diagnosis and treatment of Alzheimer disease and related disorders. *JAMA*, **278**:
   1363–1371.
4. Morris J.C., Edland S., Clark C., Galasko D., Koss E., Mohs R., van Belle G.,
   Fillenbaum G., Heyman A. (1993)   The Consortium to Establish a Registry for
   Alzheimer's Disease (CERAD). Part IV. Rates of cognitive change in the longitudinal assessment of probable Alzheimer's disease. *Neurology*, **43**: 2457–2465.
5. Stern R.G., Mohs R.C., Davidson M., Schmeidler J., Silverman J.M., Kramer-
   Ginzberg E., Searcey T., Bierer L.M., Davis K.L. (1994)   A longitudinal study of
   Alzheimer's disease: measurement, rate and predictors of cognitive deterioration. *Am. J. Psychiatry*, **151**: 390–396.
6. Galasko D., Bennett D., Sano M., Ernesto C., Thomas R., Grundman M., Ferris
   S.H. (1997)   An inventory to assess activities of daily living for clinical trials in
   Alzheimer's disease. *Alz. Dis. Assoc. Disord.*, **11**: S33–S39.
7. Green C.R., Marin D.B., Mohs R.C., Schmeidler J., Aryan M., Fine E., Davis K.L.
   (1999)   The impact of behavioural impairment on functional ability in Alzheimer's disease. *Int. J. Geriatr. Psychiatry*, **14**: 307–316.
8. Haroutunian V., Perl D.P., Purohit D.P., Marin D.B., Khan K., Lantz M., Davis
   K.L., Mohs R.C. (1998)   Regional distribution of senile plaques in nondemented elderly and cases of very mild Alzheimer's disease. *Arch. Neurol.*, **55**: 1185–
   1191.
9. Naslund J., Haroutunian V., Mohs R., Davis K.L., Davies P., Greengard P.,
   Buxbaum J.D. (2000)   Elevated amyloid β-peptides in brain: correlation with
   cognitive decline. *JAMA*, **283**: 1571–1577.
10. Haroutunian V., Purohit D.P., Perl D.P., Marin D., Khan K., Lantz M., Davis
    K.L., Mohs R.C. (1999)   Neurofibrillary tangles in nondemented elderly and
    very mild Alzheimer's disease. *Arch. Neurol.*, **56**: 713–718.
11. Davis K.L., Mohs R.C., Marin D.B., Purohit D.P., Perl D.P., Lantz M., Austin G.,
    Haroutunian V. (1999)   Cholinergic markers are not decreased in early Alzhei-
    mer's disease. *JAMA*, **281**: 1401–1406.

**3.6**
# Evaluating the Cognitive Changes of Normal and Pathologic Aging
John C. Morris[1] and William P. Goldman[1]

Increasing interest in normal and pathologic aging has sharpened focus on
defining the cognitive changes of dementia compared to those associated
with non-demented aging. Prof. Almkvist discusses available methods for
detecting these changes in relation to the characteristics of three leading

[1] *Department of Neurology, Washington University School of Medicine, 660 S. Euclid Avenue,
Campus Box 8111 MAP, St. Louis, MO 63110, USA*

dementing disorders: Alzheimer's disease (AD), cerebrovascular dementia and frontotemporal dementia.

To detect the earliest symptoms of dementia, detailed and sensitive assessment measures are required. There are no proven biological markers for dementia. The diagnosis thus rests on clinical methods that evaluate cognitive impairment, the core feature of dementia. A critical aspect for diagnosis is that the impairment must represent decline from prior cognitive abilities. The assessment of cognitive status incorporates both clinical and neuropsychologic measures.

Although brief cognitive instruments such as the Mini-Mental State Examination (MMSE) [1] are popular and require little training to administer, they have limitations as diagnostic tools. One major difficulty with diagnosing dementia based on a "cut-off" score from a brief instrument is that the score obtained does not take into account change in performance from prior functioning. In addition, these instruments may have limited longitudinal use because of high measurement error and variation in annual scores [2] and may be confounded by effects of age, education, and ethnic status [3]. Another difficulty is that proposed cut-off scores are insensitive to early-stage dementia [4]. It is inaccurate to assume, for example, that a score of 24 on the MMSE defines the lower limit of normal cognitive status in well-educated and high-functioning individuals. One alternative to these problems associated with short instruments would be to use a battery of neuropsychologic tests. These more extensive tests, however, can also be subject to ceiling effects and confounded by effects of education [5] and ethnic status [6]. Furthermore, test norms may underestimate the mean because of contamination with preclinical dementia cases [7].

A solution to these problems is to use global clinical measures of functioning, such as the Clinical Dementia Rating (CDR, [8]) or the Global Deterioration Scale [9]. Global clinical scales consider change in abilities to conduct everyday activities with respect to prior performance. Thus, these scales have face validity and are less confounded than neuropsychologic tests by age, education and ethnic status. By having an observant and reliable informant report on the current and past functioning of a patient, the time course of the disease and its influence on functioning can be determined. The observations of informants may be sensitive to the initial stages of dementia, even when neuropsychologic test performance is unimpaired [10,11]. The CDR, for example, is an ordinal scale that uses a semistructured interview of both the patient and a collateral source to assess functioning in six domains: memory, orientation, judgment and problem solving, community affairs, home and hobby, and personal care. In contrast to tests measuring only cognitive abilities, the CDR globally assesses cognitive, behavioural, and functional performance.

In the last decade, tools for dementia diagnosis have become more sophisticated. There has been a corresponding revision of the operational definition of dementia to include more subtle levels of cognitive decline and a shift in perception of what is normal for an older adult. Although cross-sectional studies report cognitive decline with increasing age [12], recent longitudinal studies [13–15] have shown that this decline is limited or non-existent in truly healthy elders, such that stable cognitive performance is possible into the ninth decade of life [13]. Thus, even mild cognitive impairment may not represent a benign, non-progressive feature of normal aging, but rather the initial manifestation of AD or other dementing disorders. The combination of sensitive clinical assessment methods, combined with the neuropsychologic test measures described by Prof. Almkvist, will enable clinicians and investigators alike to further distinguish the earliest stages of dementia from cognitively healthy aging.

## REFERENCES

1. Folstein M.F., Folstein S.E., McHugh P.R. (1975) ''Mini-Mental state''. A practical method for grading the cognitive state of patients for the clinician. *J. Psychiatr. Res.*, **12**: 189–198.
2. Clark C.M., Sheppard L., Fillenbaum G.G., Galasko D., Morris J.C., Koss E., Mohs R., Heyman A. and CERAD Investigators (1999) Variability in annual Mini-Mental State Examination score in patients with probable Alzheimer disease: a clinical perspective of data from the Consortium to Establish a Registry for Alzheimer's Disease. *Arch. Neurol.*, **56**: 857–862.
3. Mungus D., Marshall S.C., Weldon M., Haan M., Reed B.R. (1996) Age and education correction of Mini-Mental State Examination for English- and Spanish-speaking elderly. *Neurology*, **46**: 700–706.
4. Butler S.M., Ashford J.W., Snowdon D.A. (1996) Age, education, and changes in the Mini-Mental State Exam scores of older women: findings from the Nun Study. *J. Am. Geriatr. Soc.*, **44**: 675–681.
5. Doraiswamy P.M., Krishen A., Stallone F., Martin W.L., Potts N.L., Metz A., DeVeaugh-Geiss J. (1995) Cognitive performance on the Alzheimer's Disease Assessment Scale: effect of education. *Neurology*, **45**: 1980–1984.
6. Manly J.J., Jacobs D.M., Sano M., Bell K., Merchant C.A., Small S.A., Stern Y. (1998) Cognitive test performance among non-demented elderly African Americans and whites. *Neurology*, **50**: 1238–1245.
7. Sliwinski M., Lipton R.B., Buschke H., Stewart W. (1996) The effects of preclinical dementia on estimates of normal cognitive functioning in aging. *J. Gerontol. B: Psychol. Sci. Soc. Sci.*, **51B**: P217–P225.
8. Morris J.C. (1993) The Clinical Dementia Rating (CDR): current version and scoring rules. *Neurology*, **43**: 2412–2414.
9. Reisberg B., Ferris S.H., de Leon M.J., Crook T. (1982) The Global Deterioration Scale for assessment of primary degenerative dementia. *Am. J. Psychiatry*, **139**: 1136–1139.
10. Morris J.C., McKeel D.W., Jr., Storandt M., Rubin E.H., Price J.L., Grant E.A., Ball M.J., Berg L. (1991) Very mild Alzheimer's disease: informant-based clinical,

psychometric, and pathologic distinction from normal aging. *Neurology*, **41**: 469–478.

11.  Morris J.C., Storandt M., McKeel D.W., Jr., Rubin E.H., Price J.L., Grant E.A., Berg L. (1996)   Cerebral amyloid deposition and diffuse plaques in "normal" aging: evidence for presymptomatic and very mild Alzheimer's disease. *Neurology*, **46**: 707–719.

12.  Craik F.I.M., Salthouse T.A. (Eds) (1992)   *The Handbook of Aging and Cognition*, Erlbaum, Hillsdale.

13.  Rubin E.H., Storandt M., Miller J.P., Kinscherf D.A., Grant E.A., Morris J.C., Berg L. (1998)   A prospective study of cognitive function and onset of dementia in cognitively healthy elders. *Arch. Neurol.*, **55**: 395–401.

14.  Unger J.M., van Belle G., Heyman A. (1999)   Cross-sectional versus longitudinal estimates of cognitive change in non-demented older people: a CERAD study. *J. Am. Geriatr. Soc.*, **47**: 559–563.

15.  Wilson R.S., Beckett L.A., Bennett D.A., Albert M.S., Evans D.A. (1999)   Change in cognitive function in older persons from a community population: relation to age and Alzheimer disease. *Arch. Neurol.*, **56**: 1274–1279.

3.7
# Alzheimer's Disease and Other Degenerative Dementias: Need for an Early Diagnosis

Ruediger Mielke and Wolf-Dieter Heiss[1]

Human aging is joined by various physical, social and cognitive-mnestic changes, which can considerably differ inter- and intra-individually. Cognitive-mnestic changes are caused by processes in the central nervous system, but they are also determined by genetic factors, education, profession, life style, intellectual and physical activity, and especially general physical condition. Reliable norms about cognitive and mnestic functions in elder people are usually lacking. Many tests just indicate norms for a group elder than 60 years. In gerontopsychological literature, sometimes an allocation in "young olds" (65–75 years), "old olds" (75–85 years) and "eldest olds" (> 85 years) is made, in order to take into account the heterogeneity of elder people. Furthermore, there are often problems in the design of neuropsychological studies. In the cross-sectional approach, age-dependent impairments are often overestimated, while in longitudinal studies they are underestimated. Since the neurons of the central nervous system lose their ability of replication, irreversible destructive processes are accumulating in the course of the years [1]. Not only shrinkage and loss of neurons, but also changes in the neuron's energy metabolism can restrict cell function. A reduction of density of synapses and dying back of axonal

---

[1]  *Max-Planck-Institut für Neurologische Forschung, Gleueler Strasse 50, D–50931 Köln, Germany*

branching, an increase of plaques and tangles and changes in the cholinergic and dopaminergic transmitter systems have been described. However, there is little experience in the age sensitivity of the approximately 50 different transmitter systems.

Cognitive-mnestic changes are described in the elderly [2]. Intelligence deficits can be ascertained in distinguishing between crystalline and fluid intelligence [3]. Components of crystalline intelligence can remain preserved or even increase until late age, while fluid intelligence decreases [4]. This means that older people act successfully in routine situations and that their knowledge and vocabulary remain stable. In contrast, there is successive loss in the processing speed of new information. This lack of flexible adaptation to new situations and problem-solving can become crucial. Often older people complain about memory deficits. The extent of mnestic problems largely depends on age, the material to learn, and the task to solve. Memory performances are hampered, more strongly in abstract material than in everyday familiar material. There are also problems in free recall, while memory performance in recognition tasks worsens later and to a small extent only. In attention task performance, processes in selective and divided attention are especially impaired. Verbal and communicative abilities pass for being relatively stable in age, but communication can be disturbed by sensory deficiencies like hearing deficits. A decline in abstraction ability and cognitive flexibility, as well as an increased susceptibility to interference, could be verified in elder people. Deceleration of reaction time in cognitive information processing is a universal phenomenon in older people, which is considered as one of the main causes in cognitive dysfunction. Reaction time in 60-year olds compared to 30-year olds is assumed to be reduced by about 20%. Except for some subtypes of vascular dementia, cognitive decline in dementia starts slowly and sneakily, and the boundary between normal cognitive decline in age and the beginning of dementia is very difficult to define. Therefore, in different classification schemes the diagnostic uncertainty is described by terms like "age-related cognitive decline", "mild neurocognitive disorder" or "age-associated memory impairment" (AAMI). The latter, however, must be regarded very critically. The criteria of the AAMI concept could not be used for clinical diagnosis and would be inappropriate to segregate selective memory deficits in the elderly [5]. Dementia can easily be diagnosed using the operational criteria given by DSM-IV or ICD-10. However, there is a considerable need for an early diagnosis in patients with Alzheimer's disease, vascular dementia or other degenerative dementias. Due to the uncertainty of the neuropsychological evaluation in the beginning disease, the use of biological markers appears appropriate. Impairment of cognitive abilities, the hallmark in different types of dementia, will induce a reduction of neuronal energy demand and thereby cause down-regulation of gene expression for oxidative phosphorylation within neuronal mitochondria [6]. As glucose is the major substrate for brain metabolism, cerebral metabolic rates for glucose (rCMRGl) can be used to image *in vivo* energy metabolism of the brain. In this connection, position emission tomography (PET) is currently the only technology affording three-dimensional quantitative measurement of rCMRGl [7]. Other selective markers offer the ability to have a look inside specific neurochemical systems, such as N-methyl-4-piperidyl-acetate (C11– MP4A) for measuring cortical acetylcholinesterase activity as marker of the cholinergic system. Thus, at present the shift to an early differential diagnosis of the beginning of dementia vs. normal aging seems possible by modern functional neuroimaging. At this stage, meticulous neuropsychological assessment plays the role of a complementary application.

## REFERENCES

1. McGeer E.F., McGeer P.L. (1997) Aging, neurodegenerative disease and the brain. *Can. J. Aging*, **16**: 218–236.
2. La Rue A. (1992) *Aging and Neuropsychological Assessment*, Plenum Press, New York.
3. Cattell R.B. (1963) Theory of fluid and crystallized intelligence: a critical experiment. *J. Educat. Psychiatry*, **54**: 1–22.
4. Schaie K.W. (1994) The course of adult intellectual development. *Am. Psychol.*, **49**: 304–313.
5. Rosen J.T. (1990) "Age-associated memory impairment": a critique. *Eur. J. Cogn. Psychol.*, **2**: 275–287.
6. Rapoport S.I., Hatanpää K., Brady D.R., Chandrasekaran K. (1996) Brain energy metabolism, cognitive function and down-regulated oxidative phosphorylation in Alzheimer's disease. *Neurodegeneration*, **5**: 473–476.
7. Mielke R., Heiss W.D. (1998) Positron emission tomography for diagnosis of Alzheimer's disease and vascular dementia. *J. Neural Transm.*, **53**: 237–250.

3.8
## Neuropsychological and Instrumental Diagnosis of Dementia in a Clinical Context
Gordon K. Wilcock [1]

Prof. Almkvist's review is an important summary of many of the significant aspects of making a diagnosis of dementia. Interestingly, however, the

[1] *Department of Care for the Elderly, Frenchay Hospital, Bristol BS16 1LE, UK*

concept of dementia associated with Lewy bodies appears to have been excluded from the three most common dementia syndromes. Although it is quite clear to all of us that Alzheimer's disease (AD) is probably the most common cause of dementia, and that vascular and frontotemporal dementias are important and relatively frequent, the Lewy body dementias are considered by some people to be the second most common cause of dementia, and by most people in the field as probably being in the top three. Although this condition is thought by some to be a variant of AD, this is not accepted by all, and specific diagnostic criteria are now available [1].

In my view, dementia associated with Lewy bodies—which also has a number of different names, e.g. senile dementia of Lewy body type (SDLT) when it occurs in the elderly, Lewy body dementia, and others—is sufficiently important to merit specific discussion, irrespective of whether one considers it a separate condition or a subgroup of AD. It does, of course, have features in common with AD, but the clinical picture is sufficiently distinct to be able to identify many sufferers in the early stages of their disease, e.g. because of the presence of extrapyramidal features, visual hallucinations that are well formed, and the marked fluctuation in the presentation of the symptoms. Memory difficulties may be much less pronounced in the early stages than one would expect from a person with AD, but other features, e.g. attention and concentration difficulties, may be more marked. There are good clinical reasons for trying to identify this entity when it occurs, e.g. the need to use phenothiazines and similar drugs with great caution, as such patients are very sensitive to them.

Prof. Almkvist presents an excellent and in-depth discussion of the nature and role of neuropsychological testing. The test batteries that he describes are in routine use in many specialist centres and, indeed, form the basis for establishing research cohorts in many centres of excellence. Whenever it is possible, a comprehensive neuropsychological approach of this nature will not only help to establish the presence of a dementia in someone in whom the signs may be minimal, but may also help to distinguish between different underlying types of dementia. We find this very helpful in our own day-to-day management, but I know that many of my colleagues in the UK, and elsewhere in Europe, do not have the facilities to routinely avail themselves of such a comprehensive assessment battery. For many people, something simpler, e.g. the Mini-Mental State Examination, as described by Prof. Almkvist, or a similar approach, may be all that can be managed.

There has always been great difficulty in trying to assess the severely demented patient adequately, and this is becoming more important as treatments start to become available. Assessing a person with severe dementia is usually not necessary in order to establish the presence of dementia itself, but is required to assist with the diagnosis of the underlying aetiology, and also to help determine whether treatment regimes are producing any benefit. As is mentioned in Almkvist's review, test batteries for severely impaired patients are now becoming available, and this information may be particularly important to many readers.

Assessing the activities of daily living (ADL) is an important part of evaluating a person with dementia, as it is in this area that many difficulties are caused for relatives, especially elderly spouses. Many of the existing ADL assessment protocols are adapted from scales developed for other purposes. There are now, however, a number of other more recent scales specifically designed for use with people with dementia, some of them involving considerable input from carers, and people with dementia themselves, in their design and in the evaluation of their validity and reliability [2].

Prof. Almkvist makes the very important point that follow-up data is extremely helpful when managing a person with dementia. Very often a diagnosis is made at one point in time, based upon the picture presented by the patient and his family on that occasion. We, and others, have found that longer-term follow-up refines the diagnosis, and eventually some 10% or so of people receive a diagnosis different to that which they were originally given.

Prof. Almkvist very helpfully points out that a number of different neuropsychological and clinical characteristics have been suggested to help differentiate between different dementias, and also to distinguish dementia from the pseudo-dementia associated with depression. It is important not to forget that different causes of dementia may coexist, and that many people with early dementia may also have a coincidental depressive illness. The latter can be quite difficult to exclude, and often one has to resort to a trial of antidepressant treatment before being confident that there is not a depressive aspect to the patient's presentation. Vascular dementia used to be thought to result from multiple cerebral infarcts, but we now know that this is not the most common type of vascular pathology and, as Prof. Almkvist points out, there are a number of different types of vascular impairment contributing to dementia. The background has been well reviewed [3], and there are now specific assessment batteries designed to help diagnose the likely presence of vascular dementia, in an attempt to try to improve upon the Hachinski Ischaemia Scale.

The frontotemporal dementias are increasingly being recognized in most centres, and accepted as an important cause of dementia morbidity. Almkvist's review includes a very helpful account of the neuropsychological and instrumental characteristics of this type of dementia, which is a most useful starting point for readers who wish to improve their knowledge of this condition.

# REFERENCES

1. McKeith I., Galasko L.G., Kosaka K., Perry E.K., Dickson D.W., Hansen L.A., Salmon D.P., Lowe J., Mirra S.S., Byrne E.J. *et al* (1996)   Consensus guidelines for the clinical and pathologic diagnosis of dementia with Lewy bodies (DLB): report of the Consortium on DLB International Workshop. *Neurology*, **47**: 1113–1124.
2. Bucks R.S., Ashworth D.A., Wilcock G.K., Siegfried K.S. (1996)   Assessment of activities of daily living in dementia: development of the Bristol activities of daily living scale. *Age Ageing*, **25**: 113–120.
3. Amar K., Wilcock G.K. (1996)   Vascular dementia—fortnightly review. *Br. Med. J.*, **312**: 227–231.

3.9

# Neuropsychological Tests that are Helpful to the Etiological Diagnosis of Dementia

Florence Pasquier[1]

Neuropsychology contributes greatly to the diagnosis of dementia: it documents significant cognitive decline and reveals patterns of cognitive dysfunction that suggest the cause of the dementia [1]. That is why Almkvist's review is so important. Together with the medical history given by the patient and more importantly by a close informant, the somatic and psychiatric assessment, and with imaging, neuropsychological assessment is much more contributory than laboratory analyses or electroencephalogram. It is true that one problem is to infer a cognitive decline in a patient from a current performance when no premorbid functioning assessment has been performed. Follow-up is very important for confirming an ongoing decline. As pointed out in Almkvist's review, the observation of patient's behaviour is absolutely crucial: quality of answers is as important as the quantitative score.

Many tests may be used and the information they give depends on the experience of the examiner. Some tests, however, are of most interest because their design allows one to see which cognitive processes are spared and which are impaired. The choice made by Ove Almkvist is respectable, although other tests are also helpful in clinical practice.

As mentioned by Almkvist, the Weschler Adult Intelligence Scale was not designed for assessing dementia. It may document a cognitive decline, but will not establish a cognitive profile contributing to the diagnosis of the

[1] *Department of Neurology, Memory Clinic, University Hospital, 59037 Lille, France*

cause of dementia. Moreover, it is time consuming. One of the most useful instruments is the Mattis Dementia Rating Scale [2]. This test was designed as a screening instrument to detect the presence of brain pathology in impaired geriatric patients. It evaluates a broad array of cognitive functions. It is sensitive to frontal and subcortical dysfunctions. High test–retest reliability is reported by the authors, and normative data are published [3].

Memory is still a core feature of dementia and, for diagnosing the cause of dementia, it is important to distinguish between failures of (a) storage (or retention), associated with damage to limbic and especially hippocampal structures; (b) retrieval, associated with frontal-subcortical dysfunctions; and (c) episodic memory, associated with temporoparietal lesions. In our experience, the Free and Cued Selective Reminding test [4] is the best instrument for assessing memory disorders in early dementia. Performance on the test (immediate recall, free and cued recall, learning slope, recognition, delayed free and cued recall) provides a characterization of the memory impairment, which distinguishes Alzheimer's disease (AD) from subcortical dementia [5] and from frontotemporal dementia [6].

It is worth mentioning the clock face test, in which the patient is asked to draw a clock face and put the hands to indicate a certain time. This is a visuoconstructive test that has been shown to be particularly impaired in dementia with Lewy bodies (DLB), the second commonest cause of degenerative dementia, with or without Alzheimer pathology. In this test, improved performance is not noted in the "copy" compared to "draw" part of the test in DLB, in contrast to what is observed in AD, Parkinson's disease and in normal controls [7]. The test may be useful in the clinical setting to differentiate DLB and AD.

The Alzheimer's Disease Assessment Scale (ADAS–Cog) purpose was to assess patients longitudinally. This scale is not sensitive to change in very early or mild case of dementia (ceiling effect). It is not the best battery for diagnosis, but its many parallel forms avoid the test–retest effect, and it has become the standard instrument for demonstrating cognitive improvement in short-term efficacy AD drug trials, since it was used for the approval of tacrine.

The verbal fluency test assesses not only language but also semantic memory, especially the category fluency test. It is very sensitive to dementia, even at early stage, but not specific to any cause of dementia.

The upper limit of the Mini-Mental State Examination (MMSE) range for mild dementia tends to be higher and higher. At present, the indication for cholinesterase inhibitors in AD is mild and moderate dementia with MMSE score between 10 and 26.

In my opinion, the main differential diagnosis with AD is not depression, following the DSM-IV criteria, but other degenerative and vascular dementias. Depression may superficially be a differential diagnosis in some types of frontotemporal degeneration, although the affect is blank or flat in fron-totemporal dementia and not steadily sad.

In vascular dementia (VD), the Hachinski ischaemic score is good at seeing a participation of cerebrovascular disease, but is not a diagnostic criterion. It may also be high in AD with cerebrovascular pathology. A difficulty to distinguish VD from AD in certain studies is that the two conditions may be associated.

Finally, one must keep in mind that there may be overlap between two or more pathologies, and that follow-up of patients is necessary to improve diagnosis accuracy.

## REFERENCES

1. Pasquier F. (1999) Early diagnosis of dementia: neuropsychology. *J. Neurol.*, **246**: 6–15.
2. Mattis S. (1976) Mental status examination for organic mental syndrome in the elderly patients. In *Geriatric Psychiatry: a Handbook for Psychiatrists and Primary Care Physicians* (Eds L. Bellak, T.B. Karasu), pp. 77–121, Grune & Stratton, New York.
3. Schmidt R., Freidl W., Fazekas F., Reinhart B., Grieshofer P., Koch M., Eber P., Schumacher M., Polmin L., Lechner H. (1994) Mattis dementia rating scale: normative data from 1001 healthy volunteers. *Neurology*, **44**: 964–966.
4. Grober E., Buschke H. (1987) Genuine memory deficits in dementia. *Dev. Neuropsychol.*, **3**: 13–36.
5. Pillon B., Deweer B., Agid Y., Dubois B. (1993) Explicit memory in Alzheimer's, Huntington's, and Parkinson's disease. *Arch. Neurol.*, **50**: 374–379.
6. Pasquier F. (1996) Neuropsychological features and cognitive assessment in frontotemporal dementia. In *Frontotemporal Dementia* (Eds F. Pasquier, F. Lebert, P. Scheltens), pp. 49–69, ICG, Dordrecht.
7. Gnanalingham K.K., Byrne E.J., Thornton A., Sambrook M.A., Bannister P. (1997) Motor and cognitive function in Lewy body dementia: comparison with Alzheimer's and Parkinson's diseases. *J. Neurol. Neurosurg. Psychiatry*, **62**: 243–252.

3.10
## The Importance of an Early Diagnosis in Alzheimer's Disease
Agneta Nordberg[1]

Alzheimer's disease (AD) is characterized in many cases by a pre-sympto-matic period with ongoing dysfunctional brain processes for many years

[1] *Department of Clinical Neuroscience, Occupational Therapy and Elderly Care Research, Division of Molecular Neuropharmacology, Karolinska Institutet, Stockholm, Sweden*

before clinical symptoms appear. Disturbances in episodic memory appear to be an early neuropsychological sign for the disease, corresponding to a decreased activation of hippocampus and increased activation of left prefrontal cortex and left cerebellum, compared to age-matched healthy subjects, in brain activation studies performed by positron emission tomography (PET) [1].

Rapid progress has recently been made concerning understanding of the epidemiology, genetics, risk factors and neuropathophysiological processes underlying the development of AD. Some therapeutic agents have been introduced into clinical praxis which appear to have, in at least some patients, symptomatic effects and can even slow down the progression of the disease. It is plausible to assume that drugs to prevent or delay the onset and/or course of the disease will be soon available. The present conservative approach to AD requires that the patient fulfils the criteria of dementia, e.g. that the symptoms influence everyday activities and function. The clinical symptoms are thus quite evident when the diagnosis is given. Early treatment will prompt the need for early diagnosis of AD. Identification of early cognitive impairments will probably involve a population of subjects who are at increased risk. Identification of early changes is presumably best obtained at a pre-symptomatic stage. Early pre-symptomatic metabolism disturbances have been found by longitudinal studies of AD families with chromosomal aberrations [2,3]. Since the other common dementia disorders, such as frontotemporal and vascular dementia, involve other clinical characteristics, they often can be distinguished from the early forms of AD, for instance, frontotemporal dementia patients seldom show early disturbances in memory function.

Sensitive biological markers must be a prerequisite for the diagnosis of early forms of dementia disorders. Several candidates are presently evaluated, including genetic, neuroimaging (structural and functional imaging) and cerebrospinal fluid (CSF) markers (A$\beta$, tau). The increased knowledge about the genetic factors involved in AD has provided important information about the aetiology of the disease. The dominant mutations in the amyloid precursor protein (APP) gene and in the homologous presenilin 1 and 2 genes are, however, estimated to contribute to less than 20% of the prevalence of AD in the general population. Although the presence of the susceptibility gene apolipoprotein E (APOE) $\epsilon$4 allele leads to an increased risk of AD, its clinical use is limited. Functional imaging allows quantification of cerebral blood flow, glucose metabolism and neurotransmitter activities in demented patients. The technique enables pre-symptomatic detection of deficits in brain function, as well as differential diagnosis. Cognitive intact APOE $\epsilon$4 homozygotes have shown early reduction in their cortical glucose metabolism [4,5], although the presence of the APOE $\epsilon$4 allele in AD patients is not associated with specific alterations in glucose metabolism [6]. Longitudinal studies of a family carrying the Swedish APP 670/671 mutation also showed reduced glucose metabolism in the temporal lobe prior to impairment of neuropsychological tests and volume changes of the temporal lobes [3]. A reduced hippocampal volume has been reported in subjects at risk of autosomal dominant familiar AD [7]. Neocortical abnormalities in glucose metabolism have been reported to precede neuropsychological impairments in attention, abstract reasoning, visual-spatial function [8]. Left and right cerebral metabolic rate of glucose, expressed as metabolic ratios, gave an 85% diagnostic accuracy, which was improved to 91% when combined with quantitative electroencephalogram [9]. The present limitation of routine single photon emission tomography (SPECT) is that the methods do not provide quantitative measures and the resolution is not as high as PET. Improvement of suitable clinical methods will certainly make functional imaging an important and useful early diagnostic tool. Among the CSF markers, increased tau values have been measured in CSF of AD patients, but increased tau levels are also found in other forms of dementia and neurological disorders [10,11]. Decreased levels of CSF Aβ1–42 are mainly found in patients with AD [12]. Combined analysis of tau and Aβ1–42 in CSF might be a useful tool in the future to identify early cases of Alzheimer's disease [12].

Subjects with mild cognitive impairment (MCI) show cognitive deficits without functional impairments that satisfy criteria for probable AD. The rate of conversion to AD among this group of MCI patients has been estimated to be approximately 12% during a follow-up period of 4 years [13]. In a recent study of MCI subjects undergoing repeated PET investigations over 2 years, we observed that 26% of the patients converted to AD and that the deficits in glucose metabolism predicted clinical outcome in 93% of the cases [14]. Together with functional imaging, the use of CSF tau and Aβ as predictors of AD among MCI patients is promising [15]. The risk of deterioration is higher in MCI patients with severe initial metabolic impairment [16]. MCI patients will be in the future an important group of individuals to assess and treat with neuroprotective and disease-modifying drugs.

# REFERENCES

1. Bäckman L., Andersson J.L.R., Nyberg L., Winblad B., Nordberg A., Almkvist O. (1999) Brain regions associated with episodic retrieval in normal aging and Alzheimer's disease. *Neurology*, **52**: 1861–1870.
2. Kennedy A.M., Frackowiak R.S.J., Newman S.K., Bloomfield P.M., Seaward J., Roques P., Lewington G., Cunningham V.J., Rossor M.N. (1994) Deficits in cerebral glucose metabolism demonstrated by positron emission tomography in individuals at risk of familial Alzheimer's disease. *Neurosci. Lett.*, **186**: 17–20.

3. Wahlund L.O., Basun H., Almkvist O., Juhlin P., Axelman K., Shigeta M., Jelic V., Nordberg A., Lannfelt L. (1999) A follow-up study of the family with the Swedish APP 670/671 Alzheimer's disease mutation. *Dement. Geriatr. Cogn. Disord.*, **10**: 526–533.
4. Small G.W., Mazziotta J.C., Collins M.T., Baxter L.R., Phelps M.E., Mandelkern M.A., Kaplan A., Larue A., Adamson C.F., Chang L. *et al* (1995) Apolipoprotein-E type-4 allele and cerebral glucose metabolism in relation at risk for familial Alzheimer disease. *JAMA*, **273**: 942–947.
5. Reiman E.M., Caselli R.J., Yun L.S., Chen K., Bandy D., Minoshima S., Thibodeau S.N., Osborne D. (1996) Preclinical evidence of Alzheimer's disease in persons homozygous for the epsilon 4 allele for apolipoprotein E. *N. Engl. J. Med.*, **334**: 752–758.
6. Corder E.H., Jelic V., Basun H., Lannfelt L., Valind S., Winblad B., Nordberg A. (1997) No difference in cerebral glucose metabolism in Alzheimer patients with differing apolipoprotein E genotype. *Arch. Neurol.*, **54**: 273–277.
7. Fox N.C., Warrington E.K., Seiffer A.S., Agnew S.K., Rossor M.N. (1998) Presymptomatic cognitive deficits in individuals at risk of familial Alzheimer's disease. A longitudinal prospective study. *Brain*, **121**: 1631–1639.
8. Haxby J.V. Grady C.L., Koss E., Horwitz B., Heston L., Schapiro M., Friedland R.P., Rapoport S.I. (1990) Longitudinal study of cerebral metabolic asymmetries and associated neuropsychological patterns in early dementia of Alzheimer type. *Arch. Neurol.*, **47**: 753–760.
9. Jelic V., Wahlund L.O., Almkvist O., Johansson S.E., Shigeta M., Winblad B., Nordberg A. (1999) Diagnostic accuracies of quantitative EEG and PET in mild Alzheimer's disease. *Alzheimer Report*, **2**: 291–298.
10. Galasko D., Clark C., Chang L., Green R.C., Motter R., Seubert P. (1997) Assessment of CSF levels of tau protein in mildly demented patients with Alzheimer's disease. *Neurology*, **48**: 632–635.
11. Andreasen N., Minthon L., Clareberg A., Davidsson P., Gottfries J., Vanmechelen E., Vanderstichele H., Winblad B., Blennow K. (1999) Sensitivity, specificity, and stability of CSF tau in AD in a community-based patient sample. *Neurology*, **52**: 1488–1494.
12. Galasko D., Chang L., Motter R., Clark M., Kaye J., Knopman D., Thomas R., Kholodenki D., Schenk D., Lieberburg I. *et al* (1998) High cerebrospinal fluid tau and low amyloid β42 levels in the clinical diagnosis of Alzheimer disease and relation to apolipoprotein E genotype. *Arch. Neurol.*, **55**: 937–943.
13. Petersen R.C., Smith G.E., Waring S.C., Ivnik R.J., Tangalos E.G., Kokmen E. (1999) Mild cognitive impairment: clinical characterization and outcome. *Arch. Neurol.*, **56**: 303–308.
14. Jelic V., Nordberg A. (2000) Early diagnosis of Alzheimer's disease with positron emission tomography. *Alz. Dis. Assoc. Disord.*, **14** (Suppl. 1): S109–S113.
15. Andreasen N., Minthon L., Vanmechelen E., Vanderstichele H., Davidsson P., Winblad B., Blennow K. (1999) Cerebrospinal fluid tau and Aβ1–42 as predictors of development of Alzheimer's disease in patients with mild cognitive impairment. *Neurosci. Lett.*, **273**: 5–8.
16. Herlholz K., Nordberg A., Salmon E., Kellsler J., Mielke R., Halber M., Jelic V., Almkvist O., Collette F., Alberoni M. *et al* (1999) Impairment of neocortical metabolism predicts progression in Alzheimer's disease. *Dement. Geriatr. Cogn. Disord.*, **10**: 494–504.

3.11
### When Should We Use Which Diagnostic Tools?
Gabriela Stoppe[1]

Most patients with dementia are diagnosed and treated exclusively in primary care. Although there is a shared opinion that much can be managed successfully there, barriers contribute to the delivery of inadequate or untimely medical services in primary care settings [1]. As illustrated by the results of our German representative survey, there is a wide gap between expert recommendation and clinical practice in primary care [2,3].

In this situation, screening tools are of special importance and should combine easy application with high sensitivity and specificity and acceptance by the patient and caregiver [4]. As one well-known example, the Clock Drawing Test has been developed for this purpose and combines a memory task with a constructional one. Combined, for example, with the Mini-Mental State Examination (MMSE), the sensitivity for the diagnosis of dementia, especially Alzheimer's disease (AD), can be increased. The information provided by the caregiver is of special importance, too. It has been shown that informants give valid and sensitive information on incipient dementia, most probably because everyday companionship allows them to compare the individual pattern of deficits to the premorbid functioning of the person [4].

Another important issue concerning most instrumental and neuropsychological diagnostic tools is the diagnostic sensitivity in the old. Many of the neuropsychological tests still do not provide norm values up to the 80s or 90s. In addition, inter-individual variation increases with age, leading to greater overlap between demented patients and controls. Together with the common neurobiological finding that the amount of neuropathology must be larger in a younger patient of similar dementia severity, this allows the conclusion that a single point investigation, for example, of electroencephalogram or brain imaging, contributes less to the diagnosis in older than in younger patients (see, for example [5]).

This also holds true for white matter lesions on computed tomography (CT) and magnetic resonance imaging (MRI), which have been shown to increase in amount and frequency with age and vascular risk factors, especially arterial hypertension and smoking. Their presence does not automatically mean a vascular dementia or a mixed dementia [6]. With proton magnetic resonance spectroscopy it became possible to non-invasively monitor neuronal loss by a reduced concentration of $N$-acetyl-aspartate (NAA) and gliosis by an increase of myo-inositol. Contrary to (our) expectations, we

---

[1] *Department of Psychiatry, Georg-August-University, Von-Siebold-Strasse 5, 37075 Goettingen, Germany*

could not demonstrate such changes in the parietal grey and white matter of 32 patients with AD. We concluded that neuronal loss or shrinkage in AD does not go along with a reduction of neuronal density per volume unit [7].

The co-occurrence of symptoms of dementia and depression should not only induce the attempt to differentiate both syndromes. Depression is frequent in dementia. Late-onset depression, which has been known to have some special features for many years, seems to be a predictor of dementia in those cases when cognitive symptoms are part of the clinical picture [8,9]. Preliminary evidence from longitudinal studies reveals increasing conversion rates into dementia with longer follow-up.

When looking from the World Psychiatric Association (WPA) perspective, there is also a need for harmonization of common neuropsychological instruments which takes into account language and cultural variability. For example, a rural Greek person in the 80s has never heard of the "Lindbergh story" of the Cambridge Examination for Mental Disorders of the Elderly (CAMDEX), which an English senior will clearly remember. The European Harmonization Project of Instruments for Dementia (EURO–HARPID), as one initiative, is a right step in that direction and will allow cross-cultural comparisons [10].

## REFERENCES

1. Small G.W., Rabins P.V., Barry P.P., Buckoltz N.S., DeKosky S.T., Ferris S.H., Finkel S.I., Gwyther L.P., Khachaturian Z.S., Lebowitz B.D. *et al* (1997) Diagnosis and treatment of Alzheimer disease and related disorders. Consensus statement of the American Association for Geriatric Psychiatry, the Alzheimer's Association, and the American Geriatrics Society. *JAMA*, **278**: 1363–1371.
2. Stoppe G., Sandholzer H., Staedt J., Winter S., Kiefer J., Kochen M.M., Rüther E. (1994) Diagnosis of dementia in primary care: results of a representative survey in lower Saxony, Germany. *Eur. Arch. Psychiatry Clin. Neurosci.*, **244**: 278–283.
3. Stoppe G., Sandholzer H., Staedt J. Diagnostic evaluation of dementia in primary care: measurement of physicians' competence. Submitted for publication.
4. Brodaty H., Clarke H., Ganguli M. Grek A., Jorm A.F., Khachaturian Z., Scherr P. (1998) Screening for cognitive impairment in general practice: toward a consensus. *Alz. Dis. Assoc. Disord.*, **12**: 1–13.
5. Van Gool W.A., Walstra G.J.M., Teunisse S., van der Zant F.M., Weinstein H.C., van Royen E.A. (1995) Diagnosing Alzheimer's disease in elderly, mildly demented patients: the impact of routine single photon emission computed tomography. *J. Neurol.*, **242**: 401–405.
6. Stoppe G., Staedt J., Bruhn H. (1995) Fleckige Veränderungen der weissen Substanz im kranialen Computer- und Magnetresonanztomogramm: Bedeutung für die (Differential) diagnose der Demenz vom Alzheimer Typ und der vaskulären Demenz (Patchy white matter lesions in cranial computed and magnetic resonance tomography: significance for the (differential) diagnosis of Alzheimer's dementia and vascular dementia). *Fortschr. Neurol. Psychiatrie*, **63**: 425–440.

7. Bassuk S.S., Berkman L.F., Wypij D. (1998) Depressive symptomatology and incident cognitive decline in an elderly community sample. *Arch. Gen. Psychiatry*, **55**: 1073–1081.
8. Dufouil C., Fuhrer R., Dartigues J.F., Alpérovitch A. (1996) Longitudinal analysis of the association between depressive symptomatology and cognitive deterioration. *Am. J. Epidemiol.*, **144**: 634–641.
9. Stoppe G., Bruhn H., Pouwels P., Hänicke W., Frahm J. (2000) Alzheimer's disease: absolute quantification of cerebral metabolites *in vivo* using localized proton magnetic resonance spectroscopy. *Alz. Dis. Assoc. Disord.*, **14**: 112–119.
10. Verhey F.R.J., Jolles J., Houx P., vanLang N., Derix M.M.A., De Deyn P.P., Huppert F., Neri M., Pena-Casanova J., Ritchie K. *et al* (1998) European Harmonization Project of Instruments for Dementia (EURO-HARPID). *Neurobiol. Aging*, **19** (Suppl. 4): S252.

### 3.12
### Factors Affecting Diagnosis in Dementia
Andrés Heerlein[1]

In recent decades there has been a substantial increase in the prevalence of dementia across the world. The dementia syndrome affects 5–8% of individuals older than age 65, and prevalence doubles every 5 years, being 30–50% by age 85. This rising prevalence, the magnitude of the cognitive impairment and the extensive suffering for patients and family members make dementia one of the most important medical and social problems for the next century. Nonetheless, precise diagnosis and adequate treatment remain an unresolved medical issue. Despite the significant improvement in structural and functional neuroimaging technology, clinical diagnosis of dementia is still by exclusion. At present a definite etiological diagnosis can only be made on histopathological basis. Difficulties in the differential diagnosis with cognitive impairment in normal aging and with late-life depression is also a serious problem. The clinical distinction between different types of dementia and their association to specific neuropathological findings is still difficult. The proposal of new disorders, such as "vascular depression", introduces more complexity in diagnostic and etiological discussions.

Prof. Almkvist's comprehensive presentation of the neuropsychological and instrumental diagnosis of dementia shows us the central and extremely relevant role of an adequate assessment of cognitive impairment in this field. It also shows how the correlation of neuropsychological and neuroi-

[1] *Departamento de Psiquiatría, Facultad de Medicina, Universidad de Chile, Av. La Paz 1003, Santiago de Chile, Chile*

maging data can enhance our knowledge of normal and abnormal brain functioning.

Many authors agree that the identification of a clear difference between *premorbid* and *present* level of functioning and the consideration of the current cognitive state is sufficient for a reliable diagnosis. Nevertheless, several factors, such as affective state, health status, personality traits (neuroticism), anxiety, environment or culture, influence the results of cognitive tests. An example is the relationship between dementia and depression, one of the most important themes in clinical psychogeriatrics. Depression is the principal cause of pseudodementia, a very common and reversible cognitive impairment in older people. Ferran [1] found that depressive pseudodementia accounted for 18% of referrals to a presenile dementia service, but was missed by most referrers. Of patients presenting to memory clinics, 6–14% have been found to have a depressive component to their condition [2]. However, pseudodementia does not appear in ICD-10 or DSM-IV. Therefore, a reliable neuropsychological assessment of cognitive impairment should always include an accurate evaluation of the affective state as well as a report of an external informant. Furthermore, the identification of depression in older people is relevant, because this condition is very often reversible and has a high suicidal risk [3]. Despite a good general prognosis, depression in elderly people carries a high mortality and needs efficient treatment [4].

In the diagnosis of Alzheimer's disease (AD), the neuropsychological and instrumental assessment should consider the existence of clear cognitive differences between patients with early vs. late-onset dementia. Early-onset patients perform more poorly on measures of language, praxis and concentration, whereas late-onset patients perform more poorly on measures of memory and orientation [5].

At present, neuroimaging should be considered only as an adjunct to clinical diagnosis. Although some evidence from magnetic resonance imaging (MRI) studies shows that hippocampal atrophy may be a sensitive marker for AD, this atrophy is also present in normal aging and should not be considered as a diagnostic tool for AD [6]. Bergman [7] found the sensitivity for visually evaluated single photon emission tomography (SPECT) in AD to be only 29%, considering it as an inadequate test for the diagnosis of AD. Most psychiatrists agree that neuroimaging studies do not affect the subsequent management of the illness. Nevertheless, neuroimaging studies should be performed at least once in order to exclude depression or any remediable cause of cognitive impairment.

In recent years, there is a growing body of evidence linking cerebral degeneration, cerebrovascular disease and depression. Since Alexopoulos [8] proposed the "vascular depression" hypothesis, which states that vascular disease may predispose to, precipitate or perpetuate depression in older people, research has moved very fast in this field. Central to this hypothesis is an association between depression, strokes and white matter lesions. "Vascular depression" could share a common etiology with vascular dementia. However, most studies with MRI failed to demonstrate a causal relationship [9]. The inclusion of evoked potentials could be useful in the differentiation of cerebrovascular and depressive cognitive impairment [10].

In summary, the benefits of neuropsychological and instrumental diagnosis in dementia are clear. However, further studies, considering factors affecting the results of cognitive tests and the correlations between lesion location, specific depressive symptoms and deficits on neuropsychological tests, are needed.

# REFERENCES

1. Ferran J., Wilson K., Doran M., Ghadiali E., Johnson F., Cooper P., McCracken C. (1996) The early onset dementias: a study of clinical characteristics and service use. *Int. J. Geriatr. Psychiatry*, **11**: 863–870.
2. Almeida O.P., Hill K., Howard R., O'Brien J., Levy R. (1993) Demographic and clinical features of patients attending a memory clinic. *Int. J. Geriatr. Psychiatry*, **8**: 497–501.
3. Pearson J.L., Conwell Y., Lindesay J. (1997) Elderly suicide: a multinational view. *Aging Ment. Health*, **1**: 107–111.
4. Ballard C.G., Patel A., Solis M., Lowe K., Wilcock G. (1996) A one-year follow-up study of depression in dementia sufferers. *Br. J. Psychiatry*, **168**: 287–291.
5. Koss E., Edland S., Fillenbaum G. (1996) Clinical and neuropsychological differences between patients with earlier and later onset of Alzheimer's disease: a CERAD analysis, Part XII. *Neurology*, **46**: 136–141.
6. Laakso M.P., Partanen K., Riekkinnen P., Lehtovirta M., Helkala E.-L., Hallikainen M., Hanninen T., Vainio P., Soininen H. (1996) Hippocampal volumes in Alzheimer's disease, Parkinson's disease with and without dementia, and in vascular dementia: an MRI study. *Neurology*, **46**: 678–681.
7. Bergman H., Chertkow H., Wolfson C., Stern J., Rush C., Whitehead V., Dixon R. (1997) HM-PAO (CERETEC) SPECT brain scanning in the diagnosis of Alzheimer's disease. *J. Am. Geriatr. Soc.*, **45**: 15–20.
8. Alexopoulos G.S., Meyers B.S., Young R.C., Campbell S., Silberzweig D., Carlson M. (1997) "Vascular depression" hypothesis. *Arch. Gen. Psychiatry*, **54**: 915–922.
9. O'Brien J., Ames D., Schweitzer I. (1996) White matter changes in depression and Alzheimer's disease: a review of magnetic resonance imaging studies. *Int. J. Geriatr. Psychiatry*, **11**: 681–694.
10. Kalayam B. (1997) Evoked potentials in geriatric depression. *Int. J. Geriatr. Psychiatry*, **12**: 3–5.

# Pharmacological Treatment of Dementia: A Review

## Steven C. Samuels and Kenneth L. Davis

*Department of Psychiatry, Mount Sinai School of Medicine, Box 1230, One Gustave L. Levy Place, New York, NY 10029-6574, USA*

## INTRODUCTION

This paper reviews the current pharmacological choices available to clinicians treating patients with dementia. The focus is on the pharmacological treatment for Alzheimer's disease (AD). However, several other dementia subtypes are discussed, including vascular dementia (VD), dementia with Lewy bodies (DLB) and AIDS dementia. The scientific justification, mechanism of action, pharmacokinetic profile, effectiveness and safety issues for agents used to treat cognitive and non-cognitive symptoms of the various dementias are reviewed.

## PHARMACOTHERAPY FOR ALZHEIMER'S DISEASE (AD)

Clinical manifestations of AD include disturbance in the areas of memory and language, visual spatial problems and higher executive dysfunction. Non-cognitive behavioural manifestations may include changes in personality, deterioration in judgment, wandering, psychosis, mood disturbance, agitation or sleep–wake cycle abnormalities.

Pharmacological interventions in these areas are at various developmental stages. For example, cholinesterase inhibitors and the antioxidant vitamin E are the mainstays of therapy, while anti-inflammatory therapies and hormonal treatments are not the therapeutic standard of care. Pharmacotherapeutics for behavioural disturbances in demented patients are based in part on clinical trials and on treatment approaches for these conditions in non-demented patients.

*Dementia, Second Edition.* Edited by Mario Maj and Norman Sartorius.
© 2002 John Wiley & Sons Ltd..

## Food and Drug Administration (FDA)'s Requirements for Clinical Trials in AD

In the United States, the FDA has guidelines for AD therapeutics [1]. The clinical trials must be randomized, double-blind, parallel-group studies with placebo controls. Patients must fulfill established diagnostic criteria, such as those by the National Institute of Neurological and Communicative Disorders—Alzheimer's Disease and Related Disorders Association (NINCDS–ADRDA), for probable AD [2]. The trial must last at least 3 months and demonstrate superiority over placebo in the effect on memory by global clinical measures and psychometric testing. The instruments must detect a clinically meaningful change.

Behavioural, quality-of-life and functional ratings are often utilized. Commonly used primary measures include the cognitive subscale of the AD Assessment Scale (ADAS-cog) [3] and a measure of "clinical usefulness", such as the Clinician Interview Based Impression (CIBI) [4]. The Mini-Mental State Examination (MMSE) [5] is often a secondary measure of cognition. More recent studies have included ratings such as the Progressive Deterioration Scale (PDS) [6] to assess quality of life changes, and the Neuropsychiatric Inventory (NPI), to assess behavioural change [7]. Additional instruments for the assessment of activities of daily living (ADLs) include the Lawton and Brody measure of ADLs and instrumental activities of daily living (IADLs) [8], the Alzheimer's Disease Cooperative Study (ADCS) ADL measure [9] and the Disability Assessment in Dementia (DAD) [10]

### ADAS-cog

ADAS-cog is a rating of cognition, language, orientation and performance on simple tasks, word recall, word recognition, object and finger naming, following commands, constructional and ideational praxis. Possible scores range from 0 to 70; the higher score indicates greater impairment. The average 6-month change is 4 points on the ADAS for a patient with AD [11], but the rate of change is highly dependent on the severity of the condition.

### Clinical Impression Scales

Several tests have evolved that have been used in clinical trials to give a measure of clinical utility. Most allow a baseline interview with the patient and caregiver, but they differ in who provides ensuing information. For example, the CIBI [4] requires follow-up interviews to be with the patient only, while the Alzheimer's Disease Cooperative Study–Clinical Global Impression of Change (ADCS–CGIC) [12] and the Clinician Interview Based Impression of Change-plus (CIBIC-plus) [13] allow the patient and an informant to provide additional information at subsequent visits. The interview is a clinical rather than a structured one or a psychometric rating. The major domains that are discussed include performance of IADLs, psychopathology, behavioural disturbance and cognitive functioning. The developers of the ADCS–CGIC have reviewed the history of the clinical impression scales [14].

## MMSE

The MMSE is a rating of orientation, memory, concentration, language and praxis. The score is from 0 to 30, with errors resulting in a lower score. Age and education affect normative scores on the MMSE [15]. Ethnic minorities and patients with less than an eighth-grade education are at higher risk to be falsely classified as having cognitive impairment [16]. The MMSE does not reliably discriminate mild dementia (ceiling effect) or severe dementia (floor effect) [17,18].

## ADL Scales

Functional measures are a key component to provide a guidepost for response to AD treatments. The Lawton and Brody scale examines a patient's level of independence in performing ADLs and IADLs. Patients are rated on whether they are fully dependent, needing partial assistance or independent for each of the activities assessed. The ADCS ADL scale that has been validated in AD patients assesses ADLs through a large range of severity and will be used in several planned clinical trials [9]. The DAD, valid in community-dwelling AD patients, measures basic self-care and IADLs [10].

## Cholinesterase Inhibitors

Cholinergic function is decreased in AD. Neuropathological studies reveal a loss of cholinergic cortical neurons in the basal forebrain, and neurochemical investigations demonstrate decreased choline acetyltransferase (CAT), the enzyme necessary for synthesis of acetylcholine from choline and acetyl-CoA [19]. Clinical ratings of cognition (and density of amyloid plaques) have been correlated with low post-mortem measures of cholinergic function [20]. Additionally, in the healthy elderly, agents that decrease cholinergic tone (anticholinergics) have adverse effects on memory and concentration [21].

Precursor loading, post-synaptic stimulation and synaptic augmentation of acetylcholine may increase cholinergic tone. Only cholinesterase inhibitors have resulted in a clinically meaningful response for AD patients. Cholinesterase inhibitors block acetylcholinesterase and increase the availability of acetylcholine in the synaptic cleft. Early work with physostigmine showed promise in AD patients, but the main problem was inadequate duration of action [22]. Subsequent clinical trials with longer-acting cholinesterase inhibitors in a well-defined population of AD patients established the clinical utility of these agents. They are discussed in the following sections.

## Tacrine

Tacrine hydrochloride is a non-competitive inhibitor of butyrylcholinesterase and acetylcholinesterase. This agent was the first FDA approved drug for AD, but is not currently used because of its requirement for transaminase monitoring, potential for hepatic toxicity and q.i.d. dosing. The other cholinesterase inhibitors that are currently FDA approved have better risk-benefit ratios compared to tacrine. Perhaps tacrine's legacy will be that it is the agent that introduced the field to the concept that pharmacological interventions for AD could make a difference. For those who could tolerate the drug's side effects, tacrine offered some hope for patients and caregivers.

*Effects of genotype, gender and estrogen replacement therapy (ERT).* Analyses of the FDA approval trials revealed some intriguing findings in terms of the effect of apolipoprotein E (ApoE) genotype and gender on response to tacrine. Using intent-to-treat analysis, women with ApoE2–3 genotype had a larger effect size than ApoE4 genotype women. Men did not vary in response to tacrine based upon ApoE genotype [23]. In an open label trial of galanthamine or tacrine, AD patients demonstrated a differential response on the MMSE based on gender [24]. Men responded better than women at 3 months when controlling for age, baseline MMSE and ApoE4 status. This effect was no longer present at 12 months. Data from the same 30-week study revealed that women receiving estrogen replacement therapy (ERT) responded better on cognitive evaluation than women without ERT [25].

*Cost savings, delay in nursing home placement and decreased mortality.* Tacrine also demonstrated cost saving potential and this has been replicated with the other cholinesterase inhibitors [26–31]. In all of the cost saving studies, the largest potential for reducing expenditures comes from reduced time in nursing homes. Tacrine use may delay nursing home placement and decrease mortality [32]. Patients were followed for 2 years after completing the 30-week study (to determine if they had died or were in a nursing home). Patients received placebo or three ascending doses of tacrine in a placebo-controlled phase. In the open label phase of the study, all patients received medication. Patients who received >80 mg/day were less likely to be admitted to the nursing home. Patients who received >120 mg/day had a trend toward lower mortality. Although the study was not prospective and there was no control group, the dose response was intriguing. Although these results have not been replicated with tacrine, open label studies with donepezil, rivastigmine and galanthamine have suggested that the cholinesterase inhibitors may delay nursing home placement. Prospective trials are required to definitively answer this important question.

*Effect of stage of disease.*   There may be a differential response to cholinesterase inhibitors based upon AD severity. In one analysis of the 30-week tacrine trial [33], middle-stage patients, defined by MMSE score of 11–17, had a larger effect from tacrine (ADAS-cog change from baseline of 5 units) than patients with a MMSE score of 18–26 (ADAS-cog change from baseline of 2 units) [34]. Similar results were found in analysis of data from clinical trials with other cholinesterase inhibitors [35-37]. Given all the data from the cholinesterase inhibitor trials regarding expanded benefit to other dementia subtypes or more severe AD [37–43], it is expected that the indications for cholinesterase inhibitor therapy may broaden to include more severe AD, DLB and VD. These benefits appear to be a class effect rather than attributable to the purported differences in mechanism of action between these agents.

## Donepezil

Donepezil hydrochloride is a non-competitive reversible inhibitor of acetylcholinesterase to a much greater degree than butyrylcholinesterase. The agent has a long half-life, reportedly up to 104 hours in healthy adults over age 55 years, allowing for once-daily dosing [44]. When donepezil is taken with food there is no change in its bioavailability. The drug is 95% protein-bound, and hepatic metabolism is through the P450 2D6 and 3A4 isoenzymes.

*Effectiveness.*   Several trials have demonstrated the effectiveness of donepezil in mild–moderate AD [45–49]. In the 24-week double-blind placebo-controlled trial, mild–moderate AD patients were randomly assigned to placebo ($n = 162$), 5 mg/day ($n = 154$), or (titrated to) 10 mg/day ($n = 157$)

of donepezil for 24 weeks followed by a 6-week single-blind placebo washout [45]. Primary measures were the ADAS-cog and CIBIC-plus. Secondary measures were MMSE, CDR-sum boxes and a patient-rated quality of life instrument. The ADAS-cog statistically improved in 5 and 10 mg groups compared with placebo at 12, 18 and 24 weeks. The change in ADAS (difference between placebo and treatment group) at 24 weeks was 2.5 units for the 5 mg group and 2.9 units for the 10 mg group. CIBIC-plus scores were statistically superior in 5 and 10 mg groups compared with placebo at 12, 18 and 24 weeks. MMSE and CDR-sum boxes were significant better in 5 and 10 mg groups compared with placebo. The 10 mg group was not statistically superior to 5 mg group in primary or secondary outcome measures. No quality of life difference was found between treatment and placebo groups. After the 6-week washout, there was no statistical difference in ADAS-cog or CIBIC scores between groups; donepezil-treated patients returned to the level of placebo. Diarrhea, nausea and vomiting were more common in 10 than 5 mg or placebo groups. There were no significant ADL changes between groups in this study.

In a double-blind, placebo-controlled multinational study, the safety and efficacy of donepezil in probable AD patients were further established [49]. Patients received placebo, 5 mg or 10 mg/day of donepezil for 24 weeks, followed by a single-blind washout. ADAS-cog and CIBIC-plus were primary measures. CDR-sum boxes, a patient-rated quality of life scale and the modified Interview for Deterioration in Daily Living Activities in Dementia (IDDD)—an ADL scale—were also used. The 5 mg and 10 mg groups were superior to placebo in all outcome measures and a dose response was demonstrated. There were no significant laboratory abnormalities or adverse effects that led to drop-out, and the drug was well tolerated. Since this study was not a forced titration, it may have more accurately reflected dosing strategies used by clinicians outside clinical trials. However, like many clinical trials of cholinesterase inhibitors for AD, the generalizability is actually limited to the "healthy" AD patients without significant medical comorbidity.

Donepezil was compared to placebo in a 52-week multicenter double-blind randomized European trial [50]. The donepezil treated group was superior to the placebo group in measures of cognition (Gottfries-Brane-Steen, MMSE) and function (Progressive Deterioration Scale) compared to placebo at 24, 36 and 52 weeks. Of interest, adverse effects such as syncope, nausea, accidental injury (bone fracture) and pneumonia were higher in the donepezil treated group compared with placebo.

Another study examined the effect of donepezil compared to placebo on ADLs in a cohort of AD patients up to 54 weeks [51]. The donepezil treated group had a delay in decline of ADLs by 5 months compared with placebo.

The adverse events that occurred at a greater degree in the donepezil treated group included gastrointestinal side effects (nausea, diarrhea, anorexia and dyspepsia), insomnia and rhinitis. Taken together, with the other year-long study [50], the reader is reminded that the postmarketing surveillance of adverse events due to these agents is more widespread than in the FDA approval trials. The FDA site (http://www.fda.gov/medwatch/) is a useful resource when evaluating a drug's side effect profile.

Donepezil's benefit has been extended to nursing home patients with possible or probable AD on measures of cognition compared with placebo treated group over 24 weeks [52]. The mean age was 86 years and the mean MMSE was 14.4, reflecting an older and more severely demented population of subjects than previously studied. The donepezil treated group (5–10 mg/day) maintained CDR and MMSE at 24 weeks compared with placebo.

Another study examined the effectiveness of donepezil compared with placebo in more moderate to severe AD patients [37]. Donepezil demonstrated benefit in this 24-week trial in measures of cognition (MMSE, Severe Impairment Battery) and function (CIBIC-plus).

*Safety.* Donepezil is not associated with hepatotoxicity. The most common gastrointestinal side effects include nausea, emesis and diarrhea. Additionally, patients may complain of muscle cramps, headache, dizziness, syncope or flushing. Hematological side effects include anemia, thrombocytopenia and eosinophilia. No cases of agranulocytosis have been reported. Cardiac effects included bradyarrythmia and syncope. Central nervous system (CNS) effects included headache, dizziness, insomnia, weakness, drowsiness, fatigue and agitation. Side effects show a dose response. Adverse effects led to withdrawal from the 24-week study in 16% of patients in the 10 mg group, 6% of patients in the 5 mg group and 5% in the placebo group [45]. Adverse effects occurred at a higher rate when the titration from 5 mg to 10 mg was made in 1 week compared to 6 weeks. In our clinical experience, insomnia and nocturnal awakenings with donepezil are not infrequent. There is a basic science literature that supports the role of cholinergic mechanisms in sleep. Alteration of the cholinergic system has a direct effect on the suprachiasmatic nucleus, the circadian time-keeper in the brain [53]. The nicotinic acetylcholine receptors appear to mediate this process [54]. Cholinesterase inhibitors may alter sleep architecture. In healthy subjects receiving cholinesterase inhibitors, rapid eye movement (REM) sleep latency was decreased [55], REM sleep density was increased [56] and slow wave sleep was reduced [57].

Cholinesterase inhibitors, especially those with a long half-life, would be expected to alter circadian rhythms. In the clinical trial protocols with cholinesterase inhibitors, adverse effect reports about sleep need to be initiated by patient or caregiver. The sleep disturbances are probably under-reported because of the attribution of sleep disturbance to AD rather than to medication. Given that sleep and cholinergic mechanisms are related, clinicians should be careful in their attributions of sleep disturbance to AD rather than to the cholinesterase inhibitors. Investigators should design future studies to more fully explore the relationship between cholinesterase inhibitors and sleep.

*Prescription guidelines.*   The starting dosage is 5 mg/day, given at night, so that the $C_{max}$ peaks when the patient is asleep in attempt to minimize cholinergic side effects. Some patients experience increased nocturnal awakenings, sleep disturbance, agitation and sweating, possibly associated with the nightly dosing, and the $C_{max}$ of 3–5 hours. Gastrointestinal side effects may be attenuated by co-administration with food or a temporary dosage reduction to 2.5 mg at night, or change to twice-daily dosing with food. In our practice, we offer to increase the daily dose to 10 mg as tolerated after 6 weeks.

## Rivastigmine

Rivastigmine, a carbamate, is a "pseudo-irreversible" inhibitor of acetylcholinesterase, and an inhibitor of butyrylcholinesterase. Acetylcholinesterase inhibition occurs at an anionic and esteratic site. At the esteratic site, the covalent bond between the drug and the acetylcholinesterase has to be degraded by acetylcholinesterase, effectively prolonging the half-life and explaining the "pseudo-irreversible" inhibition. The site of action may be selective for the cortex and hippocampus, as rivastigmine preferentially inhibits the G1 enzymatic form of acetylcholinesterase, which predominates in the brains of AD patients. Administration with food delays absorption and reduces gastrointestinal side effects. There is essentially no P450 metabolism, and with the drug being 40% protein-bound, there is little displacement of protein-bound drugs.

*Effectiveness.*   A number of references trace the development of rivastigmine [58–62]. The most recently published clinical trial of rivastigmine for AD was a 26-week randomized, double-blind placebo-controlled study in which high-dose (6–12 mg/day, $n = 243$) and low-dose (1–4 mg/day, $n = 243$) were compared with placebo ($n = 239$) [63]. Patients met NINCDS–ADRDA criteria for probable AD. Primary outcome measures were ADAS-cog, CIBIC-plus, and the Progressive Deterioration Scale (PDS). The protocol was a slow forced titration for weeks 1–12. By week 26, cognitive deterioration occurred in the placebo group. High-dose rivastigmine was superior to placebo on the ADAS-cog ($p < 0.05$). The placebo group deteriorated by 4.15 points on the ADAS-cog at 26 weeks, a relatively high rate of deterioration compared to other clinical trials of cholinesterase inhibitors. CIBIC-plus measures showed improvement in the high-dose group compared to placebo ($p < 0.001$). Function, as measured with the PDS, demonstrated improvement in the high-dose group and deterioration in the low-dose group ($p < 0.05$). Side effects were primarily gastro-intestinal and occurred in the high-dose group. Side effects occurred pri-marily during dose escalation and led to withdrawal in 23% of the high-dose group, 7% of the low-dose group and 7% of the placebo group. Of note, inclusion criteria for these clinical trials allowed for patients with a broader range of medical comorbidities to be entered into the studies than have donepezil or tacrine trials, perhaps improving the generalizability of the findings.

In addition to the pivotal trials for FDA approval, rivastigmine may be beneficial and is reasonably tolerated in patients with DLB [42, 43, 64, 65], VD [39] or AD with vascular risk factors [41]. In addition, response to rivastigmine may be more robust in advanced AD patients compared to moderate stage patients [36]. This finding is not unique to rivastigmine and may represent a more severe cholinergic deficit with advanced AD [66]. Open label follow-up studies with rivastigmine have suggested benefit to 52 weeks on measures of cognition [67].

*Safety.* Adverse effects that occurred with rivastigmine treatment are exemplified by findings in one study [61]. Side effects that occurred in the 12 mg/day group at a level significantly greater than placebo during the titration phase were sweating, fatigue, asthenia, weight loss, malaise, dizziness (24% vs. 13% placebo), somnolence (9% vs. 2% placebo), nausea (48% vs. 11% placebo), vomiting (27% vs. 11% placebo), anorexia (20% vs. 3% placebo), and flatulence. In the maintenance phase, dizziness (14% vs. 4% placebo), nausea (20% vs. 3% placebo), vomiting (16% vs. 2% pla-cebo), dyspepsia (5% vs. 1% placebo), sinusitis (4% vs. 1% placebo) occurred statistically more in the 12 mg/day group than in the placebo group.

Weight loss of greater than 7% of baseline weight was a significant side effect associated with the use of rivastigmine, occurring more commonly in women than men. There is a bolded warning in the package insert about gastrointestinal side effects. This includes the warning that "if therapy is interrupted for longer than several days, treatment should be reinitiated with the lowest dose in order to avoid the possibility of severe vomiting and its potentially serious sequelae".

*Prescription guidelines.* Rivastigmine is not FDA-approved at the time of this writing, but it is approved in many European countries. The high prevalence of gastrointestinal side effects in the forced titration of the clinical trials makes it likely that a slower titration schedule will be recommended, based upon patient tolerability. The drug is currently dosed b.i.d.

Rivastigmine is initiated at 1.5 mg b.i.d. with food, with a titration up to 3 mg b.i.d. after waiting at least 4 weeks. After an additional 4 weeks, the dose may be further titrated to 4.5 mg b.i.d. and then, after another 4 weeks, to 6 mg b.i.d., always with a full meal. The clinical trials support the dose of 3 mg b.i.d. or greater to be therapeutic, with a dose response curve suggesting greater efficacy at the higher dosages. The higher the dose, the greater the risk of adverse effects, especially during the titration phase. If patients are unable to tolerate a dosage increase, then the next lower dosage should be attempted. If a patient does not take the rivastigmine for several days, the lowest dose should be reinstated because of the risk of adverse events, including death, if the higher dose is started without a titration [68].

*Galanthamine*

Galanthamine, an alkaloid developed from the snowdrop plant, is a reversible, competitive inhibitor of acetylcholinesterase with very little butyrylcholinesterase activity [69, 70]. In contrast to the previously reviewed cholinesterase inhibitors, galanthamine is a competitive inhibitor of acetylcholinesterase. Competitive inhibitors compete with acetylcholine at the acetylcholinesterase binding site, while non-competitive inhibitors bind to the site independent of acetylcholine. The competitive inhibitors of acetylcholinesterase are dependent on acetylcholine concentration. In areas of the brain that have high acetylcholine levels, a competitive inhibitor will be less likely to bind to the enzymatic site because acetylcholine is binding to the site. In areas of the brain where acetylcholine is low, there will be a high amount of the competitive cholinesterase inhibitor binding to acetylcholinesterase relative to acetylcholine. Consequently, competitive inhibitors will have more effect in areas with low levels of acetylcholine and less effect in areas with higher acetylcholine. This may provide an advantage to competitive inhibitors by having a selective effect in the brain areas affected in AD that have lower acetylcholine levels. In areas where acetylcholine is high, a non-competitive agent binding to the acetylcholinesterase molecule may further increase acetylcholine levels and contribute to central cholinergic side effects. In addition to acetylcholinesterase inhibition, galanthamine enhances cholinergic transmission through allosteric modulation of the nicotinic receptor, similar to how benzodiazepines affect GABA transmission [71]. The drug is less than 10% protein-bound, has 100% bioavailability, and food delays the $C_{max}$ [72]. The half-life is approximately 9 hours, allowing for b.i.d. dosing [73]. Galanthamine, metabolized through the P450 2D6 isoenzyme, has not been associated with hepatotoxicity [74]. The common side effects are cholinergic; nausea, vomiting and diarrhea are usually transient over several weeks [75, 76]. Galanthamine is available in several countries, including the United States.

*Effectiveness.* Clinical trial data support the use of galanthamine for AD patients [77–79]. The trials that led to FDA approval demonstrated galanthamine's benefit compared with placebo in measures of cognition (ADAS-cog), behaviour (NPI), ADLs (DAD) and global function (CIBIC measure). Daily doses of galanthamine of at least 16 mg were required to demonstrate benefit. Daily doses of 24 or 32 mg were superior to placebo but were associated with an increase in adverse effects. The higher dosage demonstrated benefit in behavioural measures, but was also associated with more side effects.

*Safety.* The most common adverse effects from galanthamine were gastrointestinal. They appeared related to dose and titration rate in the clinical trials. For example, in one of the clinical trials with a forced dose escalation [79], the patients took 8 mg/day for 1 week, then 16 mg/day for 1 week and then 24 mg/day for 1 week and then a subset increased to 32 mg/day while the rest either took 24 mg/day or placebo. The adverse effects with this aggressive dosing were nausea (40% with 32 mg/day, 37% with 24 mg/day, 12% with placebo), vomiting (17% with 32 mg/day, 20% with 24 mg/day, 4% with placebo), diarrhea (7% with 32 mg/day, 13% with 24 mg/day, 7% with placebo), dizziness (11% with 32 mg/day, 12% with 24 mg/day, 5% with placebo), headache (10% with 32 mg/day, 11% with 24 mg/day, 3% with placebo), anorexia (10% with 32 mg/day, 11% with 24 mg/day, 0% with placebo), weight loss (8% with 32 mg/day, 5% with 24 mg/day, 0.5% with placebo). 18% of galanthamine patients dropped out due to adverse events compared with 9% of placebo group.

The package insert for galanthamine describes the side effects from the drug (24 mg/day, 16 mg/day) or placebo when a 4-week forced titration was used. This approach of increasing the dose every 4 weeks is more similar to the method of dose escalation used in clinical practice than the 1-week forced escalation used in the other clinical trials and may better reflect the expected rate of gastrointestinal side effects. Nausea was found in 13% of the 16 mg group, 17% of the 24 mg group and 5% of the placebo group. Vomiting was present in 1% of the placebo group, 6% of the 16 mg group and 10% of the 24 mg group. Diarrhea was present in 6% of the placebo group, 12% of the 16 mg group and 6% of the 24 mg group. Anorexia was present in 3% of the placebo, 7% of the 16 mg and 9% of the 24 mg group. A decrease in weight was found in 1% of the placebo group, 5% of the 16 mg group and 5% of the 24 mg group.

*Prescription guidelines.* Galanthamine is started at 4 mg b.i.d. and may be titrated to 8 mg b.i.d. after 4 weeks. The recommended target daily dosage is at least 16 mg in divided doses. Higher doses may be achieved to a maximum of 32 mg/day with stepwise increases of 8 mg/day in divided doses at intervals no less than 4 weeks. If a patient misses several doses of medication, judicious clinical practice is to resume therapy with the lowest dose and retitrate upward in 4-week intervals.

## Metrifonate

Metrifonate is an organophosphate cholinesterase inhibitor. Although it demonstrated benefit on cognitive and non-cognitive measures for AD patients [80–81], this class of drugs has failed in AD therapeutics because of toxicity [82].

*Effectiveness and safety.* Clinical trials with metrifonate in AD demonstrated efficacy on both cognitive and non-cognitive ratings [80–81].

Safety concerns about metrifonate led to suspension of all studies. Muscle weakness occurred in some patients and the possible risk of respiratory muscle involvement leading to death was sufficient to cease clinical development of this agent [82]. Metrifonate's metabolite, dichlorvos, is similar in action to organophosphate pesticides and chemical warfare agents. Neurotoxicity from organophosphates may be acute or delayed. The delayed syndrome is one of myasthenia caused by neurotoxic esterase inhibition at the neuromuscular junction. Neurotoxic esterase inhibition by dichlorvos is thought to be responsible for the muscular weakness that occurred in the clinical trials.

## General Precautions with Cholinesterase Inhibitors

For all cholinesterase inhibitors, there is a precaution about anesthesia with succinylcholine type muscle relaxants. The succinylcholine effect may be prolonged because of plasma pseudocholinesterase inhibition [83–86]. This information should be considered in AD patients who are undergoing electroconvulsive therapy (ECT).

In addition to the potential anesthetic risk with succinylcholine, there is a theoretical risk of an interaction between cholinesterase inhibitors and cocaine or cocaine-like local anesthetics. Cocaine toxicity is associated with decreased plasma cholinesterase activity [87], and butyrylcholinesterase degrades aspirin, cocaine, mivacurium and cocaine-like local anesthetics [88, 89]. Hence, agents that inhibit butyrylcholinesterase and effectively decrease the concentration of butyrylcholinesterase may increase the potential for toxicity from cocaine or cocaine-like anesthetics.

## Choice of Cholinesterase Inhibitor for AD

The clinician is faced with the question "Which anticholinesterase inhibitor should I prescribe for my patient?". An approach for prescribing cholinesterase inhibitors that we find helpful is to compare the agents based upon effectiveness and tolerability. Although the available cholinesterase inhibitors have not been directly compared to each other in the same clinical trials, similar methodologies within the trials allow for comparison along certain domains. For example, is there significant improvement over baseline? How long does it take to return to baseline? When the drug is stopped, what happens? Is there a differential response based upon disease severity? Are there differential adverse events?

Tacrine, donepezil, rivastigmine and galanthamine all demonstrated an initial increase in ADAS-cog scores from the baseline measure. The tacrine-treated group demonstrated a maximum change of three ADAS-cog units from baseline, donepezil 2 units, rivastigmine 2 units and galanthamine 3 units, which was statistically significant.

The time to return to a baseline ADAS-cog score may give caretakers a milestone that helps them conceptualize a drug's utility. On average, patients are expected to change by 4 units on the ADAS-cog in 6 months, although there is significant individual variation [11]. Donepezil-treated patients returned to baseline by 39 weeks in an open label extension study [48]. The rivastigmine group's ADAS-cog returned to baseline by 38–44 weeks in an open label extension on doses of 2–12 mg/day [90]. Data for galanthamine shows a return to baseline after 52 weeks at doses of 24 mg/day in an open label extension [91].

Looking at the effect of medication withdrawal in a clinical trial and comparing to a placebo group may give an indication as to whether the treatment altered the course of the disease. If a medication is withdrawn and the test measures return to those of the placebo group, then there is no evidence that the treatment altered disease course, but rather that the treatment was providing symptomatic change. On the other hand, if a treatment

**TABLE 4.1** Kinetic and dynamic comparisons of cholinesterase inhibitors

| Drug name | Chemical class | Type of inhibition | Acetylcholinesterase (AC) and butyrylcholinesterase (BC) inhibition | Protein binding (%) | Hepatic metabolism | Absorption | T1/2 | Dosing |
|---|---|---|---|---|---|---|---|---|
| Tacrine | Acridine | Non-competitive, reversible Anionic site | BC > AC | 55 | P450 1A2 | Food decreases absorption | 2–4 (hours) | q.i.d. |
| Donepezil | Piperidine | Non-competitive, reversible Anionic site | AC > BC | 95 | P450 2D6 3A4 | No food effect | 70 (hours) | q.d. |
| Rivastigmine | Carbamate | Pseudo-irreversible Esteratic site (covalent bond) | G1 form of AC (more specific to brain) | 40 | Essentially none | Well absorbed, food delays absorption and decreases gastrointestinal side effects | 2 hours, but lasts 10 hours due to degradation at esteratic site by AC | b.i.d. |
| Galanthamine | Tertiary amine, phenanthrine derivative | Competitive, reversible | AC > BC | <10 | P450 2D6 | Food delays $C_{max}$ 100% bioavailability | 9 (hours) | b.i.d. |

is withdrawn and the treatment group does not return to the level of the placebo group, then the hypothesis that the treatment alters disease course may be considered.

Of the cholinesterase inhibitors discussed here, rivastigmine-treated patients' ADAS-cog scores did not return to placebo levels at the end of the double-blind trials. Allowing for extrapolation of the expected placebo decline, patients receiving open-label rivastigmine at doses of 2–12 mg/day did not reach the placebo group at 52 weeks and had a projected difference in ADAS-cog scores of approximately 5 units [92]. Donepezil-treated patients returned to placebo by 6 weeks after disconti- nuation of drug [45]. Galanthamine treated patients (24–32 mg/day) with AD did not return to baseline until the measurement at 52 weeks [93]. Compared to a historical placebo, the ADAS-cog difference was greater than 5 units [93].

Daily dosing of donepezil probably improves adherence to treatment compared with q.i.d. dosing for tacrine. B.i.d. dosing for galantha- mine or rivastigmine may have the potential for fewer nocturnal side effects. Cholinesterase inhibitors cause gastrointestinal cholinergic side effects, such as nausea and diarrhea. This can be of central or peripheral origin. In forced titration trials, the incidence of these side effects appear higher than in actual clinical use where the titration rate is slower. Addit- ionally, co-administration with food may improve the tolerability of some cholinesterase inhibitors. Galanthamine and rivastigmine's $C_{max}$ decrease when taken with food and donepezil's $C_{max}$ remains the same. Donepezil is more highly protein-bound than galanthamine, rivastigmine or tacrine. Therefore, donepezil may displace other protein-bound drugs such as warfarin, increasing the free fraction of drug, and increasing the potential for toxicity. Dosing of the drugs differs, based upon their elimina- tion half-lives. Donepezil has a long half-life, allowing for once-daily dosing, but takes a long time to reach steady state. Tacrine's half-life neces- sitates four times per day dosing, while rivastigmine and galanthamine are taken twice daily. Table 4.1 summarizes the pharmacokinetic and pharmacodynamic profiles of the acetylcholinesterase inhibitors discussed in the text.

The findings from these comparisons suggest that some cholinesterase inhibitors may alter AD course in addition to possessing palliative qualities. For example, rivastigmine-treated AD patients' performance on the ADAS-cog does not return to the levels of patients receiving placebo. Galanthamine's mechanism of action, distinct from the other cholinesterase inhibitors, involves allosteric modulation of the nicotinic receptor, and could be involved in altering AD course. Alterations in the nicotinic receptors have been found in AD [94]. Nicotine inhibits the aggregation of the β-amyloid 1–42 fragment [95] and stimulates the secretion of the non-toxic

TABLE 4.2   Adverse effects of cholinesterase inhibitors

| Drug name | Adverse effects | | | |
|-----------|-----------------|---|---|---|
| | Nausea and vomiting | Muscle weakness | Hepatic toxicity | Hematological |
| Tacrine | X | | X | X[**] |
| Donepezil | X | | | |
| Rivastigmine | X | | | |
| Galanthamine | X | | | |
| Metrifonate | X | X[*] | | |

[*] The development of metrifonate has been stopped because of muscle weakness.
[**] There has been a case report of agranulocytosis on tacrine (see text).

form of the β-amyloid precursor protein [96]. Additional evidence suggests that stimulation of the nicotinic receptors may protect cells from the toxic effects of β-amyloid [97], but does not influence the formation of the β-sheet structure [98].

Some basic work suggests additional mechanisms by which cholinesterase inhibitors may be disease-altering. Basal forebrain lesions in animals result in β-amyloid secretion in the cerebrospinal fluid (CSF), and cholinesterase inhibitors attenuate this process [99]. Cholinesterase inhibitors may influence the metabolism of β-amyloid into the non-amyloidogenic pathway, and decrease β-amyloid neurotoxicity in multiple cell lines and rat brain slices [100, 101] Acetylcholinesterase localizes in amyloid plaques and may promote the aggregation and neurotoxicity of β-amyloid [102]. This process may be blocked by cholinesterase inhibitors, possibly related to inhibition of transglutaminase induced cross-linking of β-amyloid [103].

Differential adverse effects of cholinesterase inhibitors are summarized in Table 4.2.

## Antioxidants

Oxidative stress may lead to neuronal damage and apoptosis. β-amyloid neurotoxicity may be mediated in part by free radicals [104]. Antioxidants may act as free radical scavengers, minimizing damage from lipid peroxidation and apoptosis. The brain is vulnerable to oxidative stress from many fronts. There is a demand for oxygen, an abundance of catecholamines and the possibility of auto-oxidation. Additionally, monoamine oxidase (MAO) formation of hydrogen peroxide (an oxidative compound), an abundance of iron (present in oxidative reactions) and relatively low concentration of antioxidative enzymes (superoxide dismutase (SOD), catalase, glutathione peroxidase, glutathione reductase) place the brain in a susceptible position for oxidative damage.

## Vitamin E

Several reviews have examined the role of vitamin E in AD [105–107]. Basic evidence supports the role of vitamin E in protecting cell cultures from the toxic effects of β-amyloid [108].

The absorption of vitamin E is variable by the oral route. Bile is necessary for absorption and fat enhances absorption. Vitamin E is distributed to all tissues, although adipose tissue is the major storage site. It is hepatically metabolized, 70–80% in 1 week.

The major clinical study [109] examining vitamin E in AD was a 2-year double-blind placebo-controlled trial in moderate to severe AD patients comparing vitamin E (2000 IU/day), selegeline (10 mg/day), the combination of the vitamin E and selegiline, and placebo. The outcome measures were nursing home placement, time to death, decline in well-defined ADL level and cognitive function. Neither selegiline nor vitamin E improved cognition compared to placebo. Although the trial was randomized, groups differed significantly in baseline cognition, as measured by MMSE. No difference between groups was found unless the baseline cognition was co-varied in the analysis. When this statistical manipulation was performed, the treatment groups all demonstrated benefits compared to placebo in some of the outcome measures (except cognition). There was no additive effect in the combination selegiline/vitamin E group.

*Safety.* Initial signs of toxicity are fatigue and weakness. Hepatotoxicity and ascites have been associated with vitamin E in infants. In adults, the risk of thrombophlebitis has been reported. In one study, 46 patients with an average age of 60 years had suspected or confirmed thrombophlebitis after vitamin E ingestion. The dose was less than 400 IU for two patients, 400–800 IU for 26 patients, 800 IU for 13 patients and not reported for five patients. Some patients developed thrombophlebitis again when rechallenged with vitamine E. Many of the patients had medical comorbidities that may have predisposed them to thrombophlebitis. There was no comparison group [110].

Coagulopathy is another potential adverse effect from vitamin E. The mechanism of this potential effect may be related to vitamin E's enhanced effects on oral anticoagulants, possibly secondary to interference with the effects of vitamin K on coagulation factor synthesis [111]. Patients on oral anticoagulants with a dosage change of vitamin E greater than 300 IU/day should have prothrombin time (PT) or international normalized ratio (INR) closely monitored. Dosages greater than 300 mg/day may prolong PT [112]. A case report described a 55-year old man who developed bleeding with warfarin and 1200 IU vitamin E per day for 2 months. The symptoms resolved after vitamin E was stopped, but returned after he was rechallenged with vitamin E 800 IU for 4 weeks [113]. Additional support for potential coagulopathy is based on a possible hemorrhagic stroke in the Alpha-Tocopherol, Beta-Carotene Cancer Prevention Study [114].

*Prescription guidelines.* Our practice is to prescribe vitamin E 1000 IU b.i.d to AD patients. Although the level of impairment of AD patients in the Sano study [109] was moderate to severe, we empirically start vitamin E in the mild–moderate AD patients, believing that the potential benefit outweighs the risk. For patients on anticoagulants, we start on lower doses and titrate upward, closely monitoring the INR. Quality control is not similar for vitamin E preparations as FDA approved prescription drugs. This creates the potential risk of contamination, not knowing the actual ingredients in the preparation, and other unknown risks inherent in the manufacturing process of the compound. We advise our patients to use preparations that are listed in the *United States Pharmacopeia*. In the Sano study [109], the vitamin E preparation was made exclusively for the double-blind study and is not commercially available.

## Selegiline

Selegiline is a MAO inhibitor that selectively inhibits MAO-B. Hepatic metabolism of the compound results in the production of desmethylselegiline, amphetamine and methamphetamine. Selegiline blocks free radical activity from oxidative species. Desmethylselegiline upregulates antiapoptotic molecules, glutathione and superoxide dismutase, providing additional protection [115].

In addition to having utility as an antidepressant agent, selegiline has demonstrated the ability to prevent animals from developing a parkinsonian syndrome induced by 1-methyl-4-phenyl-1, 2, 5, 6-tetrahydropyridine (MPTP). In humans, selegiline dosed at 10 mg/day may delay the emergence of disability or signs and symptoms of Parkinson's disease.

*Effectiveness and safety.* In AD, selegiline was found to be superior to placebo in delaying time to death, and decline in ADLs. There was no benefit to cognition, no significant effect on institutionalization and no additive effect with vitamin E [109]. In this clinical trial with AD patients, falls, dental events (an event that led to dental treatment) and syncope were the only categories of adverse events that differed between treatment group and placebo [109]. In routine clinical use, CNS side effects associated with selegiline may include sleep disturbance, psychosis, agitation, confusion, hypotension, anorexia and dyskinesias. Additionally, selegiline has the potential to interact with other drugs. Concurrent use of tricyclic antidepressants (TCAs), selective serotonin reuptake inhibitors (SSRIs), or miperidine should be avoided, as fatalities have been reported with these medication combinations [116–120]. Combining selegiline with bupropion has resulted in bupropion toxicity in animals, and the combination should be avoided [121]. In addition, combining selegiline and buspirone should be avoided because of the risk of hypertensive crisis [122].

*Prescription guidelines.* Selegiline is not a first-line agent for the treatment of AD. It is more costly and has a more malignant side effect profile than vitamin E. Selegiline may be offered to patients who are unable to take vitamin E because of allergy, sensitivity or coagulopathy risk, but they should be well informed that selegiline is not a standard of care for AD.

## Anti-inflammatories

A body of evidence supports the theory that inflammatory processes are involved in the pathophysiology of AD [123]. Inflammation in the brain may be neurotoxic. There is evidence of an acute phase response with elevated levels of interleukin 1 and interleukin 6 [124–126]. Complement factors are found in senile plaques and there is evidence that the complement cascade is activated by the amyloid binding to C1q [127] Both fibrillar and non-fibrillar β-amyloid appear to be involved [128]. The initial complement cascade component, C1q, interacts with β-amyloid, contributing to β-amyloid aggregation and neurotocity by activation of the complement cascade [129]. Activated microglia secrete neurotoxins and increase the production of free radicals [130, 131].

There is epidemiological support that prior use of NSAIDs may delay the onset of AD [132, 133]. Twin studies demonstrate a decreased risk of developing AD with exposure to NSAIDs [133] and longitudinal follow-up of the Baltimore Aging study cohort suggested a decreased relative risk of developing AD with increased NSAID use [134]. Patients with rheumatoid arthritis develop AD at a lower rate than the general population, possibly explained by the use of anti-inflammatory agents [132] or HLA subtype [135, 136].

Clinical trials with anti-inflammatory agents vary on a key number of methodological points. In a 6-month trial, the indomethacin-treated AD patients did not decline cognitively, while the control group declined by

8%. Limitations of the study included an unusual cognitive measure and a substantial number of drop-outs from gastrointestinal side effects [137].

In a 25-week randomized double-blind placebo-controlled trial in mild to moderate AD patients, diclofonac (a NSAID) was given with a gastroprotective agent, misoprostol [138]. Intent-to-treat analysis found no benefit in cognitive and functional measures in the treatment or placebo group and 50% of the drug treatment group withdrew.

Another class of anti-inflammatory agents is the cyclooxygenase-2 (Cox-2) inhibitors. The Cox-2 inhibitors have the potential advantage over NSAIDs of being more specific to the brain. Cox-2 is found in the hippocampus, and Cox-2 levels are elevated in hippocampal neurons in post-mortem AD patients [139]. Cox-2 levels correlate with amyloid plaque density. Animal studies demonstrate that overexpression of Cox-2 increases susceptibility to β-amyloid toxicity. There is upregulation of Cox-2 expression in AD frontal cortex. Synthetic β-amyloid peptides induced Cox-2 expression in neuroblastoma cell cultures. Further, Cox-2 may be involved in apoptosis [140]. Compared to other NSAIDs, ibuprofen, indomethacin and sulindac sulphide may preferentially inhibit the formation of Abeta42 and this mechanism may be independent of the cyclooxygenase inhibition [141]. Various Cox-2 inhibitors have been released and some are undergoing clinical trials in AD patients. Several anti-inflammatory agents have demonstrated tolerability in AD patients [142, 143], but recent results from a multicenter trial with rofexcoxib, a selective Cox-2 inhibitor, were negative, with excess gastrointestinal side effects [144]. The results of industry sponsored trials of Cox-2 inhibitors are not in the public domain.

Prednisone has been studied in AD patients in a multicenter placebo-controlled trial. No benefit was found in doses up to 10 mg/day of prednisone, and the prednisone-treated group had behavioural worsening, as measured on the Brief Psychiatric Rating Scale (BPRS) [145]. Clinical trials with colchicine and hydroxychloroquine are planned, as these agents have a theoretical rationale in AD [146, 147].

Propentofylline, an inhibitor of microglial activation, has demonstrated benefit in clinical trials with dementia patients. Patients with AD who received doses of 300–900 mg/day of propentofylline improved on global function, ADL and cognitive measures, compared to placebo [148, 149]. Propentofylline is well tolerated, with minor gastrointestinal side effects. Phase three trials have been completed in AD and VD patients [150]. The results have not demonstrated consistent benefit from this drug for AD and VD subjects [151].

We do not start patients on NSAIDs, Cox-2 inhibitors, propentofylline or other anti-inflammatory agents as standard care for AD. We do offer patients the opportunity to participate in clinical research trials with these agents. With treatments that may show benefit, but are not yet standard of care for AD, we believe in recommending that our patients consider clinical trials with the agent, if available. In fact, we are in agreement with a recent editorial suggesting that informing a patient about clinical trials for a potential treatment for their condition is an ethical obligation [152].

## Estrogen

Estrogen elicits effects on brain development, neuron survival, regeneration and plasticity [153–155]. Estrogen has demonstrated effects on the hippocampus, amygdala, locus coeruleus, pituitary and hypothalamus [156, 157]. Estrogen's mechanism of action in the brain may include enhancement of transcription and mediation of non-genomic events [158]. Clinical trial evidence suggests that patients receiving ERT may respond better to cholinesterase inhibitors (tacrine) [159]. However, the lack of randomization, variability of dosage, duration and preparation of hormonal replacement limit this conclusion.

The relationship between estrogen and brain cholinergic function may give clues to estrogen's possible effects on AD. Estrogen receptors are found in the same areas that are rich in cholinergic neurons [160]. Estrogen has role for maintenance of cholinergic neurons projecting to the hippocampus and cortex and can attenuate anticholinergic impairment [161]. Estrogen has been shown to increase CAT [162] and enhance cholinergic activity in the basal forebrain and the hippocampus [163].

Estrogen also demonstrates effects on oxidation. It is converted to catecholestrogen, eventually to semiquinones and reactive oxygen species. The reactive oxygen species and semiquinones are pro-oxidants. Estrogen also stimulates the peroxidase reaction that is necessary for oxidation. Catecholestrogen in iron redox is an antioxidant. Estrogen affects genes that inhibit the production of pathological proteins [164]. Additionally, estrogen appears to promote the non-amyloidogenic processing of amyloid precursor protein [165].

Population-based studies have examined the relationship between hormonal replacement therapy and cognitive performance or the risk of developing AD in non-demented older women. For example, a positive relationship between cognitive test performance and ERT was noted in a cohort of non-demented community-dwelling women over age 65 who were tested with the Modified Mini-Mental State (3MS) [166, 167]. Cognitive performance was the best for women who currently were receiving hormonal replacement with estrogen. Past estrogen users also had significantly higher test scores than non-users, but not as high as current users. Additionally, lower education, current depression and at least one ApoE4 allele predicted lower performance on the 3MS. Limitations of the study include the possibility of a selection bias. Women who use post-menopausal estrogen may have improved overall health status [168]. Although there have been other studies supporting the role of estrogen on cognitive function [169–173], a 15-year longitudinal study of approximately 800 women over age 65 found no relationship between duration or dosage of estrogen use and performance on neuropsychological tests of visual spatial abilities, memory or language [174].

Other studies examined the risk of developing or dying with AD. In a cohort of approximately 300 post-menopausal women, the odds of developing AD were increased in women who did not receive ERT (odds ratio 1.82). Duration of estrogen use was not discussed. The population had a relatively high prevalence of vascular dementia [175]. In another cohort of almost 9000 women in a retirement community, earlier age of menarche and longer estrogen use were associated with lower mortality rates from AD and a lower risk of developing AD (odds ratio of 0.65). A methodological limitation of the study was reliance on death certificates for AD diagnosis, reducing diagnostic sensitivity [176]. In the Baltimore Longitudinal Study of Aging, almost 500 women were followed for 16 years and approximately half were estrogen users. The relative risk of developing AD in estrogen users was 0.46 [177]. In the Italian Longitudinal Study of Aging, estrogen use was lower among the women who developed AD after controlling for age, education, number of children, age at menopause and menarche, tobacco and alcohol use [178]. In another cohort of approximately 1100 non-demented community-dwelling women, the risk of developing AD was decreased in women receiving ERT after menopause (odds ratio of 0.5). The study did not account for pre-menopausal exposure to estrogen and did not report on dosage, duration or preparation of estrogen [179]. In a small randomized, placebo-controlled trial in post-menopausal women with AD, six women received 8 weeks of transdermal 17β-estradiol, at a dosage of 0.05 mg/day, and six women received placebo. Compared to the placebo group, the transdermal estrogen group demonstrated improvements in verbal memory and attention, beginning after 1 week of treatment and lasting until the estrogen was discontinued after week 8 [180]. In a randomized placebo controlled trial sponsored by the ADCS, ERT for 1 year did not slow progression of AD or result in improved cognitive, global or functional measures in women with mild to moderate stage AD [181]. Large prospective studies, such as the Women's Health Initiative [182] and a National Institute of Aging prospective treatment study, are examining the relationship between estrogen replacement and the development or progression of AD. These efforts should help clarify the role of estrogen in AD.

Selective estrogen-receptor modulators (SERM) act as estrogen agonists in some tissues and antagonists at others. They may be cardioprotective and not have the same risk as estrogen for breast or uterine cancer [183]. They are currently being promoted as an alternative to estrogen for the treatment of post-menopausal symptoms and possibly to reduce the risk of fracture from osteoporosis, but their use is not standard [184, 185]. Some examples are raloxifene, tamoxifen, droloxifene and tiboline. No published studies have yet examined the role of these agents in the prevention or treatment of AD.

We do not routinely prescribe estrogen to women with AD, but rather encourage a discussion with the patient's gynecologist, especially in light of the recent suggestion that ERT may be associated with increased risk of ovarian cancer [186].

## Treatment of Depression in AD Patients

Once depression is diagnosed in an AD patient, aggressive treatment should be initiated, with careful monitoring of cognition. General medical conditions that may be contributing to the depression should be addressed, and medications that may be aggravating the depression should be discontinued or replaced with a more appropriate alternative [187]. Depression in AD patients is responsive to psychotherapy, pharmacotherapy, specific behavioural interventions and ECT [188–191]. Treatment with antidepressants that have high anticholinergic load must be avoided, because cognition may worsen [192].

Few clinical trials of AD patients with depression and several case reports guide antidepressant choice. One non-randomized clinical trial comparing fluoxetine to amitriptyline in depressed AD patients demonstrated efficacy for both agents, with a higher drop-out rate in the tricyclic group [193]. Clomipramine was found to improve mood but diminish cognition in a cross-over study [194]. Similarly, imipramine benefited mood but altered cognition in a depressed group of AD patients [195]. In a case series, 11 of 12 AD patients with depression and psychosis responded to a trial of SSRIs [196]. Citalopram has demonstrated efficacy for depression and affective lability in multicenter studies with depressed AD patients [197]. Not all SSRIs have demonstrated efficacy for depression in demented patients. Fluvoxamine was not effective for depression in a sample of AD and vascular dementia patients with depressive symptoms [198]. In general, SSRIs may be associated with gastrointestinal and sexual side effects [199], but have significantly less anticholinergic load than tricyclic compounds [200].

The clinician's choice of antidepressant for the AD patient should be heavily weighed against agents with adverse cognitive effects. Agents such as bupropion, venlafaxine, nefazodone and mirtazapine may be considered in addition to the SSRIs. Additionally, moclobemide, a reversible inhibitor of MAO-A, may have future role in treating demented patients who are depressed [201]. The use of TCAs should be limited to nortriptyline or desipramine, as they have less anticholinergic properties than the parent compounds, amitriptyline and imipramine. The value of serum levels to guide dosing of the TCAs in depressed AD patients is unclear, although one study reported that one-third of patients with major depression responded when nortriptyline was given so that the blood level was in the "therapeutic window" for 7 weeks [202]. There is an emerging literature testing the hypothesis that tricyclic agents may be superior to SSRIs for treating severely depressed melancholic patients, although the cohort was not a sample of depressed AD patients [203].

The clinical trials of the aforementioned agents in AD patients with depression are limited. Consequently, the empiric use of these agents is based upon treatment reviews for these agents in geriatric patients that account for the unique pharmacokinetic and pharmacodynamic profile of this population [204, 205]. Depressed elderly may take more than 6 weeks to respond to antidepressant medication [206]. The adage "start low and go slow but give enough medication for enough time" is our practice in AD patients with depression. We also believe that the discontinuation of non-essential medications may include antidepressant agents if they have been maximized and the patient has not responded.

ECT has a role in the treatment of AD patients with severe depression who have failed or been unable to tolerate medication trials [207]. Although no well-controlled trials support its role in AD patients with depression, a large body of evidence supports its safety and efficacy for depression without comorbid dementia [208]. Cognitive deficits may be minimized by decreasing the frequency of treatment from thrice to twice weekly during the index phase of treatment, considering right unilateral instead of bilateral treatment, and using appropriate doses of energy relative to seizure threshold [209].

## Treatment of Psychosis in AD Patients

Psychosis is a common feature associated with AD, occurring in 25–50% of patients. The etiology of the psychosis needs formal investigation in each patient, following the principles of a work-up for delirium. Medications or unstable medical conditions may be causative. Treatment involves removal of the offending substance or medication and optimization of comorbid illnesses. Pharmacological treatment may include antipsychotic medication. Haloperidol has been studied for this indication, and doses of 2–3 mg/day were optimal when titrated from 1 mg per day upward. The authors emphasized the narrow therapeutic window for haloperidol with a subgroup of patients developing moderate to severe extrapyramidal symptoms [210]. The atypical agent risperidone has been found to be effective in doses of 1 mg/day in a controlled trial of institutionalized demented patients [211]. Extrapyramidal side effects, somnolence and peripheral edema were the most common side effects. Olanzapine has shown benefit at doses of 5 and 10 mg per day compared to placebo in a 6-week trial for nursing home residents with AD and psychosis [212]. 15 mg/day was no better than placebo. Somnolence occurred in 6.4% of the placebo group compared with 25% of the 5 mg/day group, 26% of the 10 mg/day group and 36% of the 15 mg/day group. Gait disturbance occurred in 2.1% of the placebo group, 19.6% of the 5 mg/day group, 14% of the 10 mg/day group and 17% of the 15 mg/day group.

There is one open trial of 184 elderly patients with psychosis treated with quetiapine over 52 weeks [213]. Average age was 76 years and 78% reported to have psychosis from a medical condition such as AD. The mean dose of quetiapine was 137.5 mg/day. Of interest, over half the patients did not complete the trial. Dizziness, postural hypotension, lack of efficacy, failure to follow-up, intercurrent illness or adverse events were the most common explanations given for not completing this year-long study.

The NIMH is currently sponsoring the Clinical Antipsychotic Trials of Intervention Effectiveness (CATIE) protocol for AD, that will compare the effectiveness and sequelae of risperidone, olanzapine and quetiapine for psychosis and agitation associated with AD [214]. The results of this trial should aid clinicians with guidelines for managing psychosis in AD patients.

There are no published large controlled trials with clozapine, sertindole or ziprasidone in AD patients with psychosis.

## Effects of Cholinesterase Inhibitors on Disturbed Behaviour in AD

Anticholinergic agents can contribute to delirium with agitation, paranoid delusions and visual hallucinations. Therefore cholinergic agents are expected to be helpful to alleviate these common behavioural disturbances seen in AD patients with cholinergic deficiency. There is emerging evidence that cholinesterase inhibitors may have non-cognitive benefits for AD patients. These effects may be mediated by limbic and paralimbic structures [215]. In an analysis of the Knapp et al. trial, tacrine-treated patients in the 160 mg/day group scored better than placebo on ADAS items of cooperation, delusions and pacing [216]. A meta-analysis of double-blind placebo-controlled trials with tacrine through 1995 also supported superiority of tacrine to placebo on behavioural items of the ADAS [217]. In a double-blind placebo-controlled trial of metrifonate, a significant superiority of this drug over placebo was found using measures of depression, apathy and hallucinations [218]. The FDA approved cholinesterase inhibitors have all demonstrated effectiveness on behavioural measures for patients with dementia. Donepezil has shown benefit in an open trial of AD patients [219]. Rivastigmine has benefitted patients with psychosis associated with Parkinson's disease [220] and DLB [65]. Galanthamine has shown benefit on behavioural measures in AD [221]. Taken together, the effectiveness of the agents on the non-cognitive disturbances associated with dementia probably represents a class effect. Further investigation in this area is necessary to guide prescribing practices.

## Vaccine for AD

The field emerged excited when reports of an AD vaccine emerged. Transgenic mice immunized with β-amyloid had a substantial reduction in the amyloid burden in their brains compared to control mice [222]. This approach appeared to achieve behavioural benefit in the animals [223] and was advanced to safety trials in primates and humans. The trials were halted when human subjects developed symptoms of brain infiltration with elevated protein levels and lymphocytic infiltration [224].

## Gingko Biloba

The extract from the gingko plant (EGB 761) has demonstrated modest benefit in clinical trials in AD, but with insufficient evidence to yet withstand FDA approval for dementia [225, 226]. The compound is approved in Germany for dementia and has also been studied for age-associated memory impairment [227].

## Statins

Epidemiological evidence suggests that individuals taking statin drugs for lowering cholesterol had a decreased risk of developing AD [228–230]. When indication bias (that healthier people take statins) is addressed, the epidemiological relationship remains [231]. There does not appear to be an influence from APOE genotype, African American race, education, history of heart disease, stroke or diabetes [232]. Statins appear to reduce the Abeta levels in cell culture and guinea pigs [233]. Future trials are planned to test whether statins attenuate the progression of AD.

## Secretase Inhibitors

β-amyloid is present in plaques, one of the neuropathological hallmarks of AD, and is probably associated with the development and perhaps progression of AD. The amyloid precursor protein (APP) has several cleavage pathways, one leading to the production of Abeta which can aggregate to become neurotoxic. β- and γ-secretase are both necessary to cleave the precursor protein into β-amyloid. β- and γ-secretase inhibitors may both be potential therapeutic targets [234]. Beta-site amyloid protein-cleaving enzyme (BACE) has been identified as β-secretase [235]. BACE is a membrane associated aspartyl protease located in the lumen of golgi and endosomes. It has the highest expression in the brain and pancreas and highest enzymatic activity in the brain. BACE appears to be the rate-limiting step in the production of Abeta and BACE inhibitors could have therapeutic potential for AD. It is unclear if APP is the only substrate for BACE, whether inhibition of BACE will be non-toxic, whether the putative BACE inhibitor would be lipid soluble and small enough to reach the intracellular site of action. Finally, will BACE inhibition alter the disease course?

γ-secretases are thought to be presenilin I and/or presenilin II [236]. The γ-secretase inhibitors are in phase 1 trials. It remains unclear how many γ-secretases are present, how specific a substrate is APP for γ-secretase. Additionally, it remains unclear where and how much γ-secretase is outside the brain and, therefore, whether the consequences of γ-secretase inhibition will be deleterious.

## Glycogen Synthase Kinase-3 Inhibitors

Glycogen synthase kinase-3 beta (GSK-3 beta) is involved with the phosphorylation of tau, an event in the pathway leading to tangle formation through presumed cytoskeletal changes in microtubules [237, 238]. Valproate is an inhibitor of GSK-3 beta [239] and may be a therapeutic target in AD. Additionally, other GSK-3 beta inhibitors are being developed [240].

## Homocysteine

Homocysteine has been found to be elevated in persons with AD [241, 242]. A recent study found that homocysteine was an independent risk factor for the development of AD [243], suggesting that approaches to lower homo-cysteine levels, such as increasing oral intake of folic acid, require testing to determine whether they will successfully decrease the risk of developing AD. Some have called into question the relationship between homocysteine and AD, however, suggesting that the elevation of homocysteine is attribu-table to vascular disease, not AD pathology [244].

## PHARMACOTHERAPY FOR DEMENTIA WITH LEWY BODIES (DLB)

DLB patients may benefit from cholinesterase inhibitors. A cholinergic deficit has been shown in DLB: in fact, the relative decline in CAT is greater in DLB than in AD [245]. Patients receiving a short trial of tacrine improved in verbal initiation and digit span [246]. We explain to patients and their families that there are no current FDA-approved drugs to treat the cognitive disturbances found in DLB. We empirically offer a trial of cholinesterase inhibitors to these patients.

Over 50% of patients with DLB have depressive symptoms. There are no clinical trials to base recommendations for the treatment of depression found in DLB. We apply basic principles for treating depression in this subgroup of patients. If the depression results in functional impairment, we offer pharmacological treatment. We always recommend a comprehen-sive review of the current medications and medical comorbidities, as they may be contributing to the depressive symptoms. Pharmacotherapy is initiated at low doses with agents that have little anticholinergic potential (e.g. SSRIs, bupropion, venlafaxine, mirtazapine). We also consider ECT to be a reasonable option for depressed DLB patients who are unable or unwilling to forego a pharmacological treatment trial.

Although neuroleptic sensitivity and psychosis were proposed as core clinical features in DLB [247], the attribution of the psychosis should not automatically be made to the disease state. Concurrent medical illnesses and medications commonly cause psychosis. As an example, patients with DLB commonly have parkinsonism and are prescribed antiparkinsonism agents. These medications frequently cause psychosis. Given that neuroleptic sen-sitivity may be a finding in DLB, atypical antipsychotics should theoretically be useful in treating the psychosis. Initial case reports are disappointing, however, with 3/8 patients with DLB being unable to tolerate even low doses of olanzapine [248]. Our practice is to empirically initiate a gentle titration of an atypical antipsychotic agent for psychosis associated with DLB.

# PHARMACOTHERAPY FOR AIDS DEMENTIA

Before the routine use of zidovudine (AZT), the course of AIDS dementia was often rapid after cognitive decline emerged. Currently, patients receiving zidovudine may exhibit signs of the cognitive and motor changes for months to years before dying [249]. Additionally, health care utilization rates increase as patients with AIDS dementia live longer [250], placing even more emphasis on the development of safe and effective treatments for this condition.

Investigational treatments for AIDS dementia include adjuvant use of anti-inflammatory and neuroprotective agents [251]. This effort is based on evidence that human immunodeficiency virus (HIV) is not the direct cause of CNS damage. Loss of neurons appears related to viral infection of brain macrophages and microglia. A valuable predictor of neurological impairment following HIV infection is the absolute number of immune competent macrophages rather than the level of viral involvement in brain tissue. Additional focus has been on the role of excitatory aminoacids, cytokines, glutamate and oxidative stress.

Peptide T, an agent that presumably blocks the viral protein gp120 from binding with brain tissue, was studied to determine whether this intranasally administered compound would improve cognition in HIV-positive patients. In a double-blind placebo-controlled study, neuropsychological testing results at baseline were compared with performance after 6 months. There was no advantage in primary outcome measures. However, a subgroup of patients with relatively preserved immune function or more severe cognitive impairment demonstrated some statistical benefit in cognitive domain scores [252].

The use of psychostimulants for cognitive decline in patients with AIDS has been reviewed [253, 254]. A potential use of these drugs is for the depressive symptoms that are frequently associated with the disease. When depression is treated aggressively, cognitive improvement may also occur. Psychostimulants have been found to be beneficial in the majority of patients from several open-label trials of men with AIDS [255]. Patients in these trials often had cognitive problems associated with their depressive symptoms. Dextramphetamine doses ranged from 5 to 60 mg/day and methylphenidate doses ranged from 10 to 90 mg/day. Reported side effects included increased anxiety, dyskinesias, motor tension and possibly facial angioedema in one case. Abuse of psychostimulants and appetite suppression, although a theoretical risk, were not reported as a significant issue in these trials. The methodological limitations of these studies include no women patients, lack of blinding and small sample sizes. Generalizations must therefore be limited.

## PHARMACOTHERAPY FOR VASCULAR DEMENTIA (VD)

Once VD has been identified, thorough review should be made of the patient's medical conditions. The clinician should review with the patient and caregiver any risk factors that exist for stroke, and outline a treatment plan to control or eliminate these conditions. Cigarette smoking should be eliminated, and attention to diet and exercise regimens should be encouraged. Blood pressure control should not become overaggressive, as this may place the patient at increased risk of more brain damage from hypoperfusion. In fact, maintenance of a slightly increased blood pressure may be beneficial for cognition in VD patients [256, 257]. The use of aspirin [258] and reduction of plasma lipids may also have a role as preventive measures [259].

Previous evidence suggested a role for cholinergic enhancement [260], and now donepezil [40, 261], rivastigmine [39, 41] and galanthamine [38] suggest a potential role for cholinesterase inhibitors for VD, although caution has been advised before rushing to prescribe cholinesterase inhibitors for this condition based upon the limited evidence [262]. Pharmacological approaches for the treatment of VD have focused on the protection of the brain from ischemia. Pentoxyfylline [263] and propentofylline [264] have demonstrated some modest degree of success. Additional approaches have included reduction of intracellular calcium influx [265], glutamate antagonism and dopamine enhancement [266].

## SUMMARY

### Consistent Evidence

The current treatment approaches for dementia are based on variable degrees of scientific evidence, reflecting an incomplete comprehension of the basic pathophysiology of the various dementing disorders. In AD, cholinergic deficits have been well described and there is consistent evidence that cholinesterase inhibitors are effective for cognitive disturbances. Some cholinesterase inhibitors are better tolerated than others, but may still cause side effects that lead to drug discontinuation for an occasional patient. The treatment for AIDS dementia, DLB and VD is based upon less consistent evidence.

### Incomplete Evidence

Oxidative stress is involved in neuronal damage and apoptosis. A large-scale treatment study of vitamin E and selegiline in AD patients supports the benefit of these agents on ADL function, mortality or time to nursing home placement for moderate to severe AD patients. The study may have been limited by differences between baseline MMSE scores in the groups studied, and the treatments did not have any beneficial effect on cognition. There is incomplete evidence as to whether vitamin E is beneficial for earlier stage AD patients. Vitamin E should be used with caution to treat patients with coagulopathies or receiving anticoagulants.

Estrogen is another treatment approach for AD, with incomplete evidence supporting its use. It may be beneficial to some brain functions and may enhance the effectiveness of cholinesterase inhibitors. Preliminary evidence suggests a beneficial role of estrogen for AD patients, with the notable exception of one placebo-controlled randomized clinical trial [181]. Results from large-scale trials are required before definitive conclusions may be drawn. However, given the recent finding of increased ovarian cancer risk with ERT (186), the methodological design of studies to determine whether estrogen will benefit AD patients will require careful consideration. Theoretical and epidemiological support exists for an inflammatory response in AD. Clinical trials are underway to explore the effectiveness of various anti-inflammatory regimens. Published trials with gingko biloba suggest a modest effect in AD patients on measures of cognition. Replication of these findings with more robust results on patient functioning are required before gingko is recommended for use in clinical practice.

Epidemiological evidence suggests that statin use may be associated with decreased risk of developing AD. Large scale trials are underway or in the planning stages to determine whether these agents will prevent the conversion from mild cognitive impairment to AD or slow the progression of cognitive impairment in patients who already carry the AD diagnosis.

VD patients may benefit from pentoxyfyline or propentofylline, both vasodilator agents that inhibit adenosine uptake or phosphodiesterase. Agents that decrease calcium influx, block glutamate, and enhance cholinergic or dopaminergic function are in early stages of investigation for VD patients. Cholinesterase inhibitors have been studied in VD and suggest promise for this cohort of patients. Further studies with improved methodology may lead to the FDA indication for cholinesterase inhibitors to treat VD. Additionally, there is evidence that primary and secondary prevention measures may benefit VD patients. Vigorous attempts should be made to control or eliminate the risk factors for stroke. This effort may decrease the risk of developing VD or reduce the morbidity in patients with VD.

Depression and psychosis associated with AD, VD, DLB and AIDS dementia are significant problems that may respond to pharmacological intervention. There is preliminary evidence that cholinesterase inhibitors may offer benefit to behavioural disturbances in AD and DLB. The benefit of one agent over another is not consistently reported in the literature and the empiric choice of agents should strongly consider their side effect profile.

## Areas Still Open to Research

Cholinesterase inhibitors may alter the course of AD. They may delay nursing home placement or reduce mortality in AD patients. Future large-scale prospective studies are required to test these possibilities. After cholinesterase inhibitor therapy is stopped, AD patients may decline to the levels of a placebo group. However, open-label studies suggest that patients treated with the newer cholinesterase inhibitors may not return to the projected placebo group values even 2 years after treatment initiation. Further investigation may reveal a differential effect between agents that could correspond to differences in their mechanisms of action. As further developments in understanding the pathogenesis of AD pathogenesis emerge, so too will translation of this understanding to clinical trials. For example, the "vaccine" that appeared promising for AD by binding β-amyloid proved dangerous as humans tested with the agent developed evidence of brain inflammation. Secretase inhibitors have been synthesized and early safety and tolerability trials are beginning in AD patients.

In AIDS dementia, antiviral agents may be beneficial in delaying but not preventing cognitive decline. Therapies aimed at the virus may offer some palliation, but evidence that cognitive decline is not fully explained by direct HIV effects on the brain has led to investigation of anti-inflammatory agents, antioxidants, and neuroprotective agents as potential treatments.

## REFERENCES

1. Food, Drug and Cosmetic Reports (1992) FDA Guidance on Alzheimer's Drug Clinical Utility Assessments, FDC Reports, Washington, DC.
2. McKhann G., Drachman D. Folstein M. Katzman R. Price D., Stadlan E.M. (1984) Clinical diagnosis of Alzheimer's disease: report of the NINCDS–ADRDA Work Group under the auspices of Department of Health and Human Services Task Force on Alzheimer's Disease. *Neurology*, **34**: 939–944.
3. Rosen W.G., Mohs R.C., Davis K.L. (1984) A new rating scale for Alzheimer's disease. *Am. J. Psychiatry*, **141**: 1356–1364.
4. Knopman D.S., Knapp M.J., Gracon S.I., Davis C.S. (1994) The Clinician Interview Based Impression (CIBI): a clinician's global change rating scale in Alzheimer's disease. *Neurology*, **44**: 2315–2321.

5. Folstein M.F., Folstein S.F., McHugh P.R. (1975)   Mini-Mental State: a practical method for grading the cognitive state of patients for the clinician. *J. Psychiatr. Res.*, **12**: 189–198.

6. Dejong R., Osterlund O.W., Roy G.W. (1989)   Measurement of quality-of-life changes of patients with Alzheimer's disease. *Clin. Ther.*, **11**: 545–554.

7. Cummings J.L. (1997)   The Neuropsychiatric Inventory: assessing psychopathology in dementia patients. *Neurology*, **48** (Suppl. 6): S10–S16.

8. Lawton M.P., Brody E.M. (1969)   Assessment of older people: self-maintaining and instrumental activities of daily living. *Gerontologist*, **9**: 179–186.

9. Galasko D., Bennett D., Sano M., Ernesto C., Thomas R., Grundman M., Ferris S. (1997)   An inventory to assess activities of daily living for clinical trials in Alzheimer's disease. The Alzheimer's Disease Cooperative Study. *Alz. Dis. Assoc. Disord.*, **11** (Suppl. 2): S33–S39.

10. Gelinas I., Gauthier L., McIntyre M., Gauthier S. (1999)   Development of a functional measure for persons with Alzheimer's disease: the disability assessment for dementia. *Am. J. Occup. Ther.*, **53**: 471–481.

11. Stern R.G., Mohs R.C., Davidson M., Schmeidler J., Silverman J., Kramer-Ginsberg E., Searcey T., Bierer L., Davis K.L. (1994)   A longitudinal study of Alzheimer's disease: measurement, rate, and predictors of cognitive deterioration. *Am. J. Psychiatry*, **151**: 390–396.

12. Schneider L.S., Olin J.T., Doody R.S., Clark C.M., Morris J.C., Reisberg B., Schmitt F.A., Grundman M., Thomas R.G., Ferris S.H. (1997) Validity and reliability of the Alzheimer's Disease Cooperative Study—Clinical Global Impression of Change. The Alzheimer's Disease Cooperative Study. *Alz. Dis. Assoc. Disord.*, **11** (Suppl. 2): S22–S32.

13. Reisberg B., Schneider L., Doody R., Anand R., Feldman H., Haraguchi H., Kumar R., Lucca U., Mangone C.A., Mohr E., *et al* (1997). Clinical global measure of dementia: position paper from the International Working Group on Harmonization of Dementia Drug Guidelines. *Alz. Dis. Assoc. Disord.*, **11** (Suppl. 3): 8–18.

14. Schneider L.S., Olin J.T. (1996)   Clinical global impressions in Alzheimer's clinical trials. *Int. Psychogeriatrics*, **8**: 277–288.

15. Grigoletto F., Zappala G., Anderson D.W., Lebowitz B.D. (1999)   Norms for the Mini-Mental State Examination in a healthy population. *Neurology*, **53**: 315–320.

16. Teng E.L., Chiu H.C., Schneider L.S., Metzger L.E. (1987) Alzheimer's dementia: performance on the Mini-Mental State Examination. *J. Consult. Clin. Psychol.*, 55: 96–100.

17. Nadler J.D., Richardson E.D., Malloy P.F. (1994)   Detection of impairment with the Mini-Mental State Examination. *Neuropsychiatry, Neuropsychol. Behav. Neurol.* **7**: 109.

18. Tombaugh T.N., McIntyre N.J. (1992)   The Mini-Mental State Examination: A comprehensive review. *J. Am. Geriatr. Soc.*, **40**: 922–935.

19. Davies P., Maloney J. (1976)   Selective loss of central cholinergic neurons in Alzheimer's disease. *Lancet*, **2**: 1403.

20. Perry E., Perry R., Blessed G., Tomlinson B. (1977)   Necropsy evidence of central cholinergic deficits in senile dementia. *Lancet*, **1**: 189.

21. Katz I.R., Sands L.P., Bilker W., DiFilippo S., Boyce A., D'Angelo K. (1998)   Identification of medications that cause cognitive impairment in older people: the case of oxybutynin chloride. *J. Am. Geriatr. Soc.*, **46**: 8–13.

22. Davis K., Mohs R. (1982) Enhancement of memory processes in Alzheimer's disease with multiple-dose intravenous physostigmine. *Am. J. Psychiatry*, **139**: 1421–1424.

23. Farlow M.R., Lahiri D.K., Poirier J., Davignon J., Schneider L., Hui S.L. (1998) Treatment outcome of tacrine therapy depends on apolipoprotein genotype and gender of the subjects with Alzheimer's disease. *Neurology*, **50**: 669–677.

24. MacGowan S.H., Wilcock G.K., Scott M. (1998) Effect of gender and lipoprotein E genotype on response to anticholinesterase therapy in Alzheimer's disease. *Int. J. Geriatr. Psychiatry*, **13**: 625–630.

25. Schneider L.S., Farlow M.R., Pogoda J.M. (1997) Potential role for estrogen replacement in the treatment of Alzheimer's dementia. *Am. J. Med.*, **103** (Suppl. 3A): 46S–50S.

26. Bryant J., Clegg A., Nicholson T., McIntyre L., De Broe S., Gerard K., Waugh N. (2001) Clinical and cost-effectiveness of donepezil, rivastigmine and galantamine for Alzheimer's disease: a rapid and systematic review. *Health Technol. Assess.*, **5**: 1–137.

27. Hill J.W., Futterman R., Mastey V., Fillit H. (2002) The effect of donepezil therapy on health costs in a Medicare managed care plan. *Manag. Care Interface*, **15**: 63–70.

28. Small G.W., Donohue J.A., Brooks R.L. (1998) An economic evaluation of donepezil in the treatment of Alzheimer's disease. *Clin. Ther.*, **20**: 838–850.

29. Getsios D., Caro J.J., Caro G., Ishak K. (2001) The AHEAD Study Group. Assessment of health economics in Alzheimer's disease (AHEAD): galantamine treatment in Canada. *Neurology*, **57**: 972–978.

30. Ikeda S., Yamada Y., Ikegami N. (2002) Economic evaluation of donepezil treatment for Alzheimer's disease in Japan. *Dement. Geriatr. Cogn. Disord.*, **13**: 33–39.

31. Hauber A.B., Gnanasakthy A., Snyder E.H., Bala M.V., Richter A., Mauskopf J.A. (2000) Potential savings in the cost of caring for Alzheimer's disease. Treatment with rivastigmine. *PharmacoEconomics*, **17**: 351–360.

32. Knopman D., Schneider L., Davis K., Talwalker S., Smith F., Hoover T., Gracon S. (1996) Long-term tacrine (Cognex) treatment: effects on nursing home placement and mortality, Tacrine Study Group. *Neurology*, **47**: 166–177.

33. Knapp M.J., Knopman D.S., Solomon P.R., Pendlebury W.W., Davis C.S., Gracon S.I. (1994) A 30-week randomized controlled trial of high-dose tacrine in patients with Alzheimer's disease. The Tacrine Study Group. *JAMA*, **271**: 985–991.

34. Farlow M.R., Brashear A., Hui S., Schneider L., Unverzagt F., for the Tacrine Study Group (1995) The effects of tacrine in patients with mild versus moderate stage Alzheimer's disease. In *Research Advances in Alzheimer's Disease and Related Disorders* (Eds K. Iqbal, J. Mortimer, B. Winblad, H. Wisniewski), pp. 284–292, Wiley, Chichester.

35. Imbimbo B.P., Lucca U., Lucchelli F., Alberoni M., Thal L.J. (1998) A 25-week placebo-controlled study of eptastigmine in patients with Alzheimer disease. *Alz. Dis. Assoc. Disord.*, **12**: 313–322.

36. Farlow M.R., Hake A., Messina J., Hartman R., Veach J., Anand R. (2001) Response of patients with Alzheimer disease to rivastigmine treatment is predicted by the rate of disease progression. *Arch. Neurol.*, **58**: 417–422.

37. Feldman H., Gauthier S., Hecker J., Vellas B., Subbiah P., Whalen E., Donepezil MSAD Study Investigators Group (2001) A 24-week, randomized, double-blind

study of donepezil in moderate to severe Alzheimer's disease. *Neurology*, **57**: 613–620.

38. Erkinjuntti T., Kurz A., Gauthier S., Bullock R., Lilienfeld S., Damaraju C.V. (2002) Efficacy of galantamine in probable vascular dementia and Alzheimer's disease combined with cerebrovascular disease: a randomised trial. *Lancet*, **359**: 1283–1290.

39. Moretti R., Torre P., Antonello R.M., Cazzato G. (2001) Rivastigmine in sub-cortical vascular dementia: a comparison trial on efficacy and tolerability for 12 months follow-up. *Eur. J. Neurol.*, **8**: 361–362.

40. Mendez M.F., Younesi F.L., Perryman K.M. (1999) Use of donepezil for vascular dementia: preliminary clinical experience. *J. Neuropsychiatry Clin. Neurosci.*, **11**: 268–270.

41. Kumar V., Anand R., Messina J., Hartman R., Veach J. (2000) An efficacy and safety analysis of Exelon in Alzheimer's disease patients with concurrent vascular risk factors. *Eur. J. Neurol.*, **7**: 159–169.

42. McKeith I.G., Grace J.B., Walker Z., Byrne E.J., Wilkinson D., Stevens T., Perry E.K. (2000) Rivastigmine in the treatment of dementia with Lewy bodies. Preliminary findings from an open trial. *Int. J. Geriatr. Psychiatry*, **15**: 387–392.

43. Maclean L.E., Collins C.C., Byrne E.J. (2001) Dementia with Lewy bodies treated with rivastigmine: effects on cognition, neuropsychiatric symptoms, and sleep. *Int. Psychogeriatr.*, **13**: 277–288.

44. Ohnishi A., Mihara M., Kamakura H., Tomono Y., Hasegawa J., Yamazaki K., Morishita N., Tanaka T. (1993) Comparison of the pharmacokinetics of E2020, a new compound for Alzheimer's disease, in healthy young and elderly subjects. *J. Clin. Pharmacol.*, **33**: 1086–1091.

45. Rogers S.L., Farlow M.R., Doody R.S., Mohs R., Friedhoff L.T. (1998) A 24-week, double-blind, placebo controlled trial of donepezil in patients with Alzheimer's disease. *Neurology*, **50**: 136–145.

46. Rogers S.L., Friedhoff L.T. (1996) The efficacy and safety of donepezil in patients with Alzheimer's disease: results of a US multicentre, randomized, double-blind placebo-controlled trial. The Donepezil Study Group. *Dementia*, 7: 293–303.

47. Rogers S.L., Doody R.S., Mohs R.C., Friedhoff L.T. (1998) Donepezil improves cognition and global function in Alzheimer disease: a 15-week, double-blind, placebo-controlled study. Donepezil Study Group. *Arch. Int. Med.*, **158**: 1021–1031.

48. Rogers S.L., Friedhoff L.T. (1998) Long-term efficacy and safety of donepezil in the treatment of Alzheimer's disease: an interim analysis of the results of a US multicentre open label extension study. *Eur. Neuropsychopharmacol.*, **8**: 67–75.

49. Burns A., Rossor M., Hecker J., Gauthier S., Petit H., Moller H., Rogers S.L., Friedhoff L.T. (1999) The effects of donepezil in Alzheimer's disease—Results from a multinational trial. *Dement. Geriatr. Cogn. Disord.*, **10**: 237–244.

50. Winblad B., Engedal K., Soininen H., Verhey F., Waldemar G., Wimo A., Wetterholm A.L., Zhang R., Haglund A., Subbiah P., Donepezil Nordic Study Group (2001) A 1-year, randomized, placebo-controlled study of donepezil in patients with mild to moderate AD. *Neurology*, **57**: 489–495.

51. Mohs R.C., Doody R.S., Morris J.C., Ieni J.R., Rogers S.L., Perdomo C.A., Pratt R.D., "312" Study Group (2001) A 1-year, placebo-controlled preservation of function survival study of donepezil in AD patients. *Neurology*, **14**: 481–488.

52. Tariot P.N., Cummings J.L., Katz I.R., Mintzer J., Perdomo C.A., Schwam E.M., Whalen E. (2001) A randomized, double-blind, placebo-controlled study of the efficacy and safety of donepezil in patients with Alzheimer's disease in the nursing home setting. *J. Am. Geriatr. Soc.*, **49**: 1590–1599.

53. Liu C., Gillette M.U. (1996) Cholinergic regulation of the suprachiasmatic nucleus circadian rhythm via a muscarinic mechanism at night. *J. Neurosci.*, **16**: 744–751.

54. O'Hara B.F., Edgar D.M., Cao V.H., Wiler S.W., Heller H.C., Kilduff T.S., Miller J.D. (1998) Nicotine and nicotinic receptors in the circadian system. *Psychoneuroendocrinology*, **23**: 161–173.

55. Riemann D., Lis S., Fritsch-Montero R., Meier T., Krieger S., Hohagen F., Berger M. (1996) Effect of tetrahydroaminoacridine on sleep in healthy subjects. *Biol. Psychiatry*, **39**: 796–802.

56. Holsboer-Trachsler E., Hatzinger M., Stohler R., Hemmeter U., Gray J., Muller J., Kocher R., Spiegel R. (1993) Effects of the novel acetylcholinesterase inhibitor SDZ ENA 713 on sleep in man. *Neuropsychopharmacology*, **8**: 87–92.

57. Riemann D., Gann H., Dressing H., Muller W.E., Aldenhoff J.B. (1994) Influence of the cholinesterase inhibitor galanthamine hydrobromide on normal sleep. *Psychiatry Res.*, **51**: 253–267.

58. Forette F., Anand R., Gharabawi G. (1999) A phase II study in patients with Alzheimer's disease to assess the preliminary efficacy and maximum tolerated dose of rivastigmine (Exeloninfinity). *Eur. J. Neurol.*, **6**: 423–429.

59. Sramek J.J., Anand R., Wardle T.S., Irwin P., Hartman R.D., Cutler N.R. (1996) Safety/tolerability trial of SDZ ENA 713 in patients with probable Alzheimer's disease. *Life Sci.*, **58**: 1201–1207.

60. Anand R., Gharabawi G., Enz A. (1996) Efficacy and safety results of the early phase studies with Exelon (ENA 713) in Alzheimer's disease: an overview. *J. Drug Dev. Clin. Pract.*, **8**: 109–116.

61. Corey-Bloom J., Anand R., Veach J. (1998) A randomized trial evaluating the efficacy and safety of ENA 713 (rivastigmine tartrate), a new acetylcholinesterase inhibitor, in patients with mild to moderately severe Alzheimer's disease. *Int. J. Geriatr. Psychopharmacol.*, **1**: 55–65.

62. Anand R., Gharabawi G. (1996) Clinical development of Exelon (ENA–713): the ADENA programme. *J. Drug Dev. Clin. Pract.*, **8**: 117–122.

63. Rosler M., Anand R., Cicin-Sain A., Gauthier S., Agid Y., Dal-Bianco P., Stahelin H.B., Hartman R., Gharabawi M. (1999) Efficacy and safety of rivastigmine in patients with Alzheimer's disease: international randomised controlled trial. *Br. Med. J.*, **318**: 633–640.

64. McKeith I., Del Ser T., Spano P., Emre M., Wesnes K., Anand R., Cicin-Sain A., Ferrara R., Spiegel R. (2000) Efficacy of rivastigmine in dementia with Lewy bodies: results of a randomised placebo-controlled international study. *Lancet*, **356**: 2031–2036.

65. Grace J., Daniel S., Stevens T., Shankar K.K., Walker Z., Byrne E.J., Butler S., Wilkinson D., Woolford J., Waite J. *et al* (2001) Long-term use of rivastigmine in patients with dementia with Lewy bodies: an open-label trial. *Int. Psychogeriatr.*, **13**: 199–205.

66. Davis K.L., Mohs R.C., Marin D., Purohit D.P., Perl D.P., Lantz M., Austin G., Haroutunian V. (1999) Cholinergic markers in elderly patients with early signs of Alzheimer disease. *JAMA*, **281**: 1401–1406.

67. Farlow M., Anand R., Messina J. Jr., Hartman R., Veach J. (2000) A 52-week study of the efficacy of rivastigmine in patients with mild to moderately severe Alzheimer's disease. *Eur. Neurol.*, **44**: 236–241.
68. Babic T., Banfic L., Papa J., Barisic N., Jelincic Z., Zurak N. (2000) Spontaneous rupture of oesophagus (Boerhaave's syndrome) related to rivastigmine. *Age Ageing*, **29**: 370–371.
69. Harvey A.L. (1995) The pharmacology of galanthamine and its analogues. *Pharmacol. Ther.*, **68**: 113–128.
70. Pacheco G., Palacios-Esquivael R., Moss D.E. (1995) Cholinesterase inhibitors proposed for treating dementia in Alzheimer's disease: selectivity toward human brain acetylcholinesterase compared with butyrylcholinesterase. *J. Pharmacol. Exp. Ther.*, **274**: 767–770.
71. Maelicke A., Coban T., Storch A., Schrattenholz A., Pereira E.F., Albuquerque E.X. (1997) Allosteric modulation of Torpedo nicotinic acetylcholine receptor ion channel activity by noncompetitive agonists. *J. Recept. Signal Transduct. Res.*, **17**: 11–28.
72. Mihailova D., Yamboliev I. (1986) Pharmacokinetics of galanthamine hydrobromide (Nivalin) following single intravenous and oral administration in rats. *Pharmacology*, **32**: 301–306.
73. Bickel U., Thomsen T., Weber W., Fischer J.P., Bachus R., Nitz M., Kewitz H. (1991) Pharmacokinetics of galanthamine in humans and corresponding cholinesterase inhibition. *Clin. Pharmacol. Ther.*, **50**: 420–428.
74. Kewitz H., Davis B.M., Katz R. (1995) Safe and efficient inhibition of acetylcholinesterase in the brain for the treatment of senile dementia of Alzheimer's type. Galanthamine versus tacrine. Presented at the First European Congress of Pharmacology, Milan, July 16–19.
75. MacPherson S. (1995) Galanthamine: the new treatment of choice in Alzheimer's disease? *Inpharma*, **1002**: 3–5.
76. Szeto T. (1994) Cholinesterase inhibitors for Alzheimer's disease: towards the next generation. *Inpharma*, **939**: 9–11.
77. Raskind M.A., Peskind E.R., Wessel T., Yuan W. (2000) Galantamine in AD: a 6-month randomized, placebo-controlled trial with a 6-month extension. The Galantamine USA-1 Study Group. *Neurology*, **54**: 2261–2268.
78. Tariot P.N., Solomon P.R., Morris J.C., Kershaw P., Lilienfeld S., Ding C. (2000) A 5-month, randomized, placebo-controlled trial of galantamine in Alzheimer's disease. *Neurology*, **54**: 2269–2276.
79. Wilcock G.K., Lilienfeld S., Gaens E. (2000) Efficacy and safety of galantamine in patients with mild to moderate Alzheimer's disease: multicentre randomised controlled trial. Galantamine International-1 Study Group. *Br. Med. J.*, **321**: 445–449.
80. Becker R.E., Colliver J.A., Markwell S.J., Moriearty P.L., Unni L.K., Vicari S. (1996) Double-blind placebo-control study of metrifonate, an acetylcholinesterase inhibitor of Alzheimer's disease. *Alz. Dis. Assoc. Disord.*, **10**: 124–131.
81. Cummings J.L., Cyrus P.A., Bieber F., Mas J., Orazem J., Gulanski B. (1998) Metrifonate treatment of the cognitive deficits of Alzheimer's disease. Metrifonate Study Group. *Neurology*, **50**: 1214–1221.
82. Karalliedde L., Henry J.A. (1993) Effects of organophosphates on skeletal muscle. *Hum. Exp. Toxicol.*, **12**: 289–296.
83. Kopman A.F., Strachovsky G., Lichtenstein L. (1978) Prolonged response to succinylcholine following physostigmine. *Anesthesiology*, **49**: 142–143.

84. Sunew K.Y., Hicks R.G. (1978) Effects of neostigmine and pyridostigmine on duration of succinylcholine action and pseudocholinesterase activity. *Anesthesiology*, **49**: 188–191.
85. Baraka A. (1977) Suxamethonium-neostigmine interaction in patients with normal or atypical cholinesterase. *Br. J. Anaesth.*, **49**: 479–484.
86. Thompson M.A. (1980) Muscle relaxant drugs. *Br. J. Hosp. Med.*, **23**: 164–179.
87. Hoffman R.S., Henry G.C., Howland M.A., Weisman R.S., Weil L., Goldfrank L.R. (1992) Association between life-threatening cocaine toxicity and plasma cholinesterase activity. *Ann. Emerg. Med.*, **21**: 247–253.
88. Schwarz M., Glick D., Lowenstein Y., Soreq H. (1995) Engineering of human cholinesterases explains and predicts diverse consequences of administration of various drugs and poisons. *Pharmacol. Ther.*, **67**: 283–322.
89. Krasowski M.D., McGehee D.S., Moss J. (1997) Natural inhibitors of cholinesterases: implications for adverse drug reactions. *Can. J. Anesth.*, **44**: 525–534.
90. Knopman D. (1998) Long-term efficacy of rivastigmine tartrate in patients with Alzheimer's disease. Presented at the American Academy of Neurology Annual Meeting, Minneapolis, April 25–May 1.
91. Truyen L. (2000) Clinical implications for galanthamine's nicotinic receptor modulation. Presented at the Springfield Symposium on Advances in Alzheimer Therapy, Stockholm, April 7.
92. Anand R., Novartis (personal communication).
93. Mintzer J., Kershaw P. (2000) Galantamine provides cognitive and functional benefits over 12 months in patients with Alzheimer's disease. Presented at the 125th Annual Meeting of the American Neurological Association, Boston, October 15–18.
94. Perry E.K., Morris C.M., Court J.A., Cheng A., Fairbairn A.F., McKeith I.G., Irving D., Brown A., Perry R.H. (1995) Alteration in nicotine binding sites in Parkinson's disease, Lewy body dementia and Alzheimer's disease: possible index of early neuropathology. *Neuroscience*, **64**: 385–395.
95. Salomon A.R., Marcinowski K.J., Friedland R.P., Zagorski M.G. (1996) Nicotine inhibits amyloid formation by the beta-peptide. *Biochemistry*, **35**: 13568–13578.
96. Kim S.H., Kim Y.K., Jeong S.J. Haass C. (1997) Enhanced release of secreted form of Alzheimer's amyloid precursor protein from PC12 cells by nicotine. *Mol. Pharmacol.*, **52**: 430–436.
97. Kihara T., Shimohama S., Sawada H., Kimura J., Kume T., Kochiyama H., Maeda T., Akaike A. (1997) Nicotinic receptor stimulation protects neurons against beta-amyloid toxicity. *Ann. Neurol.*, **42**: 159–163.
98. Kihara T., Shimohama S., Akaike A. (1999) Effects of nicotinic receptor agonists on beta-amyloid beta-sheet formation. *Jpn. J. Pharmacol.*, **79**: 393–396.
99. Haroutunian V., Greig N., Pei X.F., Utsuki T., Gluck R., Acevedo L.D., Davis K.L., Wallace W.C. (1997) Pharmacological modulation of Alzheimer's beta-amyloid precursor protein levels in the CSF of rats with forebrain cholinergic system lesions. *Brain Res. Mol. Brain Res.*, **46**: 161–168.
100. Svensson A.L., Nordberg A. (1998) Tacrine and donepezil attenuate the neurotoxic effect of A beta (25–35) in rat PC12 cells. *Neuroreport*, **9**: 1519–1522.
101. Lahiri D.K., Farlow M.R., Sambamurti K. (1998) The secretion of amyloid beta-peptides is inhibited in the tacrine-treated human neuroblastoma cells. *Brain Res. Mol. Brain Res.*, **62**: 131–140.
102. Alvarez A., Alarcon R., Opazo C., Campos E.O., Munoz F.J., Calderon F.H., Dajas F., Gentry M.K., Doctor B.P., De Mello F.G. *et al* (1998) Stable com-

plexes involving acetylcholinesterase and amyloid-beta peptide change the biochemical properties of the enzyme and increase the neurotoxicity of Alzheimer's fibrils. *J. Neurosci.*, **18**: 3213–3223.
103. Zhang W., Johnson B.R., Bjornsson T.D. (1997) Pharmacologic inhibition of transglutaminase-induced cross-linking of Alzheimer's amyloid beta-peptide. *Life Sci.*, **60**: 2323–2332.
104. Pike C.J., Cotman C.W. (1996) Beta-amyloid neurotoxicity in vitro: examination of potential contributions from oxidative pathways. Presented at the Osaka Fifth International Conference on Alzheimer's disease, July 24–29.
105. Jackson C.V., Holland A.J., Williams C.A., Dikerson J.W. (1998) Vitamin E and Alzheimer's disease in subjects with Down's syndrome. *J. Ment. Defic. Res.*, **32**: 479–484.
106. Metcalfe T., Bowen D.M., Muller D.P.R. (1989) Vitamin E and Alzheimer's disease in subjects with Down's syndrome, centenarians and controls. *Neurochem. Res.*, **14**: 1209–1212.
107. Adams J.D., Klaidman L.K., Odunze I.N., Shen H.C., Miller C.A. (1991) Alzheimer's and Parkinson's disease brain levels of glutathione, glutathione disulfide and Vitamin E. *Mol. Chem. Neuropathol.*, **14**: 213–226.
108. Behl C., Davis J., Cole G.M., Schubert D. (1992) Vitamin E protects nerve cells from amyloid-β protein toxicity. *Biochem. Biophys. Res. Commun.*, **186**: 944–950.
109. Sano M., Ernesto C., Thomas R.G., Klauber M.R., Schafer K., Grundman M., Woodbury P., Growdon J., Cotman C.W., Pfeiffer E. *et al* (1997) A controlled trial of selegiline, alpha-tocopherol, or both as treatment for Alzheimer's disease. *N. Engl. J. Med.*, **336**: 1216–1222.
110. Roberts H.J. (1978) Vitamin E and thrombophlebitis. *Lancet*, **1**: 49.
111. Hansten P.D., Horn J.R. (1989) *Drug Interactions*, Lea and Febiger, Philadelphia.
112. Corrigan J.J., Ulfers L.L. (1981) Effect of vitamin E on prothrombin levels in warfarin-induced vitamin K deficiency. *Am. J. Clin. Nutr.*, **34**: 1701–1705.
113. Corrigan J.J., Marcus F.I. (1974) Coagulopathy associated with vitamin E ingestion. *JAMA*, **230**: 1300–1301.
114. Alpha-Tocopherol, Beta Carotene Cancer Prevention Study Group (1994) The effects of vitamin E and beta carotene on the incidence of lung cancer and other cancers in male smokers. *N. Engl. J. Med.*, **330**: 1029–1035.
115. Olanow C.W. (1996) Selegiline: current perspectives on issues related to neuroprotection and mortality. *Neurology*, **47** (Suppl. 3): S210–S216.
116. Sternbach H. (1991) The serotonin syndrome. *Am. J. Psychiatry*, **148**: 705–713.
117. Spiker D.G., Pugh D.D. (1976) Combining tricyclic and monoamine oxidase inhibitor antidepressants. *Arch. Gen. Psychiatry*, **33**: 828–830.
118. Insel T.R., Roy B.F., Cohen R.M., Murphy D.L. (1982) Possible development of the serotonin syndrome in man. *Am. J. Psychiatry*, **139**: 954–955.
119. Brachfeld J., Wirtshafter A., Wolfe S. (1963) Imipramine-tranylcypromine incompatibility. Near fatal toxic reaction. *JAMA*, **186**: 1172.
120. Feighner J.P., Boyer W.F., Tyler D.L., Neborsky R.J. (1990) Adverse consequences of fluoxetine–MAOI combination therapy. *J. Clin. Psychiatry*, **51**: 222–225.
121. Product Information: *Zyban (R), bupropion.* Glaxo Wellcome Inc., Research Triangle Park, 1998.
122. Product Information: *BuSpar (R), buspirone.* Bristol-Myers Squibb Company, Princeton, 1998.

123. Aisen P.S., Davis K.L. (1994) Inflammatory mechanisms in Alzheimer's disease: implications for therapy. *Am. J. Psychiatry*, **151**: 1105–1113.
124. Buxbaum J.D., Oishi M., Chen H.I., Pinkas-Kramarski R., Jaffe E.A., Gandy S.E., Greengard P. (1992) Cholinergic agonists and interleukin 1 regulate processing and secretion of Alzheimer's β/A4 protein precursor. *Proc. Natl. Acad. Sci. USA*, **89**: 10075–10078.
125. Campbell I.L., Abraham C.R., Masliah E., Kemper P., Inglis J.D., Oldstone M.B., Mucke L. (1993) Neurologic disease induced in transgenic mice by cerebral overexpression of interleukin 6. *Proc. Natl. Acad. Sci. USA*, **90**: 10061–10065.
126. Bauer J., Strauss S., Schreiter-Gasser U. (1991) Interleukin-6 and alpha-2-macroglobulin indicate an acute phase response in Alzheimer's disease cortices. *FEBS Lett.*, **285**: 111–114.
127. Eikelenboom P., Hack C.E., Rozemuller J.M., Stam F.C. (1989) Complement activation in amyloid plaques in Alzheimer's dementia. *Virchows Arch. B Cell Pathol. Incl. Mol. Pathol.*, **56**: 259–262.
128. Bergamaschini L., Canziani S., Bottasso B., Cugno M., Braidotti P., Agostoni A. (1999) Alzheimer's beta-amyloid peptides can activate the early components of complement classical pathway in a C1q-independent manner. *Clin. Exp. Immunol.*, **115**: 526–533.
129. Webster S., O'Barr S., Rogers J. (1994) Enhanced aggregation and beta structure of amyloid beta peptide after coincubation with C1q. *J. Neurosci. Res.*, **89**: 448–456.
130. Rozenmuller J.M., van der Valk P., Eikelenboom P. (1992) Activated microglia and cerebral amyloid deposits in Alzheimer's disease. *Res. Immunol.*, **143**: 646–649.
131. Giulian D., Li J., Li X., George J., Rutecki P.A. (1994) The impact of microglia derived cytokines upon gliosis in the CNS. *Dev. Neurosci.*, **16**: 128–136.
132. McGeer P.L., Schulzer M. McGeer E.G. (1996) Arthritis and anti-inflammatory agents as possible protective factors for Alzheimer's disease: a review of 17 epidemiological studies. *Neurology*, **47**: 425–432.
133. Breitner J.C., Welsh K.A., Helms M.J., Gaskell P.C., Gau B.A., Roses A.D., Pericak-Vance M.A., Saunders A.M. (1995) Delayed onset of Alzheimer's disease with nonsteroidal anti-inflammatory and histamine H2 blocking drugs. *Neurobiol. Aging*, **16**: 523–530.
134. Stewart W.F., Kawas C., Corrada M., Metter E.J. (1997) Risk of Alzheimer's disease and duration of NSAID use. *Neurology*, **48**: 626–632.
135. Aisen P.S., Luddy A., Durner M., Reinhard J.F. Jr., Pasinetti G.M. (1998) HLA-DR4 influences glial activity in Alzheimer's disease hippocampus. *J. Neurol. Sci.*, **161**: 66–69.
136. Curran M., Middleton D., Edwardson J., Perry R., McKeith I., Morris C., Neill D. (1997) HLA-DR antigens associated with major genetic risk for late-onset Alzheimer's disease. *Neuroreport*, **8**: 1467–1469.
137. Rogers J., Kirby L.C., Hempelman S.R., Berry D.L., McGeer P.L., Kaszniak A.W., Zalinski J., Cofield M., Mansukhani L., Willson P. *et al* (1993) Clinical trial of indomethacin in Alzheimer's disease. *Neurology*, **43**: 1609–1611.
138. Scharf S., Mander A., Ugoni A., Vajda F., Christophidis N. (1999) A double-blind, placebo-controlled trial of diclofenac/misoprostol in Alzheimer's disease. *Neurology*, **53**: 197–201.
139. Ho L., Pieroni C., Winger D., Purohit D.P., Aisen P.S., Pasinetti G.M. (1999) Regional distribution of cyclooxygenase-2 in the hippocampal formation in Alzheimer's disease. *J. Neurosci. Res.*, **57**: 295–303.

140. Ho L., Osaka H., Aisen P.S., Pasinetti G.M. (1998)  Induction of cyclooxygenase (COX)-2 but not COX-1 gene expression in apoptotic cell death. *J. Neuroimmunol.*, **89**: 142–149.

141. Weggen S., Eriksen J.L., Das P., Sagi S.A., Wang R., Pietrzik C.U., Findlay K.A., Smith T.E., Murphy M.P., Bulter T. *et al* (2001) A subset of NSAIDs lower amyloidogenic Abeta42 independently of cyclooxygenase activity. *Nature*, **414**: 212–216.

142. Aisen P.S., Marin D.B., Brickman A.M., Santoro J., Fusco M. (2001) Pilot tolerability studies of hydroxychloroquine and colchicine in Alzheimer disease. *Alz. Dis. Assoc. Disord.*, **15**: 96–101.

143. Aisen P.S., Schmeidler J., Pasinetti G.M. (2002) Randomized pilot study of nimesulide treatment in Alzheimer's disease. *Neurology*, **58**: 1050–1054.

144. Aisen P.S., Schafer K., Grundman M., Farlow M., Sano M., Jin S., Thomas R., Thal L., for the Alzheimer's Disease Cooperative Study (2002) Results of a multicenter trial of Rofecoxib and Naproxen in Alzheimer's disease. Presented at the 8th International Conference on Alzheimer's Disease and Related Disorders, Stockholm, July 20–25.

145. Aisen P.S., Davis K.L., Berg J., Schafer K., Campbell K., Thomas R.G., Weiner M.F., Farlow M.R., Sano M., Grundman M. *et al* (2000) A randomized controlled trial of prednisone in Alzheimer's disease. *Neurology*, **54**: 588–593.

146. Aisen P.S. (1997)  Inflammation and Alzheimer's disease: mechanisms and therapeutic strategies. *Gerontology*, **43**: 143–149.

147. Van Horn G., Arnett F.C., Dimachkie M.M. (1996)  Reversible dementia and chorea in a young woman with the lupus anticoagulant. *Neurology*, **46**: 1599–1603.

148. Marcusson J., Rother M., Kittner B., Rossner M., Smith R.J., Babic T., Folnegovic-Smalc V., Moller H.J., Labs K.H. (1997)  A 12-month, randomized, placebo-controlled trial of propentofylline (HWA 285) in patients with dementia according to DSM III-R. The European Propentofylline Study Group. *Dement. Geriatr. Cogn. Disord.*, **8**: 320–328.

149. Kittner B., Rossner M., Rother M. (1997)  Clinical trials in dementia with propentofylline. *Ann. N. Y. Acad. Sci.*, **826**: 307–316.

150. Rother M., Erkinjuntti T., Rossner M., Kittner B., Marcusson J., Karlsson I. (1998)  Propentofylline in the treatment of Alzheimer's disease and vascular dementia: a review of phase III trials. *Dement. Geriatr. Cogn. Disord.*, **9** (Suppl. 1): 36–43.

151. Kittner B. (1999) Clinical trials of propentofylline in vascular dementia. European/Canadian Propentofylline Study Group. *Alz. Dis. Assoc. Disord.*, **13** (Suppl. 3): S166–S171.

152. Marquis D. (1999)  How to resolve an ethical dilemma concerning randomized clinical trials. *N. Eng. J. Med.*, **341**: 691–693.

153. Segarra A.C., McEwen B.S. (1991)  Estrogen increases spine density in ventromedial hypothalamic neurons of peripubertal rats. *Neuroendocrinology*, **54**: 365–372.

154. Beyer C. (1999)  Estrogen and the developing mammalian brain. *Anat. Embryol.*, **199**: 379–390.

155. Mong J.A., McCarthy M.M. (1999)  Steroid-induced developmental plasticity in hypothalamic astrocytes: implications for synaptic patterning. *J. Neurobiol.*, **40**: 602–619.

156. Matsumoto A., Arai Y. (1981)  Neuronal plasticity in the deafferented hypothalamic arcuate nucleus of adult female rats and its enhancement by treatment with estrogen. *J. Comp. Neurol.*, **197**: 197–205.

157. Sibug R.M., Stumpf W.E., Shughrue P.J., Hochberg R.B., Drews U. (1991)  Distribution of estrogen target sites in the 2-day-old mouse forebrain and pituitary gland during the "critical period" of sexual differentiation. *Brain Res. Dev. Brain Res.*, **61**: 11–22.

158. Toran-Allerand C.D., Singh M., Setalo G., Jr. (1999)  Novel mechanisms of estrogen action in the brain: new players in an old story. *Front. Neuroendocrinol.*, **20**: 97–121.

159. Schneider L.S., Farlow M.R., Pogoda J.M. (1997)  Potential role for estrogen replacement in the treatment of Alzheimer's dementia. *Am. J. Med.*, **103** (Suppl. 3A): 46S–50S.

160. Blurton-Jones M.M., Roberts J.A., Tuszynski M.H. (1999)  Estrogen receptor immunoreactivity in the adult primate brain: neuronal distribution and association with p75, trkA, and choline acetyltransferase. *J. Comp. Neurol.*, **405**: 529–542.

161. Gibbs R.B., Aggarwal P. (1998)  Estrogen and basal forebrain cholinergic neurons: implications for brain aging and Alzheimer's disease-related cognitive decline. *Horm. Behav.*, **34**: 98–111.

162. Luine V., Park D., Joh T., Reis D., McEwen B. (1980)  Immunochemical demonstration of increased choline acetyltransferase concentration in rat preoptic area after estradiol administration. *Brain Res.*, **191**: 273–277.

163. Luine V.N. (1985)  Estradiol increases choline acetyltransferase activity in specific basal forebrain nuclei and projection areas of female rats. *Exp. Neurol.*, **89**: 484–490.

164. Nathan L., Chaudhuri G. (1998)  Antioxidant and prooxidant actions of estrogens: potential physiological and clinical implications. *Semin. Reprod. Endocrinol.*, **16**: 309–314.

165. Inestrosa N.C., Marzolo M.P., Bonnefont A.B. (1998)  Cellular and molecular basis of estrogen's neuroprotection. Potential relevance for Alzheimer's disease. *Mol. Neurobiol.*, **17**: 73–86.

166. Teng E.L., Chui H.C. (1987)  The modified Mini-mental State (3MS) examination. *J. Clin. Psychiatry*, **48**: 314–318.

167. Steffans D.C., Norton M.C., Plassman B.L., Tschanz J.T., Wyse B.W., Welsh-Bohmer K.A., Anthony J.C., Breitner J.C.S. (1999)  *J. Am. Geriatr. Soc.*, **47**: 1171–1175.

168. Matthews K.A., Kuller L.H., Wing R.R., Meilahn E.N., Plantinga P. (1996)  Prior to use of estrogen replacement therapy, are users healthier than nonusers? *Am. J. Epidemiol.*, **143**: 971–978.

169. Sherwin B.B. (1988)  Estrogen and cognitive functioning in surgically menopausal women. *Psychoneuroendocrinology*, **10**: 325–335.

170. Sherwin B.B., Philips S. (1990)  Estrogen and cognitive functioning in surgically postmenopausal women. *Ann. N.Y. Acad. Sci.*, **592**: 474–475.

171. Philips S., Sherwin B.B. (1992)  Effects of estrogen on memory function in surgically menopausal women. *Psychoneuroendocrinology*, **17**: 485–495.

172. Robinson D., Friedman L., Marcus R., Tinklenberg J., Yesavage J. (1994)  Estrogen replacement therapy and memory in older women. *J. Ann. Geriatr. Soc.*, **42**: 919–922.

173. Kampen D.L., Sherwin B.B. (1994)  Estrogen use and verbal memory in healthy postmenopausal women. *Obstet. Gynecol.*, **83**: 979–983.

174. Barrett-Connor E., Kritz-Silverstein D. (1993) Estrogen replacement therapy and cognitive function in older women. *JAMA*, **269**: 2637–2641.
175. Mortel K.F., Meyer J.S. (1995) Lack of postmenopausal replacement therapy and the risk of dementia. *J. Neuropsychiatry Clin. Neurosci.*, **7**: 334–337.
176. Paganini-Hill A., Henderson V.W. (1996) Estrogen replacement therapy and risk of Alzheimer disease. *Arch. Intern. Med.*, **156**: 2213–2217.
177. Kawas C., Brookmeyer R., Corrada M., Zonderman A., Bacal C., Lingle D.D., Metter E. (1997) A prospective study of estrogen replacement therapy and the risk of developing Alzheimer's disease: the Baltimore Longitudinal Study of Aging. *Neurology*, **48**: 1517–1521.
178. Baldereschi M., Di Carlo A., Lepore V., Bracco L., Maggi S., Grigoletto F., Scarlato G., Amaducci L. (1998) Estrogen-replacement therapy and Alzheimer's disease in the Italian Longitudinal Study on Aging. *Neurology*, **50**: 996–1002.
179. Tang M.X., Jacobs D., Stern Y., Marder K., Schofield P., Gurland B., Andrews H., Mayeux R. (1996) Effect of oestrogen during menopause on risk and age at onset of Alzheimer's disease. *Lancet*, **348**: 429–432.
180. Asthana S., Craft S., Baker L.D., Raskind M.A., Birnbaum R.S., Lofgreen C.P., Veith R.C., Plymate S.R. (1999) Cognitive and neuroendocrine response to transdermal estrogen in postmenopausal women with Alzheimer's disease: results of a placebo-controlled, double-blind, pilot study. *Psychoneuroendocrinology*, **24**: 657–677.
181. Mulnard R.A., Cotman C.W., Kawas C., van Dyck C.H., Sano M., Doody R., Koss E., Pfeiffer E., Jin S., Gamst A. *et al* (2000) Estrogen replacement therapy for treatment of mild to moderate Alzheimer disease: a randomized controlled trial. Alzheimer's Disease Cooperative Study. *JAMA*, **283**: 1007–1015.
182. Shumaker S.A., Reboussin B.A., Espeland M.A., Rapp S.R., McBee W.L., Dailey M., Bowen D., Terrell T., Jones B.N. (1998) The Women's Health Initiative Memory Study: a trial of the effect of estrogen therapy in preventing and slowing the progression of dementia. *Control. Clin. Trials*, **19**: 604–621.
183. Prelevic G.M., Jacobs H.S. (1997) New developments in postmenopausal hormone replacement therapy. *Curr. Opin. Obstet. Gynecol.*, **9**: 207–212.
184. Genazzani A.R., Spinetti A., Gallo R., Bernardi F. (1999) Menopause and the central nervous system: intervention options. *Maturitas*, **31**: 103–110.
185. Curtis M.G. (1999) Selective estrogen receptor modulators: a contoversial approach for managing postmenopausal health. *J. Women's Health*, **8**: 321–333.
186. Lacey J.V. Jr., Mink P.J., Lubin J.H., Sherman M.E., Troisi R., Hartge P., Schatzkin A., Schairer C. (2002) Menopausal hormone replacement therapy and risk of ovarian cancer. *JAMA*, **288**: 334–341.
187. American Psychiatric Association (1997) Practice guidelines for the treatment of patients with Alzheimer's disease and other dementias of the late life. *Am. J. Psychiatry*, **154** (Suppl.)
188. Lebowitz B.D., Pearson J.L., Schneider L.S., Reynolds C.F. III, Alexopoulos G.S., Bruce M.L., Conwell Y., Katz I.R., Meyers B.S., Monison M.F. *et al* (1997) Diagnosis and treatment of depression in late life. Consensus statement update. *JAMA*, **278**: 1186–1190.
189. Burns A. (1991) Affective symptoms in Alzheimer's disease. *Int. J. Geriatr. Psychiatry*, **6**: 371–376.
190. Harris M.J., Gierz M., Lohr J.B. (1989) Recognition and treatment of depression in Alzheimer's disease. *Geriatrics*, **44**: 26–30.

191. Benedict K.B., Nacoste D.B. (1990)   Dementia and depression in the elderly: a framework for addressing difficulties in differential diagnosis. *Clin. Psychol. Rev.*, **10**: 513–537.

192. Meyers B.S., Mei-Tal V. (1983)   Psychiatric reactions during tricyclic treatment of the elderly reconsidered. *J. Clin. Psychopharmacol.*, **3**: 2–6.

193. Taragano F.E., Lyketsos C.G., Mangone C.A., Allegri R.F., Comesana-Diaz E. (1997)   A double-blind, randomized, fixed-dose trial of fluoxetine vs. amitriptyline in the treatment of major depression complicating Alzheimer's disease. *Psychosomatics*, **38**: 246–252.

194. Petracca G., Teson A., Chemerinski E., Leiguarda R., Starkstein S.E. (1996)   A double-blind placebo-controlled study of clomipramine in depressed patients with Alzheimer's disease. *J. Neuropsychiatry Clin. Neurosci.*, **8**: 270–275.

195. Teri L., Reifler B.V., Veith R.C., Barnes R., White E., McLean P., Raskind M. (1991)   Imipramine in the treatment of depressed Alzheimer's patients: impact on cognition. *J. Gerontol.*, **46**: P372–P377.

196. Burke W.J., Dewan V., Wengel S.P., Roccaforte W.H., Nadolny G.C., Folks D.G. (1997)   The use of selective serotonin reuptake inhibitors for depression and psychosis complicating dementia. *Int. J. Geriatr. Psychiatry*, **12**: 519–525.

197. Gottfries C.G., Karlsson I., Nyth A.L. (1992)   Treatment of depression in elderly patients with and without dementia disorders. *Int. Clin. Psychopharmacol.*, **6** (Suppl. 5): 55–64.

198. Olafsson K., Jorgensen S., Jensen H.V., Bille A., Arup P., Andersen J. (1992)   Fluvoxamine in the treatment of demented elderly patients: a double-blind, placebo-controlled study. *Acta Psychiatr. Scand.*, **85**: 453–456.

199. Steffens D.C., Krishnan K.R., Helms M.J. (1997)   Are SSRIs better than TCAs? Comparison of SSRIs and TCAs: a meta-analysis. *Depress. Anxiety*, **6**: 10–18.

200. Pollock B.G., Mulsant B.H., Nebes R., Kirshner M.A., Begley A.E., Mazumdar S., Reynolds C.F. III (1988)   Serum anticholinergicity in elderly depressed patients treated with paroxetine or nortriptyline. *Am. J. Psychiatry*, **155**: 1110–1112.

201. Amrein R., Martin J.R., Cameron A.M. (1999)   Moclobemide in patients with dementia and depression. *Adv. Neurol.*, **80**: 509–519.

202. Nair N.P., Amin M., Holm P., Katona C., Klitgaard N., Ng Ying Kin N.M., Kragh-Sørensen P., Kuhn H., Leek C.A., Stage K.B. (1995)   Moclobemide and nortriptyline in elderly depressed patients. A randomized, multicentre trial against placebo. *J. Affect. Disord.*, **33**: 1–9.

203. Hirschfeld R.M. (1999)   Efficacy of SSRIs and newer antidepressants in severe depression: comparison with TCAs. *J. Clin. Psychiatry*, **60**: 326–335.

204. Pollock B.G. (1999)   Adverse reactions of antidepressants in elderly patients. *J. Clin. Psychiatry*, **60** (Suppl. 20): 4–8.

205. Salzman C. (1999)   Practical considerations for the treatment of depression in elderly and very elderly long-term care patients. *J. Clin. Psychiatry*, **60** (Suppl. 20): 30–33.

206. Georgotas A., McCue R.E., Cooper T.B., Nagachandran N., Friedhoff A. (1989)   Factors affecting the delay of antidepressant effect in responders to nortriptyline and phenelzine. *Psychiatry Res.*, **28**: 1–9.

207. Price T.R., McAllister T.W. (1989)   Safety and efficacy of ECT in depressed patients with dementia: a review of clinical experience. *Convulsive Ther.*, **5**: 1–74.

208. American Psychiatric Association Task Force on ECT (1990) *The Practice of ECT: Recommendations for Treatment, Training and Privileging.* American Psychiatric Press, Washington, DC.
209. Sackeim H.A., Prudic J., Devanand D.P., Kiersky J.E., Fitzsimons L., Moody B.J., McElhiney M.C., Coleman E.A., Settembrino J.M. (1993) Effects of stimulus intensity and electrode placement on the efficacy and cognitive effects of electroconvulsive therapy. *N. Engl. J. Med.*, **328**: 839–846.
210. Devanand D.P., Marder K., Michaels K.S., Sackeim H.A., Bell K., Sullivan M.A., Cooper T.B., Pelton G.H., Mayeux R. (1998) A randomized, placebo-controlled dose-comparison trial of haloperidol for psychosis and disruptive behaviors in Alzheimer's disease. *Am. J. Psychiatry*, **155**: 1512–1520.
211. Katz I.R., Jeste D.V., Mintzer J.E., Clyde C., Napolitano J., Brecher M. (1999) Comparison of risperidone and placebo for psychosis and behavioural disturbances associated with dementia: a randomized, double-blind trial. Risperidone Study Group. *J. Clin. Psychiatry*, **60**: 107–115.
212. Street J.S., Clark W.S., Gannon K.S., Cummings J.L., Bymaster F.P., Tamura R.N., Mitan S.J., Kadam D.L., Sanger T.M., Feldman P.D. *et al* (2000) Olanzapine treatment of psychotic and behavioral symptoms in patients with Alzheimer disease in nursing care facilities: a double-blind, randomized, placebo-controlled trial. The HGEU Study Group. *Arch. Gen. Psychiatry*, **57**: 968–976.
213. Tariot P.N., Salzman C., Yeung P.P., Pultz J., Rak I.W. (2000) Long-term use of quetiapine in elderly patients with psychotic disorders. *Clin. Ther.*, **22**: 1068–1084.
214. Schneider L.S., Tariot P.N., Lyketsos C.G., Dagerman K.S., Davis K.L., Davis S., Hsiao J.K., Jeste D.V., Katz I.R., Olin J.T. *et al* (2001) National Institute of Mental Health Clinical Antipsychotic Trials of Intervention Effectiveness (CATIE): Alzheimer disease trial methodology. *Am. J. Geriatr. Psychiatry*, **9**: 346–360.
215. Cummings J.L. (2000) The role of cholinergic agents in the management of behavioural disturbances in Alzheimer's disease. *Int. J. Neuropsychopharmacol.*, **3**: 21–29.
216. Raskind M.A., Sadowsky C.H., Sigmund W.R., Beitler P.J., Auster S.B. (1997) Effect of tacrine on language, praxis, and noncognitive behavioural problems in Alzheimer disease. *Arch. Neurol.*, **54**: 836–840.
217. Qizilbash N., Whitehead A., Higgins J., Wilcock G., Schneider L., Farlow M. (1998) Cholinesterase inhibition for Alzheimer disease: a meta-analysis of the tacrine trials. Dementia Trialists' Collaboration. *JAMA*, **280**: 1777–1782.
218. Kaufer D. (1998) Beyond the cholinergic hypothesis: the effect of metrifonate and other cholinesterase inhibitors on neuropsychiatric symptoms in Alzheimer's disease. *Dement. Geriatr. Cogn. Disord.*, **9** (Suppl. 2): 8–14.
219. Cummings J.L., Donohue J.A., Brooks R.L. (2000) The relationship between donepezil and behavioral disturbances in patients with Alzheimer's disease. *Am. J. Geriatr. Psychiatry*, **8**: 134–140.
220. Reading P.J., Luce A.K., McKeith I.G. (2001) Rivastigmine in the treatment of parkinsonian psychosis and cognitive impairment: preliminary findings from an open trial. *Mov. Disord.*, **16**: 1171–1174.
221. Olin J., Schneider L. (2001) Galantamine for Alzheimer's disease. *Cochrane Database Syst. Rev.*, 4: CD001747.
222. Schenk D., Barbour R., Dunn W., Gordon G., Grajeda H., Guido T., Hu K., Huang J., Johnson-Wood K., Khan K. *et al* (1999) Immunization with amyloid-

beta attenuates Alzheimer-disease-like pathology in the PDAPP mouse. *Nature*, **400**: 173–177.

223. Arendash G.W., Gordon M.N., Diamond D.M., Austin L.A., Hatcher J.M., Jantzen P., DiCarlo G., Wilcock D., Morgan D. (2001) Behavioral assessment of Alzheimer's transgenic mice following long-term Abeta vaccination: task specificity and correlations between Abeta deposition and spatial memory. *DNA Cell. Biol.*, **20**: 737–744.

224. Munch G., Robinson S.R. (2002) Potential neurotoxic inflammatory responses to Abeta vaccination in humans. *J. Neural Transm.*, **109**: 1081–1087.

225. Le Bars P.L., Katz M.M., Berman N., Itil T.M., Freedman A.M., Schatzberg A.F. (1997) A placebo-controlled, double-blind, randomized trial of an extract of Ginkgo biloba for dementia. North American EGb Study Group. *JAMA*, **278**: 1327–1332.

226. Le Bars P.L., Kieser M., Itil K.Z. (2000) A 26-week analysis of a double-blind, placebo-controlled trial of the ginkgo biloba extract EGb 761 in dementia. *Dement. Geriatr. Cogn. Disord.*, **11**: 230–237.

227. van Dongen M.C., van Rossum E., Kessels A.G., Sielhorst H.J., Knipschild P.G. (2000) The efficacy of ginkgo for elderly people with dementia and age-associated memory impairment: new results of a randomized clinical trial. *J. Am. Geriatr. Soc.*, **48**: 1183–1194.

228. Wolozin B., Kellman W., Ruosseau P., Celesia G.G., Siegel G. (2000) Decreased prevalence of Alzheimer disease associated with 3-hydroxy-3-methyglutaryl coenzyme A reductase inhibitors. *Arch. Neurol.*, **57**: 1439–1443.

229. Jick H., Zornberg G.L., Jick S.S., Seshadri S., Drachman D.A. (2000) Statins and the risk of dementia. *Lancet*, **356**: 1627–1631.

230. Yaffe K., Barrett-Connor E., Lin F., Grady D. (2002) Serum lipoprotein levels, statin use, and cognitive function in older women. *Arch. Neurol.*, **59**: 378–384.

231. Rockwood K., Kirkland S., Hogan D.B., MacKnight C., Merry H., Verreault R., Wolfson C., McDowell I. (2002) Use of lipid-lowering agents, indication bias, and the risk of dementia in community-dwelling elderly people. *Arch. Neurol.*, **59**: 223–227.

232. Green R.C., McNagny S.E., Jayakumar P., Cupples L.A., Benke K., Farrer L. (2002) Statin use is associated with reduced risk of Alzheimer's disease. Presented at the 8th International Conference on Alzheimer's Disease and Related Disorders, Stockholm, July 20–25.

233. Fassbender K., Simons M., Bergmann C., Stroick M., Lutjohann D., Keller P., Runz H., Kuhl S., Bertsch T., von Bergmann K. *et al* (2001) Simvastatin strongly reduces levels of Alzheimer's disease beta-amyloid peptides Abeta 42 and Abeta 40 in vitro and in vivo. *Proc. Natl. Acad. Sci. USA*, **98**: 5856–5861.

234. Dovey H.F., John V., Anderson J.P., Chen L.Z., de Saint Andrieu P., Fang L.Y., Freedman S.B., Folmer B., Goldbach E., Holsztynska E.J. *et al* (2001) Functional gamma-secretase inhibitors reduce beta-amyloid peptide levels in brain. *J. Neurochem.*, **76**: 173–181.

235. Vassar R., Bennett B.D., Babu-Khan S., Kahn S., Mendiaz E.A., Denis P., Teplow D.B., Ross S., Amarante P., Loeloff R. *et al* (1999) Beta-secretase cleavage of Alzheimer's amyloid precursor protein by the transmembrane aspartic protease BACE. *Science*, **286**: 735–741.

236. Xia W., Zhang J., Perez R., Koo E.H., Selkoe D.J. (1997) Interaction between amyloid precursor protein and presenilins in mammalian cells: implications

for the pathogenesis of Alzheimer disease. *Proc. Natl. Acad. Sci. USA*, **94**: 8208–8213.

237. Flaherty D.B., Soria J.P., Tomasiewicz H.G., Wood J.G. (2000) Phosphorylation of human tau protein by microtubule-associated kinases: GSK3beta and cdk5 are key participants. *J. Neurosci. Res.*, **62**: 463–472.

238. Sang H., Lu Z., Li Y., Ru B., Wang W., Chen J. (2001) Phosphorylation of tau by glycogen synthase kinase 3beta in intact mammalian cells influences the stability of microtubules. *Neurosci. Lett.*, **312**: 141–144.

239. Chen G., Huang L.D., Jiang Y.M., Manji H.K. (1999) The mood-stabilizing agent valproate inhibits the activity of glycogen synthase kinase-3. *J. Neurochem.*, **72**: 1327–1330.

240. Martinez A., Alonso M., Castro A., Perez C., Moreno F.J. (2002) First non-ATP competitive glycogen synthase kinase 3 beta (GSK-3beta) inhibitors: thiadiazolidinones (TDZD) as potential drugs for the treatment of Alzheimer's disease. *J. Med. Chem.*, **45**: 1292–1299.

241. Clarke R., Smith A.D., Jobst K.A., Refsum H., Sutton L., Ueland P.M. (1998) Folate, vitamin B12, and serum total homocysteine levels in confirmed Alzheimer disease. *Arch. Neurol.*, **55**: 1449–1455.

242. Vermeer S.E., van Dijk E.J., Koudstaal P.J., Oudkerk M., Hofman A., Clarke R., Breteler M.M. (2002) Homocysteine, silent brain infarcts, and white matter lesions: The Rotterdam Scan Study. *Ann. Neurol.*, **51**: 285–289.

243. Seshadri S., Beiser A., Selhub J., Jacques P.F., Rosenberg I.H., D'Agostino R.B., Wilson P.W., Wolf P.A. (2002) Plasma homocysteine as a risk factor for dementia and Alzheimer's disease. *N. Engl. J. Med.*, **346**: 476–483.

244. Miller J.W., Green R., Mungas D.M., Reed B.R., Jagust W.J. (2002) Homocysteine, vitamin B6, and vascular disease in AD patients. *Neurology*, **58**: 1471–1475.

245. Perry E.K., Haroutunian V., Davis K.L., Levy R., Lantos P., Eagger S., Honavar M., Dean A., Griffiths M., McKeith I.G., *et al* (1994) Neocortical cholinergic activities differentiate Lewy body dementia from classical Alzheimer's disease. *Neuroreport*, **15**: 747–749.

246. Lebert F. (1998) Tacrine efficacy in Lewy body dementia. *Int. J. Geriatr. Psychiatry*, **13**: 516–519.

247. McKeith I.G., Perry E.K., Perry R.H. (1999) Report of the second dementia with Lewy body international workshop: diagnosis and treatment. Consortium on Dementia with Lewy Bodies. *Neurology*, **53**: 902–905.

248. Walker Z., Grace J., Overshot R., Satarasinghe S., Swan A., Katona C.L., McKeith I.G. (1999) Olanzapine in dementia with Lewy bodies: a clinical study. *Int. J. Geriatr. Psychiatry*, **14**: 459–466.

249. Sidtis J.J., Gatsonis C., Price R.W., Singer E.J., Collier A.C., Richman D.D., Hirsch M.S., Schaerf F.W., Fischl M.A., Kieburtz K. *et al* (1993) Zidovudine treatment of the AIDS dementia complex: results of a placebo-controlled trial. AIDS Clinical Trials Group. *Ann. Neurol.*, **83**: 343–349.

250. Starace F., Dijkgraaf M., Houweling H., Postma M., Tramarin A. (1998) HIV-associated dementia: clinical, epidemiological and resource utilization issues. *AIDS Care*, **10** (Suppl. 2): S113–S121.

251. Lipton S.A., Gendelman H.E. (1995) The dementia associated with the acquired immunodeficiency syndrome. *N. Engl. J. Med.*, **332**: 934–940.

252. Heseltine P.N., Goodkin K., Atkinson J.H., Vitiello B., Rochon J., Heaton R.K., Eaton E.M., Wilkie F.L., Sobel E., Brown S.J. (1998) Randomized double-

blind placebo-controlled trial of peptide T for HIV-associated cognitive impairment. *Arch. Neurol.*, **55**: 41–51.

253. Brown G.R. (1995) The use of methylphenidate for cognitive decline associated with HIV disease. *Int. J. Psychiatry Med.*, **25**: 21–37.

254. Masand P.S., Tesar G.E. (1996) Use of stimulants in the medically ill. *Psychiatr. Clin. N. Am.*, **19**: 515–548.

255. Fernandez F., Adams F., Levy J.K., Holmes V.F., Neidhart M., Mansell P.W. (1988) Cognitive impairment due to AIDS-related complex and its response to psychostimulants. *Psychosomatics*, **29**: 38–46.

256. Meyer J.S., Judd B.W., Tawaklna T., Rogers R.L., Mortel K.F. (1986) Improved cognition after control of risk factors for multi-infact dementia. *JAMA*, **256**: 2203–2209.

257. Gorelick P.B., Brody J.A., Cohen D.C., Freels S., Levy P., Dollear W., Forman H., Harris Y. (1993) Risk factors for dementia associated with multiple cerebral infarcts: a case-control analysis in predominantly African American hospital-based patients. *Arch. Neurol.*, **50**: 714–720.

258. Meyer J.S., Rogers R.L., McClintic K., Mortel K.F., Lotfi J. (1989) Randomized clinical trial of daily aspirin therapy in multi-infarct dementia. *J. Am. Geriatr. Soc.*, **37**: 549–555.

259. Walzl M., Walzl B., Lechner H. (1994) Results of a two-month follow-up after a single heparin-induced extracorporeal LDL precipitation in vascular dementia. *J. Stroke Cerebrovasc. Dis.*, **4**: 179–182.

260. Chandra B. (1992) Treatment of multi-infarct dementia with citicholine. *J. Stroke Cerebrovasc. Dis.*, **2**: 232–233.

261. Pratt R.D., Perdomo C.A. (2002) Cognitive and global benefits of donepezil in vascular dementia: results from study 308, a 24-week, randomized, double-blind, placebo-controlled trial. Presented at the 7th International Geneva/Springfield Symposium on Advances in Alzheimer Therapy, Geneva, April 3–6.

262. Schneider L.S. (2002) Galantamine for vascular dementia: some answers, some questions. *Lancet*, **359**: 1265–1266.

263. European Pentoxifylline Multi-Infarct Dementia (EPMID) Study Group (1996) European pentoxifylline multi-infarct dementia study. *Eur. Neurol.*, **36**: 315–321.

264. Marcusson J., Rother M., Kittner B., Rossner M., Smith R.J., Babic T., Folnegovic-Smalc V., Moller H.J., Labs K.H. (1997) A 12-month, randomized, placebo-controlled trial of propentofylline (HWA 285) in patients with dementia according to DSM III-R. *Dement. Geriatr. Cogn. Disord.*, **8**: 320–328.

265. Pantoni L., Carosi M., Amigoni S., Mascalchi M., Inzitari D. (1996) A preliminary open trial with nimodipine in patients with cognitive impairment and leukoaraiosis. *Clin. Neuropharmacol.*, **19**: 497–506.

266. Nadeau S.E., Malloy P.F., Andrew M.E. (1988) A crossover trial of bromocriptine in the treatment of vascular dementia. *Ann. Neurol.*, **24**: 270–272.

# Commentaries

**4.1**
## Alzheimer's Disease is Treatable
Pierre N. Tariot[1]

There is much to treat in dementia. To begin with, it is widely recognized that up to 90% of patients with dementia will experience significant behavioural or psychological signs and symptoms at some point in the course of illness. They include depressive and anxious features, hallucinations, delusions, agitation and aggression, apathy, withdrawal, and vegetative signs and symptoms. These signs and symptoms can be subjectively distressing, lead to dangerous interactions, and result in the use of appropriate or inappropriate psychotropic medications. They are a major cause of caregiver burden. In brief, these manifestations are common, morbid, but also classifiable, quantifiable and treatable.

Most consensus statements emphasize the use of non-pharmacologic approaches first for these behavioural manifestations, including careful investigation for possible delirium as well as social or environmental interventions that capitalize on the patients' residual strengths [1]. Psychotropics should be reserved for cases where other, simpler interventions have been attempted and deemed inadequate.

In their Olympian summary, Samuels and Davis focus on two aspects of the somatic treatment of psychopathology in Alzheimer's disease (AD), "depression" and "psychosis". The cautious reader is urged to bear in mind that the definition of syndromal depression in dementia is a topic of debate, since there is a wide range of depressive signs and symptoms that can occur and fluctuate spontaneously, and placebo response in clinical trials is high. Controlled clinical trials are modest in number and impact: most are cited in Samuels and Davis' review, except for those by Katona *et al* [2], regarding paroxetine and imipramine and Roth *et al* [3], regarding moclobemide. On balance, these trials show a small or no advantage for antidepressants over placebo, and it is not clear to what extent efficacy should be expected. No specific class of antidepressants has been shown to be superior to any others. Adverse effects in patients with dementia appear to be similar to those observed in other patient groups. We can

[1] *Department of Psychiatry, Monroe Community Hospital, 435 E. Henrietta Road, Rochester, NY 14620, USA*

look forward to more definitive trials in the future that apply more strict diagnostic criteria as well as criteria for a response.

The authors also address the issue of pharmacologic treatment of psychosis in patients with AD, avoiding definitional confusion about the concept and spectrum of psychotic features in patients with AD. The review does not mention several key references regarding the use of conventional antipsychotics (e.g. [4–6]). In the aggregate, studies indicate modest efficacy of conventional agents, with a high likelihood of toxicity, which usually limits their use. There is therefore great interest in the impact of the atypical antipsychotics. The important paper of Katz *et al* [7] is referenced, but not the more recent data from DeDyn *et al* [8], also regarding risperidone, or the fairly large open experience trial with quetiapine [9]. There are new data, available so far only in abstract form, regarding the use of olanzapine [10]. In the aggregate, the data suggest efficacy of atypicals as a class for treatment of psychotic features in dementia, although there are no prospective trials yet specifically addressing this issue (all have included patients with mixed behavioural features). There are no head-to-head studies of atypical antipsychotics, so that it is difficult to indicate superiority within this class. The limited data regarding comparison of atypicals with conventional antipsychotics come from the study of DeDyn *et al* [8], suggesting modest superiority of risperidone over haloperidol in terms of tolerability and efficacy. It will be useful to clarify both the issue of class superiority and within-class superiority in the future.

Behavioural signs and symptoms that go beyond depressive or psychotic features have also been the object of considerable therapeutic investigations. These generally focus on "agitation", which may be defined simplistically as inappropriate verbal, vocal or motor activity unexplained by apparent needs or confusion.

The available data indicate that antipsychotics as a group can show benefit for agitation, either associated or not with psychotic features. The literature regarding non-antipsychotic medications includes five placebo-controlled studies of different anticonvulsants, a small number of studies of antidepressants, fewer yet regarding anxiolytics, and a variety of other agents with less foundation [11]. The evidence suggests, but does not prove, that alternatives to antipsychotics can be deployed. As data accrue regarding these different therapeutic approaches, we will have a clear sense of exactly how and when they should be deployed. In the meantime, clinicians are forced to deal with real world patients, and may be guided to a certain extent by consensus guidelines, in the absence of definitive data [1].

We also have relatively new tools to treat the dementia itself. Cholinesterase inhibitors were developed primarily for relief of cognitive dysfunction in AD. They are the only class of agents to have consistently demonstrated efficacy in well-controlled multicenter trials, and that are approved by numerous national regulatory authorities. A wide range of other compounds have been tested in experimental animals, but the majority of these have had only modest, non-significant or inconsistent effects in clinical trials. Samuels and Davis do an impressive job in summarizing the literature regarding the impact of cholinesterase inhibitor therapy. Further, they help shift the discussion away from a focus on short-term benefit, which certainly does occur in a substantial minority of patients, to subtler but equally important questions. The duration of beneficial effect of this class of agents has not been fully delineated, because the length of trials have usually been 3–6 months. Data are emerging from long-term open studies suggesting that progression of disease assessed by worsening of cognitive function, functional status, or global ratings of dementia appears to be ameliorated by chronic cholinergic therapy. Positive data from 1-year placebo-controlled trials are pending. The point is not proven, but clinicians and advocates will be well served to pay attention to the real possibility that the trajectory of AD can be favourably affected by this class of agents, in addition to the well-established short-term benefit. Put differently, given the fact that there is a substantial likelihood of easily discernible short-term benefit, and mounting evidence of possible long-term benefit, it is becoming increasingly hard to justify not treating patients with AD.

As the role of cholinesterase inhibitors becomes well established, treatment research goals have shifted from symptomatic improvement to modification of clinical course or even delay of onset of AD [12]. Basic and preclinical evidence suggests the potential benefit of treatments such as vitamin E and selegiline, supported by limited clinical trials data. The presumed mechanism of action involves antioxidative properties, although selegiline may have other disease-modifying properties (e.g. neurotrophic). There is evidence suggesting a role for estrogens in the maintenance of normal brain function, as well as evidence suggesting that the loss of estrogen may play a role in cognitive decline and the development of AD. Epidemiologic studies and very small controlled clinical trials suggest that estrogen replacement therapy may possibly delay the onset of AD, although the point is not proven. Finally, epidemiologic data suggest that anti-inflammatory medications may influence the time of onset of AD. This is supported by reasonable scientific evidence indicative of a role of altered inflammatory processes in AD. Clinical trials data are limited in extent. As Samuels and Davis point out, the early returns on treatment of AD with anti-inflammatory agents are not particularly encouraging, although numerous trials are still ongoing. Their role in prevention or delay has yet to be delineated.

The long wait for meaningful therapeutics for the dementias is over. The steady drumbeat of new treatment developments is setting the pace for advances in the recognition, diagnosis and management of dementia. We know a great deal about how to manage the behavioural manifestations. The first and second generation cholinesterase inhibitors are available and new ones are coming to market rapidly. Agents with the potential to modify the course of dementia or delay onset are actively being developed, and definitive studies will give us powerful information about the extent to which disease modification or delay will become a reality. This disease and these data require our attention.

## REFERENCES

1. American Psychiatric Association (1997) Practice guideline for the treatment of patients with Alzheimer's disease and other dementias of late life. *Am. J. Psychiatry*, **154** (Suppl.).
2. Katona C.L.E., Hunter B.N., Bray J. (1998) A double-blind comparison of the efficacy and safety of paroxetine and imipramine in the treatment of depression with dementia. *Int. J. Geriatr. Psychiatry*, **13**: 100–108.
3. Roth M., Mountjoy C.Q., Amrein R. and the International Collaborative Study Group (1996) Moclobemide in elderly patients with cognitive decline and depression. An international double-blind, placebo-controlled trial. *Br. J. Psychiatry*, **168**: 149–157.
4. Schneider L.S., Pollock V.E., Lyness S.A. (1990) A meta-analysis of controlled trials of neuroleptic treatment in dementia. *J. Am. Geriatr. Soc.*, **38**: 553–563.
5. Devanand D.P., Marder K., Michaels K.S., Sackeim H.A., Bell K., Sullivan M.A., Cooper T.B., Pelton G.H., Mayeux R. (1998) A randomized, placebo-controlled dose comparison trial of haloperidol for psychosis and disruptive behaviours in Alzheimer's disease. *Am. J. Psychiatry*, **155**: 1512–1520.
6. Kirchner V., Kelly C.A., Harvey R.J. (1999) Thioridazine for dementia (Cochrane review). In *The Cochrane Library*, Issue 1, Update Software, Oxford.
7. Katz I.R., Jeste D.V., Mintzer J.E., Clyde C., Napolitano J., Brecher M. for the Risperidone Study Group (1999) Comparison of risperidone and placebo for psychosis and behavioural disturbances associated with dementia: a randomized, double-blind trial. *J. Clin. Psychiatry*, **60**: 107–115.
8. DeDeyn P.P., Rabheru K., Rasmussen A., Bocksberger J.P., Dautzenberg P.L.J., Eriksson S., Lawlor B.A. (1999) A randomized trial of risperidone, placebo, and haloperidol for behavioural symptoms of dementia. *Neurology*, **53**: 946–955.
9. McManus D.Q., Arvanitis L.A., Kowalcyk B.B., for the Seroquel Trial 48 Study Group (1999) Quetiapine, a novel antipsychotic: experience in elderly patients with psychotic disorders. *J. Clin. Psychiatry*, **60**: 292–298.
10. Street J., Clark W.S., Gannon K.S., Mitan S., Kadam D., Sanger T., Tamura R., Tollefson G.D. (1999) Olanzapine reduces psychosis and behavioural disturbances associated with Alzheimer's disease. *Int. Psychogeriatrics*, **11** (Suppl. 1): 139.
11. Tariot P.N. (1999) Treatment of agitation in dementia. *J. Clin. Psychiatry*, **60**: 11–20.
12. Tariot P.N., Loy R., Schneider L.S. The pharmacological wager: prospects for delaying the onset or modifying the progression of Alzheimer's disease. Submitted for publication.

4.2
## Treatment of Dementia: Where Do We Go from Here?
Davangere P. Devanand[1]

Samuels and Davis provide a comprehensive and balanced review of the available data on a variety of treatments for patients with dementia, though there are a few minor omissions, e.g. *Ginkgo biloba* is widely used and there are some supporting, though limited, data. I will raise a few points about issues that arise from the extant research database, and discuss where we go from here.

*What is the right cognitive instrument to use?* To assess change, the Clinical Dementia Rating (CDR) sum of boxes and the Clinician Interview Based Impression (CIBI) are excellent global measures. The cognitive subscale of the Alzheimer's Disease Assessment Scale (ADAS–Cog) has become the most widely used scale to assess cognitive change in pharmacotherapy trials in dementia, and research with the cholinesterase inhibitors has established its utility for this purpose. However, there are few data comparing the use of other potentially useful scales or neuropsychological tests in such trials. This is not an argument against the ADAS–Cog; rather, as research expands into the use of other compounds and non-Alzheimer's dementias become the target with some of these newer agents, it is possible that other neuropsychological tests and rating instruments will be more sensitive to treatment-induced change. For example, there are data suggesting that nicotinic compounds may improve attention and arousal to a greater degree than memory test performance, and targeted neuropsychological tests are needed to pick up this type of change [1]. Interestingly, the research database comparing the utility of different activities of daily living (ADL) and behavioural scales in clinical trials in dementia is much greater than what is available with respect to cognitive assessment.

*Effect size and cost-effectiveness.* The major limitation of the current crop of available treatments for dementia is that the magnitude of the effect size, regardless of compound, is small. Many physicians have become disenchanted with the cholinesterase inhibitors, because the clinical effects have turned out to be much smaller in magnitude than what they had imagined. So these drugs, which can be effective, even if modestly and in subgroups of patients with dementia, appear to be under-used as a result. Perhaps one lesson from this experience is that overselling the effect size can boost medication use in the short run, but backfire in the long run,

---

[1] *Department of Biological Psychiatry, New York State Psychiatric Institute, Box 72, 722 W. 168th Street, New York, NY 10032, USA*

when physicians become disappointed and stop prescribing the agent altogether.

Cost-effectiveness becomes crucial when the effect size is small. As Samuels and Davis point out, there are data suggesting that the use of cholinesterase inhibitors can be cost-effective. However, there are many ways in which both costs and effectiveness can be measured, and the debate about the cost-effectiveness of medications with small effect sizes remains to be fully resolved.

*Mild cognitive impairment.* Many of the same agents used to treat dementia are now being studied to treat patients with mild cognitive impairment, i.e. patients who fall between "normal" and "dementia". Clinically, this is a very heterogeneous group of patients, but the trials to date have tended to focus on patients with CDR 0.5, "questionable dementia", whose clinical presentation and neuropsychological test performance often suggest very early Alzheimer's disease. If the scope of sample selection is extended beyond this narrow group of patients, it would be interesting to see if potentially broad-spectrum agents like vitamin E and estrogen have an advantage over other agents that are selective for memory loss. This issue is assuming growing importance because, as the population ages, many people would prefer to take one or two agents that work against aging-related changes in a variety of organs and not restrict themselves to a cognitive enhancer.

*Treatment of psychiatric symptoms in dementia.* Most clinicians use psychotropic agents to treat depression or psychosis or behavioural dyscontrol in dementia. However, with the possible exception of the use of antipsychotic medications to treat psychosis and behavioural dyscontrol, the data supporting the use of psychotropic medications in dementia is very limited. In this context, the finding that cholinesterase inhibitors may be effective in treating psychopathology in dementia is intriguing. The data suggest that these agents may improve apathy and depression more than behavioural dyscontrol, but there have been no direct comparisons between cholinesterase inhibitors and any psychotropic medication. Clinically, it is common to see patients on cholinesterase inhibitors develop frank psychotic features, as well as severe agitation and aggressive behaviour. Therefore, in the absence of direct comparison trials between cholinesterase inhibitors and psychotropics, it is premature to recommend them as a primary treatment for any symptoms of psychopathology in dementia. From a clinical perspective, identifying and following specific target symptoms of psychopathology can sometimes be more useful than relying on rating scales.

There have been few treatment studies of non-Alzheimer's dementias, such as Lewy body disease, both in the cognitive and non-cognitive treatment domains. The improved accuracy in clinical and investigative diagnostic methods should facilitate the conduct of such studies in the future.

*New directions.* In addition to pursuing current therapies alluded to in the review, new directions include preventing amyloid accumulation or blocking tau protein aggregation. Recent basic science developments suggest that these notions [2], which seemed very distant only a few years ago, may well turn into reality in the near future, thereby transforming the treatment of dementia as we know it.

## REFERENCES

1. Newhouse P.A., Potter A., Levin E.D. (1997) Nicotinic system involvement in Alzheimer's and Parkinson's diseases. Implications for therapeutics. *Drugs Aging*, **11**: 206–228.
2. Vassar R., Bennett B.D., Babu-Khan S., Kahn S., Mendiaz E.A., Denis P., Teplow D.B., Ross S., Amarante P., Loeloff R. *et al* (1999) Beta-secretase cleavage of Alzheimer's amyloid precursor protein by the transmembrane aspartic protease BACE. *Science*, **286**: 735–741.

4.3

## The Future of Alzheimer's Pharmacotherapeutics

Elaine R. Peskind[1]

Samuels and Davis provide a scholarly review of the cholinesterase inhibitors and antioxidants, including vitamin E. This commentary briefly discusses some other emerging issues in Alzheimer's disease (AD) pharmacotherapeutics.

*Ginkgo biloba.* Extracts of the leaf of the *Ginkgo biloba* tree have been used in traditional Chinese medicine for thousands of years for their believed benefits to the brain. Preclinical data suggest that such extracts may have antioxidant, anti-inflammatory, and stimulant properties. Because of ginkgo's popular appeal as a "natural remedy" and its widespread use by older persons, both with and without dementia, to promote cognition, placebo-controlled trials have been undertaken. A recent large-scale, double-blind,

[1] *Veterans Affairs Puget Sound Health Care System, S-116 Mirecc, 1660 S. Columbian Way, Seattle, WA 98108, USA*

randomized trial of EGb 761, a standardized concentrated extract of *Ginkgo biloba*, was evaluated for safety and efficacy in a 52-week trial in patients with AD and vascular dementia [1]. Very small but statistically significant differences favouring *Ginkgo biloba* were found on the Alzheimer's Disease Assessment Scale–Cognitive subscale (ADAS–Cog), but no difference was found on a clinical global impression of change. The very high dropout rate and other questions regarding design of the study and interpretation of the results necessitate replication before ginkgo can be considered a treatment for the cognitive deficits of AD. In addition, significant safety issues are raised by ginkgo's potential effects on blood-clotting mechanisms, and by the lack of federally-regulated safeguards for both drug potency and purity. At this time, ginkgo can not be recommended as safe and effective treatment for the cognitive deficits of AD.

*Estrogen replacement therapy (ERT).* The epidemiologic evidence suggesting that ERT may be effective in the treatment of AD is discussed in detail by Samuels and Davis. However, recent data from a large, multicenter, randomized trial performed by the Alzheimer's Disease Cooperative Study (ADCS) indicate no benefit with respect to either symptomatic improvement or slowing of progression in women patients who have already developed AD [2]. ERT may still be beneficial for delaying onset of AD in postmenopausal women; data from large, randomized primary prevention trials are not yet available. At this time, it appears that the diagnosis of AD itself is not an indication for ERT. However, other well-demonstrated health benefits of ERT should still be considered in individual women with AD (reviewed in [3]).

*Anti-inflammatory agents.* Similar epidemiologic data to those for estrogen have suggested a 50% reduction in relative risk of AD in persons who have received 2 or more years of treatment with non-steroidal anti-inflammatory drugs (NSAIDs) (reviewed in [4]). Such a protective effect was not observed for aspirin or acetaminophen. Recent data from an ADCS multicenter study of the anti-inflammatory steroid prednisone failed to demonstrate efficacy in improving cognition or delaying progression in AD [5]. Large, multicenter, randomized trials of NSAIDs, including the selective COX-2 inhibitors, are currently underway. Because NSAIDs are associated with significant risk of peptic ulcer disease and hypertension, they are not at this time recommended for AD patients who have no other indication for these agents.

*Utilizing the immune system to alter β-amyloid (AB) deposition.* In a novel approach [6], mice with an amyloid precursor protein (APP) transgene, which highly overexpress APP and have profound amyloid plaque deposition by 18 months of age, were immunized with Aβ 1–42. Immunization early in life largely prevented formation of amyloid plaques and abnormal neurites and decreased the inflammatory response. Immunization at 11 months of age, when substantial plaque deposition has already occurred, resulted in drastic reductions in progression of amyloid plaque formation, reduction in abnormal neurites, and a slowed inflammatory response.

Many questions remain regarding the utility of this approach for human disease. The APP-overexpressing mouse is only a partial model of AD; although these mice develop abundant amyloid pathology, they do not develop neurofibrillary tangles, undergo neuronal loss, or have behaviour changes suggestive of a dementing disorder. In addition, the mouse strain used in these experiments is not immunocompetent; similar immunization strategies in humans may be limited by the development of antigenic tolerance or induction of an autoimmune response. These caveats having been made, this approach may present significant therapeutic potential, and initial safety studies in humans will soon be undertaken.

*Protease inhibitors.* Cleavage of APP at the $\beta$-cleavage site is a critical step in the formation of amyloidogenic A$\beta$. The recent identification of the $\beta$-secretase, termed BACE (or $\beta$-site APP-cleaving enzyme) [7], presents a new target for AD pharmacotherapeutics. Design of protease inhibitors which prevent $\beta$-cleavage may potentially prove beneficial for treatment and possibly prevention of AD.

*Alteration of risk factors.* AD has been demonstrated to be associated with elevations of serum and cerebrospinal fluid homocysteine (8–10), even in the presence of normal vitamin $B_{12}$ and folate levels [11]. Possible mechanisms for a role of homocysteine in the pathobiology of AD include: vascular damage; increased platelet, monocyte, and polymorphonuclear cell adhesiveness; generation of oxidative free radicals; and excitotoxicity via agonist activity at the NMDA receptor. Supplementation with folate and vitamins $B_6$ and $B_{12}$ results in a 30% reduction in homocysteine levels and has been proposed as a strategy to alter the risk and/or slow progression of AD.

Cerebrovascular and cardiovascular disease are additional risks for the expression of AD. Neurobiologic evidence supporting the use of lipid lowering agents for treatment or prevention of AD includes a protective effect of statins against neurotoxic effects of A$\beta$ *in vitro* [12].

# REFERENCES

1. LeBars P.L., Katz N.M., Berman N., Itil T.M., Freedman A.M., Schatzberg A.F. (1997) A placebo-controlled, double-blind, randomized trial of an extract of *Ginkgo biloba* for dementia. North American EGb Study Group. *JAMA*, **278**: 1327–1332.

2. Mulnard R.A., Cotman C.W., Kawas C., van Dyck C.H., Sano M., Doody R., Koss E., Pfeiffer E., Jin S., Gamst A. *et al* (2000)   Estrogen replacement therapy for treatment of mild to moderate Alzheimer's disease: a 1-year randomized controlled trial. *JAMA*, **283**: 1007–1015.
3. McNagny S.E. (1999)   Prescribing hormone replacement therapy for menopausal symptoms. *Ann. Intern. Med.*, **131**: 605–616.
4. McGeer E.G., McGeer P.L. (1999)   Brain inflammation in Alzheimer's disease and the therapeutic implications. *Curr. Pharmacol. Res.*, **5**: 821–836.
5. Aisen P.S., Davis K.L., Berg J., Schafer K., Campbell K., Thomas R., Weiner M.F., Farlow M.R., Sano M., Grundman M. *et al* (2000)   A randomized controlled trial of prednisone in Alzheimer's disease. *Neurology*. **54**: 588–593.
6. Schenk D., Barbour R., Dunn W., Gordon G., Grajeda H., Guido T., Hu K., Huang J., Johnson-Wood K., Khan K. *et al* (1999)   Immunization with amyloid-beta attenuates Alzheimer-disease-like pathology in the PDAPP mouse. *Nature*, **400**: 173–177.
7. Vassar R., Bennett B.D., Babu-Khan S., Kahn S., Mendiaz E.A., Denis P., Teplow D.B., Ross S., Amarante P., Loeloff R. *et al* (1999) Beta-secretase cleavage of Alzheimer's amyloid precursor protein by the transmembrane aspartic acid protease BACE. *Science*, **286**: 735–741.
8. Clarke R., Smith A.D., Jobst K.A., Refsum H., Sutton L., Ueland P.M. (1998)   Folate, vitamin $B_{12}$, and serum total homocysteine levels in confirmed Alzheimer disease. *Arch. Neurol.*, **55**: 1449–1455.
9. Miller J.W. (1999)   Homocysteine and Alzheimer's disease. *Nutr. Rev.*, **57**: 126–129.
10. Gottfries C.G., Lehmann W., Regland B. (1998)   Early diagnosis of cognitive impairment in the elderly with the focus on Alzheimer's disease. *J. Neural Transm.*, **105**: 773–786.
11. McCadon A., Davies G., Hudson P., Tandy S., Cattell H. (1998)   Total serum homocysteine in senile dementia of Alzheimer type. *Int. J. Geriatr. Psychiatry*, **13**: 235–239.
12. Simons M., Keller P., De Strooper B., Beyreuther K., Dotti C.G., Simons K. (1998)   Cholesterol depletion inhibits the generation of beta-amyloid in hippocampal neurons. *Proc. Natl. Acad. Sci. USA.*, **95**: 6460–6464.

4.4

## Outcome Measures and Ethical Issues in the Pharmacotherapy of Alzheimer's Disease

Gunhild Waldemar[1]

The advent of pharmacological treatment for Alzheimer's disease (AD) has already been of significant importance to patients, caregivers and clinicians. Although a symptomatic effect on functional measures has been demonstrated for several cholinesterase inhibitors, a number of clinical and ethical

[1] *Memory Disorders Research Unit, Department of Neurology N2082, University Hospital Rigshospitalet, 9, Blegdamsvej, DK-2100 Copenhagen, Denmark*

issues are still unsolved. In their thorough review, Samuels and Davis discuss recent advances in pharmacotherapy for AD, with a main emphasis on cholinesterase inhibitors. This commentary focuses on the challenges of defining relevant outcome and efficacy measures for a gradually progressive disorder like AD. It then deals with practical and ethical issues in the adaptation of efficacy measures from clinical trials to clinical practice. In closing, the commentary considers ethical perspectives in the drug treatment of cognitive disorders.

*Outcome measures.* The demonstration of the efficacy of cholinesterase inhibitors depends on statistically significant improvement in a cognitive measure and a global functional measure when compared with placebo. The limitation of this design is that it measures symptomatic improvement and not delayed progression. With the advent of drugs with other mechanisms of action which may potentially alter the course of the disease, there is a need for methods to demonstrate slowing of the disease process. The International Working Group on Harmonization of Dementia Drug Guidelines [1] has suggested two clinical trial protocols for the demonstration of slowing of disease: the randomized start and the randomized withdrawal design. The latter was commented on by Samuels and Davis in their comparison of cholinesterase inhibitors. For a drug to have modified the biological progression of the disease, the slope of the efficacy curve for the withdrawal group should be at least parallel with that of the placebo group. If the lines converge, the drug has an effect on symptomatic progression only [1]. There may be differences in the time for the withdrawal group to reach the level of the placebo group, and in this context it is a limitation of most drug trials that the randomized withdrawal period has lasted for only a few weeks. There are no published clinical data which prove that cholinesterase inhibitors modify the biological progression of disease. However, preliminary data from a Nordic long-term double-blind placebo-controlled donepezil study [2] suggest that the significant symptomatic improvement on functional measures lasts for at least 1 year, confirming the observations in previous open-label continuation studies. The use of biological markers for measurements of disease progression will be crucial in future drug trials of disease modifying agents. However, the relevant chemical and brain imaging markers still need further methodological development.

Even when considering symptomatic improvement only, there are a number of unsolved questions in the definition of outcome. How much is required for a symptomatic effect to be clinically relevant? In a disease with relentless progression of symptoms, what is a clinically relevant duration of symptomatic effect? Will patients benefit from treatment even when there is no initial improvement on functional scales? Are all patients responders? If not, how can we define a responder? The results of ongoing trials will provide us with evidence-based answers to some of these still unsolved issues.

*From clinical trial to clinical practice.* Samuels and Davis discuss the considerations associated with the choice of the cholinesterase inhibitor for an AD patient, but the clinician is faced with many other practical questions. Which patients are eligible for a treatment trial? How can treatment effect be monitored in the clinical office? When should treatment be stopped? Now that medication is becoming more widely available, many patients will be seen by their general practitioners. The wide array of functional scales used by a team of clinicians in clinical trials will not be feasible in general practice. Suggestions for a smaller battery of scales vary, and many clinicians rely on a "holistic impression" obtained from unstructured interviews of patients and caregivers. There is a need for validation of brief and feasible monitoring and evaluation programs for patients receiving drug treatment for AD. Harvey [3] reviewed a sample of guidelines for the drug treatment of AD, and found substantial variations in recommendations, which were most often based on consensus opinion rather than evidence. Recommendations varied as to dosage adjustments, scales to be used for monitoring and criteria to continue or to discontinue treatment.

In the recent dementia guidelines from a European Federation of Neurological Societies (EFNS) Task Force Working Group [4], it was recommended that a therapeutic trial with an acetylcholinesterase inhibitor be considered in patients with mild to moderate AD. If a trial is given, there should be a caregiver who can assist in administering the treatment. Therapeutic and side effects should be monitored periodically and discontinuation of treatment be considered when there are no signs of benefit. Treatment with vitamin E, or other anti-dementia drugs, was not recommended on a routine basis. Vitamin E is not registered for use in AD, and the results of the 2-year randomized placebo-controlled trial [5] were equivocal, with a statistically significant benefit over placebo only after post-hoc correction for an accidental bias in the pre-treatment randomization of patients.

*Ethical issues.* In clinical practice, the prescription of drug treatment with a cognitive enhancer must go hand-in-hand with other (non-pharmacological) therapies, with careful information to the patient and caregiver, with careful discussions with the patient and caregiver on the range of treatment possibilities and on the range of possible treatment effect, and with support to the caregiver when needed. The advent of drug treatment has raised new ethical issues in AD management: while cognitive enhancement is often a valid goal, it shall not dominate over quality of life. Some patients regain insight along with renewed anxiety on treatment with cognitive enhancing medication [6]. We have not given enough attention to the point at which medication should be stopped or not initiated. These and other ethical issues will be even further augmented when future drug treatments for mild cognitive impairment and disease modifying agents for AD come into clinical practice.

## REFERENCES

1. Anonymous (1997) Protocols to demonstrate slowing of Alzheimer disease progression. Position paper from the International Working Group on Harmonization of Dementia Drug Guidelines. The Disease Progression Sub-group. *Alz. Dis. Assoc. Disord.*, **11** (Suppl. 3): 50–53.
2. Winblad B., Engedal K., Soininen H., Verhey F., Waldemar G., Wimo A., Wetterholm A.L., Zhang R., Haglund A., Subbiah P. (1999) Donepezil enhances global function, cognition and activities of daily living compared with placebo in a double-blind trial in patients with mild to moderate Alzheimer's disease. *Int. Psychogeriatrics*, **11** (Suppl. 1): 138.
3. Harvey R.J. (1999) A review and commentary on a sample of 15 UK guidelines for the drug treatment of Alzheimer's disease. *Int. J. Geriatr. Psychiatry*, **14**: 249–256.
4. Waldemar G., Dubois B., Emre M., Scheltens P., Tariska P., Rossor M. (2000) Diagnosis and management of Alzheimer's disease and related disorders: the role of neurologists in Europe. *Eur. J. Neurol.* **7**: 133–144.
5. Sano M., Ernesto C., Thomas R.G., Klauber M.R., Schafer K., Grundman M., Woodbury P., Growdon J., Cotmann C.W., Pfeiffer E. *et al* (1997) A controlled trial of selegiline, alpha-tocopherol, or both as treatment for Alzheimer's disease. *N. Engl. J. Med.*, **336**: 1216–1222.
6. Post S.G., Whitehouse P.J. (1998) Emerging antidementia drugs: a preliminary ethical view. *J. Am. Geriatr. Soc.*, **46**: 784–787.

4.5

## From Bench to Bedside: How to Treat Dementia

Serge Gauthier[1]

The review on pharmacological treatment of dementia by Samuels and Davis illustrates the value of the "bench to bedside" principle of Walter Penfield. Indeed, the cholinergic hypothesis was developed from brain biopsy and post-mortem measurements of reduced choline acetyl transferase activity in the brains of patients with Alzheimer's disease (AD), complemented by animal models of lesions in selected nuclei and nerve tracts leading to central cholinergic depletion and behavioural deficits, and

[1] *Alzheimer's Disease Research Unit, McGill Centre for Studies in Aging, 6825 Lasalle Blvd., Verdun, Quebec, H4H 1R3, Canada*

human pharmacologic experimentation in young and old volunteers. It was thus predicted that cholinergic supplementation in patients with AD would lead to improvement in some of their symptoms.

The observable improvement in randomized clinical trials (RCT) and in clinical practice using cholinesterase inhibitors (CIs) as monotherapy is real [1]. Unfortunately, the amount of benefit for individual patients is not predictable *a priori* from clinical or biological features, and each patient in mild to moderate stages of AD should be offered a therapeutic trial with a CI after control of concomitant disorders such as depression, with careful follow-up to determine tolerance and efficacy [2]. Furthermore, the improvement above the starting point is transient, in the order of 9 months, as demonstrated by the 1-year Nordic placebo-controlled study using donepezil [3], since CIs were developed primarily for symptomatic control via transmitter replacement. Trial designs to prove disease modification using amyloid anti-aggregating, antioxidants and anti-arthritic drugs will differ from the parallel placebo-controlled 3–6 month pivotal studies followed by open-label extensions used with CIs [4]. Combination studies with CIs and disease-modifying drugs will also have to be done to confirm their safety and additive benefit [5]. In reference to Samuels and Davis' practice of adding vitamin E 2000 IU a day to CIs, there is no consensus as to the value of this combination, at least among experts in Canada [6].

We still have unanswered questions about the value of CIs in non-cognitive aspects of dementia. The "draft guidelines" issued by the Food and Drug Administration in 1990 [7] have helped move the field of RCT in AD forward, although the statement that behavioural manifestations of AD were "pseudospecific" has delayed the interest in non-cognitive aspects of dementia by industry. A systematic effort at harmonization of dementia drug guidelines has been spearheaded by Peter Whitehouse [8], and has led to major initiatives towards trial designs and outcome variables, applicable not only to AD but also to vascular dementia [9]. The International Psychogeriatric Association has also been proactive in defining behavioural and psychological signs and symptoms of dementia [10]. Finally, investigators are now reanalysing the data generated from pivotal RCT to understand better the response of neuropsychiatric symptoms to CIs [11].

As more CIs become available for regular prescription use by physicians caring for patients with AD, the issues raised by Samuels and Davis about effectiveness and safety will be quite relevant. As for selecting a serotonin reuptake inhibitor, the ease of use (particularly with patients living alone), tolerability (particularly in small body weight women) and familiarity of the clinician with a given compound will play an important role. The clinical relevance of pharmacological characteristics, such as selectivity for acetylcholinesterase vs. butyrylcholinesterase, and reversibility vs. pseudo-irreversibility of enzyme inhibition has not been established [12].

Clinicians caring for patients with AD should feel optimistic about the possibility of improving symptoms, from depression to cognition and behaviour, as well as delaying loss of functional autonomy, using the best drugs available to them. This is not a substitute for careful diagnosis and follow-up, but rather an important component of the global management of dementia.

## REFERENCES

1. Gauthier S. (1999)   Do we have a treatment for Alzheimer disease? Yes. *Arch. Neurol.*, **54**: 738–739.
2. Gauthier S. (in press)   Cholinesterase inhibitors in the treatment of dementia. In *Yearbook of Alzheimer's Disease and Related Disorders* (Eds S. Gauthier, J.L. Cummings), Dunitz, London.
3. Winblad B., Engedal K., Soininen H., Verhey F., Waldemar G., Wimo A., Wetterholm A.L., Zhang R., Haglund A., Subbiah P. (1999)   Donepezil enhances global function, cognition, and activities of daily living compared to placebo in a one year, double-blind trial in patients with mild to moderate Alzheimer's disease. *Int. Psychogeriatrics*, **11** (Suppl. 1): 138.
4. Gauthier S. (1998)   Clinical trials and therapy. *Curr. Opin. Neurol.*, **11**: 435–438.
5. Murali Doraiswam P., Steffens D.C. (1998)   Combination therapy for early Alzheimer's disease: what are we waiting for? *J. Am. Geriatr. Soc.*, **46**: 1322–1324.
6. Patterson J.S., Gauthier S., Bergman H., Cohen C.A., Geightner J.W., Feldman H., Hogan D.B. (1999)   The recognition, assessment and management of dementing disorders: conclusions from the Canadian Consensus Conference on Dementia. *Can. Med. Ass. J.*, **160** (Suppl. 12): S1–S15.
7. Leber P. (1990)   *Guidelines for Clinical Evaluation of Antidementia Drugs*, US Food and Drug Administration, Washington, DC.
8. Whitehouse P. (1997)   The International Working Group on Harmonization of Dementia Drug Guidelines: past, present, and future. *Alz. Dis. Assoc. Disord.*, **11** (Suppl. 3): 2–5.
9. Erkinjuntti T., Sawada T., Whitehouse P. (1999)   The Osaka Conference on Vascular Dementia. *Alz. Dis. Assoc. Disord.*, **13** (Suppl. 3): S1–S3.
10. Finkel S.I. (1996)   New focus on behavioural and psychological signs and symptoms of dementia. *Int. Psychogeriatrics*, **8** (Suppl. 3): 215–216.
11. Mega M.S., Masterman D.M., O'Connor S.M., Barclay T.R., Cummings J.L. (1999)   The spectrum of behavioural responses to cholinesterase inhibitor therapy in Alzheimer's disease. *Arch. Neurol.*, **56**: 1388–1393.
12. Gauthier S. (1999)   Acetylcholinesterase inhibitors in the treatment of Alzheimer's disease. *Exp. Opin. Invest. Drugs*, **8**: 1511–1520.

4.6
## Some Limitations in the Drug Treatment of Alzheimer's Disease
Brian E. Leonard[1]

Samuels and Davis have comprehensively reviewed the choices of drugs that are currently available in the United States for the treatment of Alzheimer's diseas (AD). In addition, they have briefly considered drug treatments for Lewy body and vascular dementia, and AIDS-associated dementia. The review will be particularly useful to practising physicians, as the authors have included details of the pharmacokinetic profiles of the drugs discussed, their clinical effectiveness and their safety. However, there are several areas of potential therapeutic importance that are omitted from the review and will be considered in this commentary.

Drug development for the treatment of AD has focused on cholinergic agents, which have been based on defects in the cholinergic system that are associated with age-related cognitive decline, described by Bartus and co-workers [1]. These pioneering studies demonstrated that muscarinic receptor antagonists such as scopolamine induced a memory deficit in young monkeys that resembled those changes seen in aged monkeys. Similar learning and memory deficits were also shown to occur in humans treated with scopolamine, which laid the basis to the hypothesis that a defect in the cholinergic system was responsible for the cognitive decline associated with ageing. The subsequent discovery that there was a marked degeneration of the forebrain cholinergic system in patients with AD [2] laid the foundation for the use of drugs that enhanced cholinergic function for the treatment of this condition. Experimental studies in marmosets, in which lesions of the medial septum and basal forebrain (the main cholinergic regions in the brain) resulted in cognitive impairment [3], gave further support to the cholinergic hypothesis.

Despite the seductive nature of this hypothesis, there is evidence that loss of the basal forebrain cholinergic neurons does not result in impaired learning and memory, at least in those experimental procedures used to model human cognitive function. Cholinergic depletion produced by lesions of the basal forebrain is frequently much greater than those seen even in the most advanced cases of AD. Furthermore, such experimentally induced neuronal loss results in a disruption of attention rather than memory as such [4], and experimental studies show that selective forebrain lesions fail to produce the full spectrum of cognitive deficits observed in AD, even though they mimic the defects in attention that commonly occur in the disease [5]. Thus, animals with selective forebrain lesions may provide a model system in which drugs may be tested for the correction of

[1] Pharmacology Department, National University of Ireland, Galway, Ireland

attentional defects, but they do not model cognitive decline and memory deficits that characterize the disease. This is confirmed in clinical studies in which tacrine was shown to ameliorate attentional deficits in AD [6], but which failed to show that the drug improved the memory of these patients. This may account for the limited efficacy of cholinergic agonists and anticholinesterases in the symptomatic treatment of AD patients.

Another aspect which requires attention when extrapolating from experimental studies to patients concerns the impact of the cognitive status of the patient on the drug response. The basic assumption which continues to drive drug development is the principle of the "magic bullet", in which it is assumed that the correction of the primary neurochemical defect by a drug will improve all aspects of cognition. With regard to the central cholinergic system, for example, there is experimental evidence to show that drug-induced increases in acetylcholine release only occur when the cholinergic system is activated; the cholinergic pathways remain "silent" unless cognitively dependent neuronal inputs activate the cholinergic system [7]. These observations could be important in differentiating between patients who respond, or fail to respond, to cholinomimetic treatments, as the cognitive variables which contribute to the efficacy of these drugs are seldom considered. Clinical evidence to support this view is provided by the effects of mental exercise on cognitive function in both elderly and demented patients [8].

In addition to the use of anticholinesterases in the treatment of patients with AD, research has also been directed to selective agonists of cholinergic receptors in the brain, in particular the M1 receptors. The use of the older muscarinic agonists, such as bethanechol and arecoline, was precluded by their short half-lives, low brain penetrability and high incidence of side effects. Several novel drugs (for example, PD 151832) are now in development which possess selectivity for the M1 receptors, are orally active and display a large separation between their pharmacological effects and their side effects [9]. A potentially important sequel to the discovery of such drugs lies in the experimental observation of a possible link between muscarinic receptor stimulation and the production of soluble amyloid precursor protein (APP), a process which could lead to a reduction in β-amyloid peptide (β A4). These studies have shown that M1 and M3 activation increases soluble APP synthesis [10]. If these observations are confirmed by *in vivo* studies and subsequent clinical trials, the application of cholinergic agonists could be of considerable therapeutic value in the future.

The role of nicotinic receptors may also be of importance in the aetiology of AD. There is evidence that the density of the post-synaptic nicotinic receptors is decreased in the brains of AD patients, even though the post-synaptic muscarinic receptors are largely preserved [11]. Thus, the restoration of nicotinic receptor function may be useful in the treatment of some of the cognitive defects, and there is some evidence from the studies of the effects of transdermal nicotine patches in patients to support this view [12]. Although the side effects and addiction liability have precluded the clinical development of nicotine agonists, the discovery of subtypes of the nicotine receptor, some of which do not participate in the expression of the nicotine cue [13], may be an important finding for the future development of such drugs.

In their review, Samuels and Davis have provided evidence that postmenopausal estrogen deficiency may contribute to cognitive dysfunction, a condition which may be attenuated by estrogen replacement. There is also evidence that estrogen replacement in the normal aged has beneficial effects on cognitive function. The possible link with the cholinergic system is provided by the experimental observations that estrogens enhance the activity of the high-affinity choline transporter in the brain and, in addition, increase choline acetyl transferase (leading to increased acetylcholine synthesis) in the forebrain [14]. There is also evidence that estrogens may help to prevent degenerative changes in the forebrain cholinergic neurons. Thus, estrogen receptors are known to be co-localized with neurotrophin receptors, which may act to preserve these neurons from age-related degenerative changes [15]. Estrogen replacement following the menopause may therefore have a protective effect, not only due to the enhancement of cholinergic function but also by increasing the activity of trophic factors that protect against neuronal loss. Somewhat surprisingly, little research appears to be published whereby modified estrogens that lack the harmful side effects associated with the conventional drugs are being developed for treating the cognitive decline associated with normal ageing and dementia. This indirect approach to enhancing nerve growth factor function could be more therapeutically acceptable, as there is evidence that the direct application of peptides with nerve growth factor activity causes severe side effects in patients with dementia [16].

In conclusion, the development of drugs to treat the main symptoms of AD has largely focused on cholinergic replacement therapy, with relatively modest success. Preclinical research has undoubtedly been hampered by the inadequacy of animal models, as well as the unpredictability of the clinical trials and the limited value of the diagnostic procedures currently available. Although the production of transgenic mice which overexpress β-amyloid is an interesting development in animal modelling, it still has to be proven that this abnormal protein is the main cause of AD. This area has been reviewed recently by Heininger [17]. Clearly there is still a long way to go before effective drugs are discovered that will prevent the broad degenerative changes in the brain that characterize AD, but already there are useful developments which may lead to a better control of the symptoms of the disease, particularly if the treatments are started early. The development of sensitive diagnostic tests would undoubtedly aid this progress.

# REFERENCES

1. Bartus R.T., Johnson H.R. (1976) Short-term memory in the rhesus monkey: disruption by the anticholinergic scopolamine. *Pharmacol. Biochem. Behav.*, **5**: 39–46.
2. Whitehouse P.T., Price D.L., Struble R.G., Clark A.W., Coyle J.T., DeLong M.R. (1982) Alzheimer's disease and senile dementia: loss of neurons in the basal forebrain. *Science*, **215**: 1237–1239.
3. Ridley R.M., Baker H.F., Drewett B., Johnson J.A. (1985) Effects of ibotenic acid lesions of the basal forebrain on serial reversal learning in marmosets. *Brain Res.*, **628**: 56–64.
4. Voytko M.L., Olton D.S., Richardson R.T., Gorman L.K., Tobin T.R., Price D.L. (1994) Basal forebrain lesions in monkeys disrupt attention but not learning and memory. *J. Neurosci.*, **14**: 167–186.
5. Parasuraman R., Haxby J.V. (1993) Attention and brain function in Alzheimer's disease: a review. *Neuropsychology*, 7: 242–272.
6. Sahakian B.J., Owen A.M., Morant N.J., Eagger S.A., Boddington S. (1993) Further analysis of the cognitive effects of tacrine in Alzheimer's disease: assessment of attentional and mnemonic function using CANTAB. *Psychopharmacology*, **110**: 395–401.
7. Starter M., Bruno J.P. (1994) Cognitive functions of cerebral acetylcholine lesions from studies on the transsynaptic modulation of activated efflux. *Trends Neurosci.*, **17**: 17–22.
8. Bird M., Luszcz M. (1993) Enhancing memory performance in Alzheimer's disease: acquisition assistance and cue effectiveness. *J. Clin. Exp. Neuropsychol.*, **15**: 921–932.
9. Jaen J.C., Johnson G., Moos W.H. (1992) Cholinomimetics and Alzheimer's disease. *Bioorg. Med. Chem. Lett.*, **2**: 777–780.
10. Nitsch R.M., Slack B.E., Wurtman R.I., Growdon J.H. (1992) Release of Alzheimer amyloid precursor derivatives stimulated by activation of muscarinic acetylcholine receptors. *Science*, **258**: 304–307.
11. Schroeder H., Giacobini E., Struble R.G., Zilles K., Maclicke A. (1991) Nicotinic cholinoceptive neurons of the frontal cortex are reduced in Alzheimer's disease. *Neurobiol. Aging*, **12**: 259–262.
12. Wilson A.L., Langley L.K., Morley J., Bauer T. (1995) Nicotine patches in Alzheimer's disease: pilot study on learning, memory and safety. *Pharmacol. Biochem. Behav.*, **51**: 509–514.
13. Brioni J.D., Kim D.J.B., O'Neill A.B. (1996) Nicotine cue: lack of effect of the alpha 7 nicotinic receptor antagonist methylcaconitine. *Eur. J. Pharmacol.*, **301**: 1–5.
14. Singh M., Meyer E.M., Millard W.J., Simpkins J.W. (1994) Ovarian steroid deprivation results in a reversible learning impairment and compromised cholinergic function in female rats. *Brain Res.*, **644**: 305–312.
15. Sohrabye F., Green L.A., Miranda R.C., Toran-Allevand C.D. (1994) Reciprocal regulation of oestrogen and NGF receptors by their ligands in PC12 cells. *J. Neurobiol.*, **25**: 974–988.
16. Olson L. (1994) Neurotrophins in neurodegenerative disease: theoretical issues and clinical trials. *Neurochemistry*, **25**: 1–3.
17. Heininger K. (1999) A unifying hypothesis of Alzheimer's disease. 2. Pathophysiological processes. *Hum. Psychopharmacol.*, **14**: 525–581.

4.7
## Issues Regarding the Pharmacotherapy of Dementia
Krista L. Lanctôt[1]

The review by Samuels and Davis provides an overview of treatments for both cognitive and non-cognitive symptoms of dementia. While this practical review generates excitement that there are now treatments for dementia, it clearly highlights the need for additional research in targeted areas.

*Issues in pharmacoeconomics.* Tacrine and other cholinesterase inhibitors may decrease caregiving costs, as outlined in the review. Arguments that these medications delay institutionalization and are therefore cost-saving do not consider the economic impact on the family caregiver. There are many issues to be considered. Valuing the treatment outcome is difficult. Our own willingness-to-pay survey has suggested that even the small symptomatic relief from cholinesterase inhibitors is valuable to family caregivers [1]. Conversely, there may be increased use of medical resources, lost wages and additional utilization of home care, respite care and community resources. Quality of life of the caregiver may also suffer. When the societal perspective is adopted and both direct and indirect costs are measured, cost-effectiveness models suggest that donepezil may be cost-neutral [2–4]. However, these models are hampered by inadequate information. None of the cost or utility information was collected during the clinical trials. The models all used cognitive data from short-term clinical trials to predict long-term economic savings. Cognitive measures may be a poor predictor of economic outcome. There is still a need to demonstrate conclusively that current treatments deliver relevant health outcomes at a cost that is justified with respect to both alternative treatments and alternative uses of resources. Prospective economic evaluations of symptomatic treatments for dementia are warranted.

*Pharmacotherapy of behavioural disturbances.* The review mentions that current treatments for the behavioural and psychological symptoms of dementia (BPSD) arise from clinical trials and from extrapolation from other psychiatric illnesses. This information forms the basis for current treatment recommendations. Current treatment algorithms [5] categorize patients clinically by the presence of a given symptom, with or without an underlying cause (e.g. aggression due to psychosis). Unfortunately, these recommendations are not supported by current evidence. The first problem

[1] *Department of Psychiatry and HOPE Research Centre, Sunnybrook and Women's College Health Sciences Centre, 2075 Bayview Avenue, Toronto, Ontario M4N 3M5, Canada*

is demonstration of efficacy. Conventional antipsychotics have the largest body of literature supporting their use. In fact, randomized controlled trials of conventional antipsychotics show limited efficacy and an important placebo response rate [6]. This lack of efficacy may partially reflect methodological issues with these older trials [6]. Other psychotropic medications, such as antidepressants, atypical antipsychotics, beta-blockers, hormones, lithium, benzodiazepines and anticonvulsants have also been assessed [7]. Second, specific drug-responsive behaviours for each medication are unknown, and may not exist. Overlapping drug-responsive behaviours have been reported for each medication evaluated [7,8]. Since many of the behaviours themselves overlap, selecting on the basis of the presence of a single behaviour will not provide homogeneity of the patient population. Furthermore, the cause of most behaviours is unknown. Therefore, treatment suggestions based on behaviours are not evidence-based and may not be useful to the clinician.

Rational treatment is limited by the fact that the neurobiology of BPSD is not well understood. It has been suggested that alterations in neurotransmitters other than acetylcholine may be responsible for many non-cognitive symptoms [7,9]. For example, our own work suggests that agitated aggression in severe Alzheimer's disease may be related to hyperresponsivity of the serotonergic system [10]. A neurotransmitter-based approach will offer information that, for now, can be more closely linked with treatment options. Novel ligands for neuroimaging make this increasingly feasible. This approach may eventually lead to the identification of behavioural subtypes which may be better linked to treatment outcome.

*Behavioural disturbances in dementia with Lewy bodies (DLB).* As stated in the review, patients with DLB may benefit from cholinesterase inhibitors, as demonstrated by cognitive improvement following tacrine. In theory, behavioural disturbances may also benefit from cholinesterase inhibitors. For example, hallucinations in DLB have been linked to cholinergic dysfunction [11,12]. When we treated seven patients diagnosed with DLB with donepezil to determine its effect on managing behavioural disorders [13], five patients showed improvement in behavioural symptoms. Hallucinations were improved in three of five patients with these symptoms, and delusions were improved in four of four patients. Responders also showed marked improvement in agitation, depression, apathy and irritability. Effective treatment of behavioural disturbances associated with DLB may be limited by side effects. In this case series, four patients reported side effects and two discontinued therapy. The neurobiology of other dementias such as DLB is not well understood, hampering treatment efforts.

# REFERENCES

1. Lanctôt K.L., Oh P.I., Risebrough N., Herrmann N. (1999) Cost–benefit analysis of cholinesterase inhibitors in Alzheimer's disease. *Clin. Pharmacol. Ther.*, **65**: 169.
2. Neumann P.J., Hermann R.C., Kuntz K.M., Araki S.S., Duff S.B., Leon J., Berenbaum P.A., Goldman P.A., Williams L.W., Weinstein M.C. (1999) Cost–effectiveness of donepezil in the treatment of mild or moderate Alzheimer's disease. *Neurology*, **52**: 1138–1145.
3. O'Brien B.J., Goeree R., Hux M., Iskedjian M., Blackhouse G., Gagnon M., Gauthier S. (1999) Economic evaluation of donepezil for the treatment of Alzheimer's disease in Canada. *J. Am. Geriatr. Soc.*, **47**: 570–578.
4. Stewart A., Phillips R., Dempsey G. (1998) Pharmacotherapy for people with Alzheimer's disease: a Markov-cycle evaluation of five years. *Int. J. Geriatr. Psychiatry*, **13**: 445–453.
5. Alexopoulos G.S., Silver J.M., Kahn D.A., Frances A., Carpenter D. (Eds) (1998) Treatment of agitation in older persons with dementia: expert consensus guidelines. *Postgrad. Med.*, Special Issue: 1–88.
6. Lanctôt K.L., Best T.S., Mittmann N., Liu B.A., Oh P.I., Einarson T.R., Naranjo C.A. (1998) Efficacy and safety of neuroleptics in behavioural disorders associated with dementia. *J. Clin. Psychiatry*, **59**: 550–561.
7. Herrmann N., Lanctôt K.L. (1997) From transmitters to treatment: the pharmacotherapy of behavioural disturbances in dementia. *Can. J. Psychiatry*, **42** (Suppl. 1): 51S–64S.
8. Cummings J.L., Back C. (1998) The cholinergic hypothesis of neuropsychiatric symptoms in Alzheimer's disease. *Am. J. Geriatr. Psychiatry*, **6**: S64–S78.
9. Esiri M.M. (1996) The basis for behavioural disturbances in dementia. *J. Neurol. Neurosurg. Psychiatry*, **61**: 127–130.
10. Lanctôt K.L., Herrmann N., Eryavec G., van Reekum R., Naranjo C.A. (1997) Central serotonergic function is related to agitated aggression in Alzheimer's disease. *Clin. Pharmacol. Ther.*, **63**: 222.
11. Perry E.K., Marshall E., Kerwin J., Smith C.J., Jabeen S., Cheng A.V., Perry R.H. (1991) Evidence of monoaminergic–cholinergic imbalance related to visual hallucinations in Lewy body dementia. *J. Neurochem.*, **55**: 1454–1456.
12. Perry E.K., Perry R.H. (1995) Acetylcholine and hallucinations: disease-related compared to drug-induced alterations in human consciousness. *Brain & Cognition*, **28**: 240–258.
13. Lanctôt K.L., Herrmann N. (2000) Donepezil for behavioural disorders associated with Lewy bodies: a case series. *Int. J. Geriatr. Psychiatry* **15**: 338–345.

4.8
## Treatment of Cognitive and Non-cognitive Disturbances in Dementia
William Samuel[1] and Dilip V. Jeste[1]

Dementia has many possible causes, the most frequent being Alzheimer's disease (AD). A high proportion of AD patients have non-cognitive behavioural disturbances, such as agitation (80%), psychosis (30–50%), or depression (20–30%). Jeste and Finkel [1] maintain that psychosis in patients with AD is a distinct entity, different from primary psychotic disorders such as schizophrenia, and has its own set of diagnostic criteria. A comprehensive review of pharmacological therapies in dementia which gives careful attention to potential problems and pitfalls is a very welcome addition to the literature in this area.

In AD and the closely-related dementia with Lewy bodies (DLB), acetylcholinesterase (AChE) inhibitors offer the most effective available therapy for cognitive impairment and may also improve psychosis and agitation [2]. Their usefulness is, however, often limited by undesirable side effects such as hepatotoxicity (most prominent with tacrine), muscle weakness (metrifonate) or intense gastrointestinal disturbance (rivastigmine, galanthamine). All of these substances may prolong the action of succinylcholine anesthesia or potentiate the action and toxicity of cocaine or anesthetics of similar chemical structure. The AChE inhibitor with the most favourable balance between cognitive improvement and undesirable side effects appears to be donepezil, which seems also to have a particularly beneficial effect on cognition, as well as agitation, and psychosis, in DLB as compared to "pure" AD patients [3]. The greater responsiveness of DLB patients to donepezil could be due to their greater absolute deficit in neocortical choline acetyltransferase activity, found in some studies [4].

Until recently, the most common treatment for psychosis and agitation in dementia patients has been conventional or "typical" neuroleptics such as haloperidol. Yet, these drugs have been found to be only modestly more effective than placebo and can produce the particularly problematic side effect of tardive dyskinesia, a potentially persistent movement disorder seen in 30% of elderly patients so treated [5]. Fortunately, the newer atypical antipsychotics offer an alternative means of managing dementia complicated by psychosis or severe agitation. Two large-scale multisite trials of risperidone in nursing home patients and one similar study of olanzapine reported that these drugs were significantly more effective than placebo while having a relatively low risk of side effects. Quetiapine also appears to be efficacious and safe in elderly patients with psychotic disorders,

[1] *Geriatric Psychiatry Division, University of California, San Diego, VA San Diego Healthcare System, 116A-1, 3350 La Jolla Village Drive, San Diego, CA 92161, USA*

including psychosis associated with dementia [6]. It is nonetheless apparent that even the atypical antipsychotics have a risk of certain adverse effects in elderly individuals with dementia and, therefore, need to be prescribed in much lower dosages than those administered to younger adults [5]. The literature on the use of psychotropic medications other than antipsychotics for the treatment of psychosis and agitation in dementia is limited, but suggests that anticonvulsants and antidepressants may be useful in non-psychotic agitation in this patient population.

Returning to the topic of treatments for the cognitive impairment in AD, there have been several reports of an inflammatory component of the disease process in brain tissue. Large-scale retrospective studies have found that exposure to non-steroidal anti-inflammatory drugs (NSAIDs) reduces the risk of developing AD [2], but they are not routinely prescribed for this purpose due to concern for occasionally severe gastrointestinal side effects. For female patients, estrogens offer a comparable mix of potential benefits and hazards. Post-menopausal estrogen therapy for at least 1 or 2 years seems to reduce the likelihood of developing AD, but treating already-demented female patients with estrogens may or may not significantly improve their cognition [2]. While estrogen supplementation in combination with progestins offers general health benefits to post-menopausal women, there is a downside of mildly increased risk of endometrial and breast cancer. Among AD patients of both sexes, other sources of endocrine dysfunction, such as hypothyroidism, must also be considered and ruled out. Treatable nutritional deficiencies (e.g. of vitamin $B_{12}$) must be corrected, and there is evidence of a mild therapeutic benefit from high daily doses of vitamin E [7]. Due to a relative excess of cortisol over dehydroepiandrosterone (DHEA) production by the adrenals that is sometimes seen in AD, DHEA and other anti-cortisols have been proposed as both prophylactic and therapeutic agents [8], but there is so far no strong evidence of their effectiveness. An unconventional therapy, *Gingko biloba*, mildly improved cognition in AD patients in at least one placebo-controlled trial, perhaps due to an anti-platelet effect which maintains blood flow through small vessels in the brain that are vulnerable to thrombotic occlusion with age [9]. Perhaps the most exciting new development in AD therapy is the discovery of the β-secretase that cleaves the amyloid precursor protein (APP) molecule at one end of the segment that forms β-amyloid. Excess amyloid deposition in the brain is the leading contender for being the ultimate cause of AD, and blockade of this process through inhibition of β-secretase or by immuno-modulatory techniques could offer a potential cure for the disease [10].

One must always consider other causes of dementia besides AD, including the pseudodementia of psychiatric depression, which can be ameliorated by conventional antidepressants [2]. Impaired cognition due to a large stroke or the additive effect of several small ones, called vascular dementia, appears to be fairly common in the elderly. The main treatment here is management of stroke risk factors and prophylaxis with an anti-platelet agent. If the brain suffers no further insults, the cognitive deficit should not progress, as it does in AD. The dementia characteristic of normal pressure hydrocephalus is, in theory, treatable with a ventriculoperitoneal shunt, although this diagnosis is difficult to confirm and the treatment is fraught with potential complications. The dementia associated with multiple sclerosis (MS) is thought to be due mainly to the cumulative effect of thousands of axonal transections during the course of the disease and is best treated prophylactically with immunomodulatory agents (interferon-$\beta$ 1a and 1b or glatiramir acetate) approved for use in MS by the United States Food and Drug Administration (FDA) [11]. The severity of dementia often seen in human immunodeficiency virus (HIV) infection correlates with the degree of viremia in the central nervous system (CNS). Treatment is best directed prophylactically against viral replication using the various FDA-approved agents now available [12]. An older, more familiar CNS infection, neurosyphilis, is commonly looked for as a treatable cause of dementia but rarely found in the post-antibiotic era.

In conclusion, dementia has a variety of causes and has both psychiatric and cognitive manifestations. Treatments for psychiatric symptomatology may be applied to any of the dementia subtypes, whereas treatments for cognitive impairment are often disease-specific. In general, the psychiatric manifestations of any of these dementia syndromes will likely diminish to the degree that cognition can be maintained or improved.

## ACKNOWLEDGEMENTS

This work was supported, in part, by the National Institute of Mental Health grants MH43693, MH49671, MH45131, MH42522, MH01452, and by the Department of Veterans Affairs.

## REFERENCES

1. Jeste D.V., Finkel S.I. (2000) Psychosis of Alzheimer's disease: diagnostic criteria for a distinct syndrome. *Am. J. Geriatr. Psychiatry*, **8**: 29–34.
2. Samuel W., Alford M., Hofstetter C.R., Hansen L. (1997) Dementia with Lewy bodies versus pure Alzheimer disease: differences in cognition, neuropathology, cholinergic dysfunction, and synapse density. *J. Neuropathol. Exp. Neurol.*, **56**: 499–508.
3. Samuel W., Caligiuri M., Galasko D., Lacro J., Marini M., McClure F.S., Warren K., Jeste D.V. (2000) Better cognitive and psychiatric response to donepezil in patients prospectively diagnosed as dementia with Lewy bodies: a preliminary study. *Int. J. Geriatr. Psychiatry*. **15**: 794–802.

4.  Samuel W., Galasko D., Thal L.J. (1997)   Alzheimer's disease: biochemical and pharmacological aspects. In *Behavioral Neurology and Neuropsychology* (Eds T.E. Feinberg, M.J. Farah), pp. 551–569, McGraw-Hill, New York.
5.  Jeste D.V. Rockwell E., Harris M.J., Lohr J.B., Lacro J. (1999)   Conventional vs. newer antipsychotics in elderly patients. *Am. J. Geriatr. Psychiatry*, 7: 70–76.
6.  Jeste D.V., Lacro J.P., Nguyen H.A., Petersen M.E., Rockwell E., Sewell D.D., Caligiuri M.P. (1999)   Incidence of tardive dyskinesia with risperidone versus haloperidol. *J. Am. Geriatr. Soc.*, 47: 716–719.
7.  Sano M., Ernesto C., Thomas R.G., Klauber M.R., Schafer K., Grundman M., Woodbury P., Growdon J., Cotman C.W., Pfeiffer E. *et al* (1997)   A controlled trial of selegiline, alpha-tocopherol, or both as treatment for Alzheimer's disease. *N. Engl. J. Med.*, 336: 1216–1222.
8.  Sapse A.T. (1997)   Cortisol, high cortisol diseases and anti-cortisol therapy. *Psychoneuroendocrinology*, 22: S3–S10.
9.  Oken B.S., Storzbach D.M., Kaye J.A. (1998)   The efficacy of gingko biloba on cognitive function in Alzheimer disease. *Arch. Neurol.*, 55: 1409–1415.
10. Relkin N.R. (1999)   Enzyme found that puts the "beta" in beta-amyloid. *Neurol. Alert*, 18: 27–28.
11. van den Noort S., Holland N.J. (Eds) (1999)   *Multiple Sclerosis in Clinical Research*, Demos, New York.
12. Chang L., Ernst T., Leonido-Yee M., Witt M., Speck O., Walot I., Miller E.N. (1999)   Highly active retroviral therapy reverses brain metabolite abnormalities in mild HIV dementia. *Neurology*, 53: 782–789.

4.9

# Are There Concerns About the "Real World" Effectiveness and Safety of Medications for Alzheimer's Disease?

Lon S. Schneider[1]

Samuels and Davis point out some of the important gaps in our knowledge of treatment effectiveness for dementia and Alzheimer's disease (AD) in particular. For example, the aims of the cholinesterase inhibitor trials, nearly always sponsored by industry, are to assess clinical efficacy in order to obtain marketing approval, and not to assess actual clinical value or effectiveness in the community. To this end, rather sensitive cognitive tests are used, differences on which show only modest mean effects on scores. It is difficult as well to assess the impact of cholinesterase inhibitors on daily function. As illustrated by Samuels and Davis, many instruments for rating activities of daily living have been used, some of them proprietary, but differences due to medication, when they occur, are often very small and their correlation with actual clinical function remains speculative.

[1] *Keck School of Medicine, University of Southern California, 1975 Zonal Ave. KAM 400, Los Angeles, CA 90033, USA*

Moreover, the basis on which we assess the usefulness of cholinesterase inhibitors is largely with clinical trials data that are submitted to regulatory authorities, and are comprised of that small proportion of AD patients who are relatively healthy, live with a caregiver and, at an average age of about 72, are significantly younger than the vast majority of people who actually have AD [1].

The use of patients who are not representative of the overall population of AD patients is a continuing and largely unrecognized problem, if for no other reason than that safety data cannot be adequately generalized. For example, the prescribing information for donepezil indicates very little safety concern beyond mild gastrointestinal effects, based largely on two clinical trials in medically healthy AD patients. The cautionary statement, however, mentions muscle cramping, fatigue and insomnia occurring with a greater than 5% incidence and at twice the frequency of placebo, and a low level of accidents and dizziness. Otherwise, the prescribing information implies that side effects are mild. Perhaps not surprisingly, the publications do not mention these side effects [2]. Further concern about cholinesterase inhibitors emerge when it is realized that metrifonate is associated with neurotoxicity, respiratory depression and bradycardia, and that other cholinesterase inhibitors may be associated with these effects as well as weight loss [3].

Of potential concern is that new clinical trials of donepezil, the most widely prescribed cholinesterase inhibitor, reveal a substantial incidence of asthenia, syncope, vertigo and bone fractures, occurring in 5–8% of patients and at twice the rate of placebo over the course of 1 year (slightly less for bone fractures) [4]. Unfortunately, there was no assessment of the incidence of bradyarrhythmias. In another study of nursing home patients [5], who were, of course, over a decade older than the typical outpatients included in trials, and who had a much greater frequency of concomitant medical illnesses, 19% of donepezil-treated patients compared to 10% of placebo patients suffered significant weight loss over a 6-month period, losing a mean of 3 kg. In addition to weight loss, asthenia, anorexia, myasthenia and abdominal pain occurred at nearly twice the rate of placebo and over 5% of the time. Again, although results are neither fully reported nor understood, they are a cause for concern about the actual "real-world" safety of cholinesterase inhibitors when used in the community. These potentially unrecognized and significant adverse effects are in addition to Samuels and Davis' observations on how cholinesterase inhibitors may affect sleep, cause insomnia, nocturnal awakenings and daytime agitation, and yet may be unrecognized by physicians. The possibility exists that the longer a patient is taking a cholinesterase inhibitor, the greater are his or her risks, thus complicating the decision on how long to treat. It is time to do the necessary research and to factor safety into the efficacy question with these medications.

Antioxidants may have salutary effects in a variety of conditions. Indeed, oxidative stress and damage is only part of the neurodegeneration story in AD, and is not specific to it. Unfortunately, there is only one trial suggesting the efficacy of vitamin E or selegiline at delaying the clinical progression of the illness, and in more severely impaired patients. Moreover, both vitamin E and selegiline over the course of approximately 1.4 years had equivalent numbers of patients with significant side effects. It is quite surprising to observe that on the basis of a single study physicians have markedly changed their prescribing behaviour to use more vitamin E, especially so when there seems to be no measurable cognitive effect from either vitamin E or selegiline. This again speaks to the need for more highly effective treatments and the need to better understand this aspect of neurodegeneration.

The anti-inflammatory and estrogen replacement stories are remarkable in their similarities. As Samuels and Davis describe, a substantial body of observational and epidemiologic evidence suggests that either of these two classes of drugs delay the onset of AD or essentially reduce risk for developing it. These observations were enriched by a substantial preclinical literature demonstrating anti-inflammatory, neuroprotective and neurotrophic effects as well. On this basis, clinicians have prescribed anti-inflammatories and estrogen replacement to many patients with AD, long before clinical trials were completed.

Surprisingly, in the clinical trials cited by Samuels and Davis in patients who already had mild to moderate AD, neither anti-inflammatories nor estrogen replacement was effective. Indeed, placebo was more effective than the active drugs on some measures. In effect, some physicians changed their prescribing practices on the basis of a belief and a scientific paradigm, before the clinical evidence was in. At present, we can best understand the effects of anti-inflammatories and estrogen replacement as substances that may have a preventative function for younger people who do not have AD, but not as a symptomatic or therapeutic medication in patients who already have the illness.

Samuels and Davis discuss the critical and interesting issue of the effect of cholinesterase inhibitors on disturbed behaviour, by pointing out that in studies using a certain scale there were measurable mean differences in aspects of behaviour such as depression, apathy, hallucinations and agitation. But these small differences are of unclear clinical significance in patients who were not significantly disturbed to begin with. Further confounding these observations is that in several trials there is a significant incidence of agitation and hallucinations due to the cholinesterase inhibitor, even as "improvement" in agitation is reported as a positive outcome [6]. So it would appear on the one hand that scale scores are somewhat improved overall, but on the other, there are patients whose behaviour becomes worse on cholinesterase inhibitors.

## REFERENCES

1. Schneider L.S., Olin J.T., Lyness S.A., Chui H.C. (1997) Eligibility of Alzheimer's disease clinic patients for clinical trials. *J. Am. Geriatr. Soc.*, **45**: 923–928.
2. Rogers S.L., Farlow M.R., Doody R.S., Mohs R., Friedhoff L.T. (1998) A 24-week, double-blind, placebo-controlled trial of donepezil in patients with Alzheimer's disease. Donepezil Study Group. *Neurology*, **50**: 136–145.
3. Schneider L.S., Giacobini E. (1999) Metrifonate: a cholinesterase inhibitor for Alzheimer's disease therapy. *CNS Drugs*, **5**: 14–27.
4. Winblad B., Engedal K., Soininen H., Verhey F., Waldemar G., Wimo A., Wetterholm A.-L., Haglund A., Subbiah P. (1999) Donepezil enhances global function, cognition and activities of daily living compared with placebo in a one-year, double-blind trial in patients with mild to moderate Alzheimer's disease. Presented at the Ninth Congress of the International Psychogeriatric Association, Vancouver, August 15–20.
5. Tariot P., Perdomo C.A., Whalen E., Sovel M.A., Schwam E.M. (1999) Age is not a barrier to donepezil treatment of Alzheimer's disease in the long-term care setting. Presented at the Ninth Congress of the International Psychogeriatric Association, Vancouver, August 15–20.
6. Raskind M., Cyrus P., Ruzicka B., Gulanski B.I. for the Metrifonate Study Group (1999) The effects of metrifonate on the cognitive, behavioural, and functional performance of Alzheimer's disease patients. *J. Clin. Psychiatry*, **60**: 318–325.

### 4.10
### Phytoneuropsychotropics in Alzheimer's Disease: Treatment and/or Prevention
Turan M. Itil[1]

The somatic treatment of dementia is reviewed in detail in the excellent paper by Samuels and Davis. Instead of repeating some of the issues already described in the review, I would like to comment on two herbal products that are definitely not the first choice in the treatment of Alzheimer's disease (AD), but may become important drugs for prevention.

*Ginkgo biloba.* This is one of the world's oldest living plant species. Known to traditional Chinese medicine for more than 3500 years, it is used as a therapeutic for heart and lung disorders [1]. *Ginkgo* preparations have been available over-the-counter in Europe since the mid-1960s for the treatment of peripheral and central vascular diseases, hearing and vision disorders. In 1994, the German Health Authorities, which are equivalent to the Food and

[1] *New York Institute for Medical Research, New York University Medical Center, 41 Park Avenue, New York, NY 10016, USA*

Drug Administration (FDA) in the USA, approved the standard extract of *Ginkgo biloba* (SeGb) as safe and effective in dementia syndromes, including AD and multi-infarct dementia.

*Ginkgo biloba* became famous overnight among medical professionals in the USA when the results of our multicenter trial were published and subsequently presented at an international media convention at the National Press Club in Washington [2]. This multicenter, double-blind, placebo-controlled parallel group trial indicated that the standard extract of *Ginkgo biloba* (EGb-761®), in comparison to placebo, produced statistically significant, but clinically only "modest" therapeutic effects in patients with AD and multi-infarct dementia, without having any significant or serious side effects. While the quality and quantity of the therapeutic effects were similar to those seen in studies with tacrine, the side effects were less noticeable. Compared to donepezil, SeGb, in daily dosages of 120 mg, produced a lesser degree of clinical appreciable therapeutic effects, but with a lesser degree of side effects. As in tacrine and donepezil trials, SeGb was more effective in patients with lesser degree of illness. Based on the therapeutic results—29% showed improvement on the Alzheimer's Disease Assessment Scale (ADAS-Cog) of at least four points—we interpreted that SeGb would delay the progression of the dementia by approximately 6 months. The findings of quantitative pharmaco-electroencephagraphy (EEG) studies indicated that the 240 mg dose was significantly more effective on the central nervous system (CNS) than the previously recommended daily dose of 120 mg [3]. Indeed, another large clinical trial conducted by Kanowski *et al* [4] showed a more significant therapeutic effect of 240 mg of SeGb on AD than that of 120 mg daily dose of our study. The therapeutic effect of *Ginkgo biloba* was hypothesized to be the result of synergistically acting multiple compounds of SeGb involved in the counteraction of the inflammation and oxidative stress, providing membrane protection and neurotransmitter modulation. This would result in the improvement of the speed of information processing [5]. The therapeutic effects of *Ginkgo biloba* may be similar to vitamin E and most likely dissimilar to the marketed anti-AD drugs with potent cholinesterase inhibiting properties.

Based on our own as well as other studies [6], *Ginkgo biloba* has therapeutic effects on memory disturbances. However, because of the lesser degree of therapeutic efficacy than that of donepezil and the unknown mode of action, *Ginkgo biloba* should not be the first choice of treatment of dementia. Even in benign memory disturbance, a person should not treat him- or herself with extract of *Ginkgo biloba* or any over-the-counter product. He or she should go to an expert to have a thorough medical, psychological, brain function and performance evaluation. If the diagnosis of AD is established, a marketed, prescription drug, that is proven to be safe and effective, must be initiated. *Ginkgo biloba* or vitamin E may be combined with standard drugs, if necessary.

*Huperzine-A (Hup-A).* This an alkaloid compound was discovered in Chinese herbal medicine and used in China for centuries to treat fever and inflammation. Just recently, the purified compound has been used as a prescription drug for the treatment of memory disturbances and senility. Although Hup-A has no antipyretic or anti-inflammatory properties, it appears to be an important inhibitor of acetylcholinesterase [7]. It affords almost absolute specificity for acetylcholinesterase, having very little efficacy on butyrylcholinesterase, in marked contrast to compounds like tacrine.

Most of the basic scientific data concerning pharmacological effect suggest clinical anti-dementia properties of Hup-A. However, the published clinical studies are much less convincing that Hup-A has therapeutic effects on AD. There are no published bioavailability trials and/or double-blind, placebo-controlled clinical trials with adequate sample size.

We conducted a series of Phase I to Phase II clinical studies in the USA with Hup-A using our method of quantitative pharmaco-EEG. In a safety study, 30 healthy volunteers received $50 \mu g$ daily of Hup-A up to 30 consecutive days. No significant clinical side effects or abnormal findings were established [8]. In other studies, healthy volunteers as well as subjects with age-associated cognitive dysfunctions received single dosages of 100 and $200 \mu g$ of Hup-A alone or in combination with 120 mg of SeGb. Again, there were no clinical side effects. $100 \mu g$, but particulary $200 \mu g$ Hup-A, produced significant pharmacological effects on human brain function, as it was evident by the increase of slow and decrease of alpha frequencies in computer-analyzed EEG measurements. The effects were classified by the drug data base in some subjects as "antidepressant", in others as "anxiolytic" and in some others as "cognitive activator". In the same population, 46% of the subjects showed strong cognitive activating pharmacological effects with 240 mg of SeGb, and in a lesser degree with 120 mg (33% of the subjects). $200 \mu g$ of Hup-A alone produced a much smaller degree (16%) of cognitive activator effects. In 50% of the subjects, Hup-A produced antidepressant – anxiolytic type CNS effects. However, when 120 mg of SeGb were combined with only $100 \mu g$ of Hup-A, the subjects showed more cognitive activating pharmacological effects than those seen after $200 \mu g$ of Hup-A alone (33% of the subjects). Thus, we hypothesized that the combination of *Ginkgo biloba* and Hup-A produced synergistic pharmacological effects, which may result in important therapeutic effects in AD and other dementias [9]. According to our studies and the results of the basic studies, we also hypothesize that a combination of *Ginkgo biloba* and Hup-A may be a promising preventive treatment. Safety profiles of both compounds, along with the economy, will certainly make them both eligible candidates for a secondary prevention program.

## REFERENCES

1. Newall C.A., Anderson L.A., Phillipson J.D. (Eds) (1997) *Herbal Medicines: a Guide for Health Care Professionals*, Pharmaceutical Press, London.
2. Le Bars P., Katz M.M., Berman N., Itil T.M., Freedman A.M., Schatzberg A.F. (1997) A placebo-controlled, double-blind, randomized trial of an extract of *Ginkgo biloba* for dementia. *JAMA*, **278**: 1327–1332.
3. Itil T.M., Eralp E., Tsambis E., Itil K.Z., Stein U. (1996) Central nervous system effects of *Ginkgo biloba*, a plant extract. *Am. J. Ther.*, **3**: 63–73.
4. Kanowski S., Herrmann W.M., Stephan K., Wierich W., Horr R. (1996) Proof of efficacy of the *Ginkgo biloba* special extract (EGb 761) in outpatients suffering from mild to moderate primary degenerative dementia of the Alzheimer's type or multi-infarct dementia. *Pharmacopsychiatry*, **29**: 47–56.
5. Packer L. Haramaki N. Kawabata T., Marcucci L., Maitra I., Maguire J.J., Droy-Lefaix M.-T., Sekaki A.H., Gardes-Albert M. (1995) *Ginkgo biloba* extract (EGb 761). In *Effects of Ginkgo biloba Extract (EGb 761) on Aging and Age-Related Disorders* (Eds Y. Christen, Y. Courtois, M.T. Droy-Lefaix), pp. 23–47, Elsevier, Paris.
6. DeFeudis F. V. (1998) *Ginkgo biloba Extract (EGb 761): from Chemistry to the Clinic*, Ullstein Medical Verlagsgesellschaft GmbH and Co., Wiesbaden.
7. Tanczxg X.C., Zhu X.D., Lu W.H. (1988) Studies on the nootropic effects of huperzine A and B: two selective AChE inhibitors. In *Current Research in Alzheimer Theory: Cholinesterase Inhibitors* (Eds E. Giacobini, R. Becker), pp. 289–293, Taylor and Francis, New York.
8. Ahmet I., Itil T.M., Kunitz A. Chronic administration of huperzine A in healthy subjects. Submitted for publication.
9. Itil T.M. Central nervous system effects of huperzine A alone and in combination with *Ginkgo biloba* and its clinical implications. Submitted for publication.

# 5

# Psychosocial Interventions for Dementia: A Review

## Franz Baro

*Catholic University of Leuven, Psychiatric Centre Sint-Kamillus, Broeders van Liefde, Krijkelberg 1, B–3360 Bierbeek, Belgium*

## INTRODUCTION

This review starts with a section on the most common psychosocial interventions for patients with dementia: reality orientation therapy, reminiscence, validation therapy, behaviour modification, sensory stimulation and motor activity. Then it covers individual and group psychotherapeutic approaches to those patients and support interventions for the principal carers. Finally, it addresses the quality of life issues that must be considered in the development of a comprehensive approach to helping both patients and their families.

## REALITY ORIENTATION THERAPY

Almost certainly, reality orientation therapy existed before 1958, but it was in that year that James Folsom set up a structured programme with that name in the USA. The methods and implementation were further developed and subsequently used worldwide. Originally designed for people who are disoriented as well as neglected, it has been applied to many other populations [1].

Three major components of reality orientation therapy are usually identified [2]. The first is the 24-hour, continual process (sometimes called "informal" or "basic") whereby staff present current information to the patient in every interaction, reminding him or her of time, place, persons, events, etc. and responding to all questions. The environment is structured with signs and cues to help the person.

*Dementia, Second Edition.* Edited by Mario Maj and Norman Sartorius.
© 2002 John Wiley & Sons Ltd.

As a supplement, intensive sessions of reality orientation (variously called "classes", "intensive" or "formal" reality orientation, and "groups") are held daily for half an hour to an hour with three to six patients depending on the level of impairment. According to this level, the group sessions are divided into basic, standard and advanced. The basic group repeats simple information on day, weather, names, etc. The standard group uses sensory stimulation and past/present discussion. The advanced group has a wide range of activities.

The final traditional component of reality orientation therapy is the use of one of a number of prescribed attitudes (attitude therapy) to be used by all care staff with a particular person. This attitude is chosen according to the person's personality and needs, in order to facilitate staff consistency.

It should be noted that reality orientation therapy is based on interaction between staff and patient and provides, of course, many opportunities for prompting and social reinforcement of desired behaviour as in a behavioural approach. It also involves environmental changes, through the use of memory aids, signs, etc. The person is shown where to find the answer to the question. In the group and outside, the person is enabled to succeed, thus functioning and feeling better.

Reminiscence, stimulation and even validation techniques have been incorporated in sensitive applications of reality orientation therapy for some time. Also, positive attitudes of both staff and institutions are involved. Communication implies listening as well as talking, with respect for the older person with dementia. Clearly, there is much common ground between reality orientation therapy and other psychosocial approaches [2].

Controlled trials offer solid evidence that reality orientation sessions are associated with improved scores on measures of verbal orientation. This improvement is rarely associated with basic 24-hour reality orientation [3]. It seems to be a very restricted form of learning; general cognitive change does not occur but some reports suggest improvements in new learning ability [4]. Behaviouural changes are much more elusive, but many anecdotal reports point to an increased sense of well-being.

Reality orientation therapy, as perhaps the most studied of psychosocial approaches, has been subject to numerous critiques over the years [2]. Especially, its emphasis on verbal learning by repetition (at least in the classroom setting) has been particularly identified as a limitation of the approach, with cognitively impaired older people being thought to respond better to a more systematic, multi-model approach, including non-verbal material.

Actually, in current use, reality orientation therapy has developed to a point where it requires another name, having all but abandoned the classroom format and now having a positive influence in areas outside verbal orientation. More specifically, reality orientation therapy seems to provide a reassuring foundation in reality for those who are unable to provide it for themselves [5].

## REMINISCENCE

Since Butler's [6] seminal work on life review, reminiscence is seen as a positive activity, rather than as a negative attitude of old people. Also, persons with dementia retain an ability to recall the distant past, often in detail, far longer than they can remember and recall the recent past; therefore they should find it easier to talk about their pasts than to talk about the here and now.

There are several forms of reminiscence work, such as life review, simple reminiscence, life history, and life story. There is still considerable confusion as to the aims, target population and techniques of reminiscence therapy.

Life review is seen as a task to be accomplished in the last phase of life. Acceptance is the goal of a successful life review; despair is the consequence of a life seen as worthless. Life review therapy is an active attempt to make sense of distressing memories; it should be undertaken with the person's consent, with a clear aim, by properly trained and supervised therapists. Generally speaking, it is a more appropriate approach for older people without dementia. Garland [7] provides an account of life review therapy. A study examining the effects on veteran and novice participants of a life review program, designed for nursing home residents with Alzheimer's disease (AD) or severe cognitive dysfunction, has shown that there is an impact on the level of disorientation, social interaction and self-esteem. There is some evidence that the improvements may be stored in memory and triggered when the program is repeated [8].

The focus of simple reminiscence, by comparison, is on providing pleasure, communication and socialization. This form of reminiscence may be individual or group-based, structured or free-flowing, spontaneous or prompted, general or specific. Sad memories may emerge, but support is available from the therapist. Reminiscence work is appropriate for people with dementia. Norris [9] provides an overview of reminiscence techniques and their practical applications. The 1998 book *Reminiscence in Dementia Care* [10] gives a stimulating account of reminiscence work as a means of improving the quality of life of older people with dementia and of those who care for them.

Another form of reminiscence is the life history work. This approach involves the compilation of a detailed life history, from which a care-plan is evolved, aiming at more personalized interactions, activities and environments. Particularly in a group setting, awareness of participants' life histories is important, to ensure that appropriate support can be given if distressing memories are being raised [11].

Life story work, as opposed to life history, consciously includes contemporary aspects of the life of the person with dementia. Life story material combines written information, photographs, postcards, videos, newspaper cuttings and other significant images. Its aim is to see "the person behind the illness" in caring for people with dementia. It provides a sense of continuity between the past and the present and may assist a person to overcome inevitable change. It only works if the staff are honestly interested in learning from the older person [12].

Empirical research on reminiscence with people with dementia is scarce, despite many positive anecdotal reports (e.g. [13,14]). Reminiscence work seems to provide a meaningful and stimulating activity for people with even a severe dementia, greater staff knowledge of the residents, and enjoyment of sessions [15,16]. Small, structured groups seem to be most effective for people with dementia [17].

Some people do not enjoy reminiscence, because their past has been full of troubles or because reflecting on a happy past acts as a reminder of all that has been lost in the present [18]. It must be re-emphasized that simple reminiscence is practised purely for pleasure, whereas life review aims to solve painful memories in order for the individual to come to terms with the present [19].

Some persons will not reminisce at all, as they find the present totally fulfilling [20]. Other persons will produce confabulation or pseudo-reminiscence, making it difficult but not impossible to grasp the sense of their stories [21]. People will also differ in how much they wish to speak about personal matters in a group setting, and members should never be prompted or pressured to do so. These and other factors of importance that should be considered in running reminiscence groups are outlined by Holden and Woods [2] and Woodrow [14].

## VALIDATION THERAPY

Validation therapy was developed in the USA by Naomi Feil [22] as a way of communicating with disoriented elderly persons by validating and supporting their feelings in whatever time or location is real to them, even though this may not correspond to the present reality. For example, many people with dementia talk of their parents, as if they were still alive. This should be seen as an expression of need, not simply as a sign of confusion. They feel a deep need for protection in a perplexing environment; this need returns to the parents, the original attachment figures [23]. Confronting such persons with the present reality ("the truth") often leads to the person withdrawing and even becoming hostile.

The aim of validation therapy is to restore dignity and prevent the retreat into vegetation, through the provision of an empathic, non-judgemental listener, who accepts the person's view of reality. At the core of this approach is the recognition of the individuality of the person with dementia, the importance of what has gone on previously in the person's life, and the need to resolve "unfinished business" before the end of their life. Painful feelings from the past that are expressed, acknowledged and validated are expected to decrease in strength; whereas if ignored or not expressed they are expected to heighten.

Feil [24] describes in detail the techniques involved, the exclusion criteria, and the general or personal issues to be tackled. The core technique is to recognize the person's communication of feelings and emotions and to acknowledge and validate these, verbally and non-verbally. This technique can be applied on a one-to-one basis, as well as in a group setting. The specific techniques include many aspects of non-verbal communication (use of touch, eye contact, tone of voice, etc.) as well as using music, rituals and roles. Group members are encouraged to take on responsibilities within the group (e.g. hostess, song leader), intended to reflect the person's background and needs.

A number of anecdotal reports attest to the effectiveness of validation therapy in individual as well as group applications. A pilot study by Bleathman and Morton [25] has documented the surprising ability of moderately demented group members to share feelings and problems, and the depth of interactions during the sessions.

Carrying out validation successfully is demanding and draining; it is recommended to seek support and supervision [2].

Validation therapy has attracted some criticism. Putting emphasis on past life and unresolved conflicts, it may overlook current sources of devaluation [26]. Also, it may encourage staff to collude with delusion [27]. The emphasis on "unfinished business" could lead to the assumption that if one can learn to cope with life's problems in an adaptive way, dementia can be avoided; there is no evidence to support this notion [2]. It is re-emphasized that, in contrast to other psychosocial approaches, validation merely acknowledges and validates individual feeling; it is not deemed necessary to update past experiences.

## BEHAVIOUR MODIFICATION

Stokes and Goudie [28] provided a practical account of behavioural approaches to working with problems common in dementia care, such as wandering, screaming and aggression. Miller and Morris [29] identified four areas where learning is relatively well preserved in patients with AD: classical conditioning, operant conditioning, implicit memory, and verbal learning and retention. If any learning is possible for the dementing person, then the behavioural approach will facilitate the learning process. It will indicate the environmental conditions needed for new behaviour to be learned, or for existing behaviour to be maintained.

Applied behaviour modification is—unfortunately so—demonstrated whenever attempts by residents in nursing homes to be independent in self-care are ignored by staff, as it often happens, whilst dependent behaviour is systematically reinforced [30]. A more positive example, given by Sandman [31], is based on the preservation of implicit memory. When dementia sufferers were involved in a significant event standing out from the usual routine (e.g. a picnic), and subsequently asked about details of the day, such as who they met, they showed better recall for items from these special days whilst being significantly impaired on items from ordinary days. By making the experience as rich and meaningful as possible, memories associated with it will be enhanced. Another therapeutic application concerns noisemaking, one of the most disturbing behaviour disorders associated with dementia. Interventions used by Doyle *et al* [32] were contingent reinforcement of quiet behaviour and environmental stimulation tailored to individual preferences. A number of long-term care residents with severe dementia showed a clear reduction in noise during the intervention period.

Holden and Woods [2] offer an interesting review of applied studies of behavioural approach to self-care, speech difficulties, mobility, social interaction, participation in activities, continence, challenging behaviour, and excess disabilities. There is still little systematic research on the use of behaviour modification *per se* with patients clearly diagnosed as having dementia, and the positive results are limited. To be successful, a behavioural approach involves a careful individual assessment (e.g. shouting or screaming may be a way of expressing pain, echoing noise made by others, self-stimulation, attention seeking, suffering delirium, etc.) as well as an individual package of interventions. Given this person-centred approach, the authors are in favour of the consistent application of reward techniques.

The fundamental principle in encouraging change is the use of a reward for desirable behaviour and no reward for inappropriate behaviour. Such an approach is often mistakenly equated with "artificial" and "mechanical", but good interpersonal relationships with staff are of prime importance as motivational force. Moreover, cold or punishing relationships have to be excluded on ethical grounds; programmes using punishment have lent themselves too readily to abuse, especially in institutions or carers under pressure from poor resources.

## SENSORY STIMULATION

Elderly people with dementia may experience reduced sensory input for several reasons: first, by virtue of deterioration in sensory acuity; second, their environment can be monotonous and lacking in sensory stimulation; third, the person can withdraw and reject stimulation, as a means of coping with an unwanted experience (e.g. constant playing of radio or TV, noisy group sessions, aggressive staff). The lack of stimulation often leads to increase in confusion, wandering at night, etc.

A number of studies have shown that anxiety in patients with dementia is lower immediately following expressive physical touch and verbalization. Therefore, it behoves family members as well as caregivers to use expressive physical touch and verbalization when caring for these patients, since it is cost-effective, simple to learn and practice, and effective in improving and maintaining patients' quality of life [33].

Programmes offering a range of social, physical and psychosocial stimulation (including occupational therapy, domestic and recreational activities) have reported positive effects and become a widely accepted aspect of good practice [34]. The focus of attention has now shifted to consideration of more specific forms of stimulation or activity (e.g. music, pets, children).

Whilst no differences in reaction to touch and smell were detected, a study by Norberg et al [35] indicated a definite positive response to music in severely demented patients. In a less impaired group of demented patients, "Big Band" music from the 1920s and 1930s clearly improved the mood, social interaction and recall of personal information [36]. Music therapy in dementia seems to have a universal appeal [37].

Examining the effects of preferred music in decreasing occurrences of aggressive behaviour during bathing episodes, individuals aged 55–95 with severe Alzheimer's type dementia were randomly scheduled for observation during bath time under either a control (no music) condition or an experimental condition in which recorded selections of preferred music were played via audiotape recorder. Following a 2-week (10 observations) period, conditions were reversed; a total of 20 observations were recorded for each individual [38]. During the music condition decreases were significant for identified aggressive behaviours; caregivers frequently reported improved affect and a general increase in cooperation with the bathing task.

A programme bringing school-age children together with older people with dementia prompted a significant increase in interaction and activity [39]. Such stimulation needs careful handling—the attraction wears off rapidly when the children are too noisy and lively, or run around out of control.

Visitors with a dog had a positive impact on interaction levels, mobility and dependency in demented people [40,41], but the improvements were not maintained on subsequent days. The presence of the pets is needed to elicit the changes.

An innovative programme, originating in the Netherlands, is called "Snoezelen"—a contraction of two Dutch words, meaning "sniffing and dozing". Using gentle touch and music, relaxing armchairs, cushions, pleasant smells, soap bubbles, coloured lights and visual effects, "snoezelen" improved mood and decreased agitation, although with little carry-over beyond the session [42].

## MOTOR ACTIVITY

Most activity programmes include some form of motor activity, except where there is a reluctance to involve older, frailer people. There have been some indications of cognitive improvement, but it was difficult to link any benefit with certainty to the physical exercise component of the total programme [43].

There is sufficient evidence to show that inactivity is a major weakening factor. There is also evidence that structured physical activity (such as brisk walking, movement to music, throwing a ball, light bending and stretching exercises) can produce changes of a physical nature in older people in general, but much weaker evidence was found that cognitive function in people with dementia might be enhanced [44,45]. It is suggested that physical exercise should be performed during the daytime or early evening in order to improve sleep quality, with the late evenings offering quieter activities in preparation for sleep.

Examining the acquisition and long-term retention of a gross motor skill, Dick-Muehlke *et al* [46] found AD patients able to learn and retain a tossing task as well as healthy controls. Only subjects receiving constant practice showed these changes; there was no benefit from varied practice. These results suggest that people with dementia have the potential to relearn basic activities of daily living involving a significant motor component (e.g. dressing), but only under constant practice conditions (that is, practice must involve invariant repetitions of a movement pattern rather than variations of the skill to be acquired). A recent study [47] has also shown that patients with AD who were apraxic had normal motor learning. Such results suggest that ideomotor praxis and motor learning are at least partly dissociable.

Burgio *et al* [48] successfully applied a prompt and praise procedure to increase independence in walking. The improvement was evident as soon as the behavioural intervention began and was generally maintained at a 4-month follow-up. Not only did most patients walk further, but most progressed to more independent means of mobility, e.g. needing less staff assistance, using fewer prosthetic aids, not using a wheelchair, etc. An important component of the intervention appeared to be the opportunity it provided to the patient to walk; therefore efforts were made to teach the staff to adopt the intervention procedure.

Relaxation programmes offer another example of the effects of motor activity on health and well-being in older people with dementia. An interesting study by Welden and Yesavage [49] provides support for the usefulness of relaxation techniques with this population. Twenty-four matched pairs of patients with dementia attended either a relaxation-training group or a current affairs discussion group for an hour three times a week over a 3-month period. Relaxation instructions included progressive muscle relaxation and a self-hypnosis technique. Subjects attending relaxation sessions showed improvement on ratings of behavioural function compared with the control group. In addition, just over 40% of those taught relaxation techniques no longer required sleeping medication, whereas none of the control group was able to discontinue.

Other conventional relaxation techniques (such as hand/foot massage, aromatherapy, gentle music, one-to-one encouragement of slow deep breathing, etc.) were equally effective in calming patients with dementia [50]. In fact, the above-mentioned sensory stimulation approach, named "snoezelen", has a strong relaxation component [42]. Also, expressive physical touch with verbalization was effective in producing a relaxation response as well as in decreasing episodes of dysfunctional behaviour [33]. On the other hand, two nursing interventions using therapeutic touch and, even more, hand massage, were effective in producing a relaxation response in persons with dementia who had a history of agitation behaviours, but they did not decrease agitation behaviour [51].

Physical exercise cannot ignore psychological and emotional needs. Man is a functional "mind–body" unit. Psychomotor functions are fundamentally important. They encompass a wide variety of movement-mediated activities. Droës and Van Tilburg [52] compared psychomotor therapy with general therapy in demented patients. In this study, psychomotor therapy refers to a group therapeutic method with supportive and behavioural elements, in which movement activities are employed in coping with adaptive problems. The results showed a positive influence of psychomotor therapy on emotional-behavioural problems such as dissatisfaction, aggression and restlessness at night.

Studying the psychomotor competence of demented elderly, Hendrickx and De Lausnay [53] have developed an innovative motor–cognitive approach. Every individual's life situation has, at any moment, a complex structure with three basic dimensions: non-conscious motor-cognitive, partially conscious emotional-affective, and conscious intellectual-cognitive. The motor-cognitive dimension is determined by the direct and spontaneous relation between, on the one hand, the action body that turns to the world and, on the other hand, the perception and action field that is pre-structured by the position and the approaching activity of the action body. Objects and events that are not part of this action field do not exist in the subjective experience and therefore fail to influence the person's behaviour. Systematic motor-cognitive observation gives a valid insight in the constraints of the perception and action field of the demented individual.

The motor-cognitive interpretation strongly contributes to better understanding of relationships between functional changes in the course of the dementia and inverse corresponding development sequences. Often the motor-cognitive stages of dementia can be translated into developmental age equivalents, thus allowing standardized assessment and structured interventions that optimize remaining capabilities.

The relevance of this "retrogenesis" model for dementia management has to be explored and eventually amended, but there is little doubt that the model can offer useful understanding of the general and specific care needs of the patient. Knowledge of retrogenesis and the developmental age of the older person with dementia can form the nucleus for the development of nascent science of disease management [54].

## INDIVIDUAL PSYCHOTHERAPY

The myth persists that older people are not "psychologically minded" and that they cannot change. Psychotherapies have been offered to older adults less often than to younger people. This may be related to ageist attitudes towards older people, perpetuating negative stereotypes about later life and predicting inevitable decline and the impossibility of change. In recent years there has been a dramatic surge of interest in work with older people. Socioeconomically it is an important developing area. Along with psychoeducational work with families of dementia sufferers, individual psychotherapy for persons with dementia is emphasized in terms of quality care, in interaction with cognitive-enhancing drug treatment.

Meaningful psychotherapy with persons with dementia has traditionally been considered difficult, if not impossible, given their lack of awareness. Communication is frequently limited to simple concrete subjects and closed-ended questions, especially in the later stages of AD. A study of facial expression of demented patients has shown how difficult it is to find a balance between imputing too much meaning into the patients' sparse and unclear cues and ignoring the possibility that there is some meaning to be interpreted [55].

The use of broad opening statements or questions, establishing commonalties, speaking as equals, sharing of self-facilitated expression of feeling, and recognizing themes with salience for the individual have been recommended to maintain communication with demented persons [56]. Investigation of the effects of emotional involvement has shown that fear reinforces memory retention of distressing episodes (e.g. a devastating earthquake) in subjects with AD, but does not enhance retention of their factual content and context, despite repeated exposure to the information [57].

Given the complexities of work with people with dementia, individual psychotherapies have not followed the traditional pathways: supportive, insight-oriented, cognitive-behavioural. Insight-oriented psychotherapy, for instance, has not been commonly used, because persons with dementia may have difficulty in memory, awareness, verbalizing and reflecting. Also, sad memories may emerge, leading to the person being withdrawn, depressed, even hostile.

The study of insight in dementia has been relatively neglected [58]. The relationship between level of insight and severity of dementia was studied in a large sample of patients with AD, largely with mild to moderately severe dementia, who were enrolled in the Consortium to Establish a Registry for Alzheimer's Disease (CERAD) [59]. This study confirms the generally accepted belief that patients with AD experience a progressive loss of insight as the severity of dementia increases (see also [60,61]).

Another follow-up study showed patients with AD to have significantly greater unawareness of cognitive deficit than patients with vascular dementia [62]. Both groups had significantly greater unawareness of cognitive deficit than a geropsychiatric and a geriatric control group. These results support the premise that, independent of dementia severity, unawareness of cognitive deficit is disease-specific.

The term "cognitive psychotherapy" or "cognitive therapy" refers to a group of interventions which adopt a communication-oriented approach towards improving cognitive functioning. Therapies such as reality orientation, validation, reminiscence and life review are thus included to some extent within the category of cognitive therapy. Existing research offers contradictory evidence as to the practical application and usefulness of such therapies. The relationship between these therapies is complex and overlapping, as it is unlikely that they are practised in a pure form. The research methodology is still weak. Increased job satisfaction could be held accountable for promoting these therapies.

On the other hand, there is little doubt that people with dementia are able to express their views and feelings to a much greater degree and for a longer period of time than has generally been thought to be possible. Many moving accounts of a year-long process of psychotherapy with one person with dementia have been published (e.g. [63,64]).

In recent years there have been developments in the application of dynamic psychotherapy [65], counselling [28] and cognitive-behavioural therapy [66] to older people with dementia. These developments reflect the earlier recognition and diagnosis of dementing conditions, resulting in a growing number of individuals with a clear awareness of what is happening to them. As yet, detailed studies of these approaches with these patients are not available.

The narrative approach to psychotherapy with people with dementia [67] provides a good example of meaningful psychotherapy. A person with dementia has so much to try and make sense of; among his or her experiences may be an overwhelming sense of loss, uncertainty and threat, all of which is lived out within the context of cognitive difficulties and a changed social world. It should therefore be no surprise that within the stories that people with dementia tell about the past and the present a therapist can see echoes of these losses and threats. These stories can be understood as a way of exploring the present and thus making sense out of it. Sometimes the stories that people with dementia tell are of occasions in the past when they had been important people, such as a teacher, a nurse and a mother; this valued identity is often in painful contrast with their current identity as dependent and often devalued people. The telling of stories thus allows the narrator to present him- or herself in a variety of different "identities", experiences and emotional meanings. This process is not easy, nor is it always possible.

Related to this narrative approach, as well as to validation, is resolution therapy, based on counselling methods [28]. There is less emphasis on the painful past and more on identifying the current feelings, using counselling skills—empathic listening, warmth, acceptance, etc. Having identified the feelings, the next stage is to acknowledge them, verbally and non-verbally, and to modify the environment and the pattern of care to respond to unmet needs.

Learning from experience and from critiques of specific approaches, Holden and Woods [2] are in favour of developing an integrated approach, able to satisfy the diversity of individual needs, responses and preferences shown by people with dementia. The first and fundamental feature of an integrated approach is that it should be based on an explicit set of values regarding the elderly person with dementia (such as the King's Fund principles [68]). Any approach can be potentially harmful if applied with "malignant" attitudes that devalue the elderly person [69]. The second feature is a careful, thorough holistic assessment of the person; the third feature is an individualized care-plan with clear, realistic, regularly reviewed goals.

## GROUP PSYCHOTHERAPY

The apparent increase in sociability and ability to converse noticed in many persons with dementia participating in group approaches (such as reminiscence, validation or reality orientation sessions) may result from the provision of a more stimulating group environment [70]. Groups are advantageous, first, in that they provide an opportunity for people to talk with one another within a socially stimulating environment. Second, a group enables persons with dementia to develop some sense of belonging to a group (group identity). Third, a group provides a structured situation in which staff can directly help these persons to re-learn or adapt to difficulties. Moreover, it is evident that, in order to maximize resources, group meetings may be preferable; they are often cheaper and easier to organize.

It is clear that therapists must have a working knowledge of the group process and of interaction between people in order to practise effectively. Heron [71] defined six dimensions of group facilitation: planning (where aims and objectives are set); meaning (where explanation is given to group actions); confronting (where individuals or the group as a whole are challenged); feeling (how is emotional release to be handled?); structuring (how is the group to be structured over a period of time?); valuing (whereby a supportive atmosphere is created).

For a group to work, it requires a shared interest, activity or purpose. Therapists should be very clear about the purpose of the group and the commitment they are making. They have to establish a consistent setting and time in order to provide continuity. Topics can be decided by the therapist or, as the group matures and becomes more autonomous, by the group members themselves. It is imperative that suitable members are chosen for the group. People of similar cognitive ability should be matched. Individuals with moderate to severe dementia will restrict the facilitator's ability to cope with a large group. At all times, the therapist has the responsibility of maintaining a safe and securing environment. The professionals, likely to be faced with this important but demanding task of group therapy, should get appropriate training and support. A useful guide to setting up groups has been produced by Bender and Norris [72].

Specialist services bring people with dementia together in two kinds of groups. The first kind is "therapeutic", where participants engage in psychosocial therapy. The second kind of group is more "pragmatic"; recipients meet in pragmatic groups because they share a need, which is professionally defined (e.g. day care).

In pragmatic groups, recipients are likely to spend more time with other clients than with staff [73]. Will this kind of social interaction improve or diminish self-esteem and well-being? Will diversity be stimulating or difficult to tolerate? When does healthy assertiveness become aggressive behaviour? What can staff do to promote good interactions? There are no easy answers. Pragmatic groups exist mainly because of lack of resources, and the quality of social interactions in these groups are often neglected.

Overviewing the variety of therapeutic groups available, it seems difficult to classify them according to traditional criteria (such as supportive, insight-oriented, cognitive-behavioural), exactly as already pointed out in relation to individual psychotherapies with dementing people. For instance, most if not all groups commonly used for people with dementia are supportive. Their basic aim is to help the dementing person succeed; indeed, dementia brings so many experiences of failure that every opportunity must be grasped to reverse this damaging trend.

Holden and Woods [2] offer a wealth of ideas for stimulating and purposeful group activities (e.g. music to reinforce orientation, reminiscence theatre, games with children). They suggest breaking down group activities into those suitable for each level of ability. The basic group aims at the lowest level of ability; its activities have to open up communication with the person. In the standard group, the person is drawn into contributing to the group. In the advanced group, the group initiates its own programs. At times, special groups based around a shared difficulty will be formed (e.g. language deficits) and a program designed to meet this specific need.

## GROUP LIVING

One might speculate that people with dementia would be adversely affected by large groups. In smaller groups it becomes easier to develop positive patient-to-patient interaction. This concept has attracted much interest and has been implemented in many residential homes for older people in the UK and elsewhere. Group living combines changes to the care regime with changes to the physical environment. Group living homes are divided into living units of 8–12 members. Each group shares a range of self-care activities. Anecdotally, results were promising [74], with residents reporting greater life satisfaction and staff greater job satisfaction; rejection of the less able seemed to occur less frequently in smaller groups. Relatives, volunteers and neighbours were said to come into the homes more. However, the physical changes in themselves do not always provide a positive change of regime, whereas, on the other hand, a number of large homes are adopting positive changes without the group living format.

In Sweden, group living homes have developed quite differently; typically they consist of a group of four flats in an ordinary housing block, in which eight people with dementia live, each having their own room and possessions, with 24-hour staff cover for the unit as a whole. The Swedish group living homes are a cost-effective alternative to institutional care, but they are unable to manage aggressive behaviour, severe physical disabilities, and severe dementia [75]. Comparing a group of people with dementia moved from institutional care with a control group who remained, it was found that cognitive and mood changes favoured the group living residents over a 6-month period, although both groups declined over a full year [76].

## THERAPEUTIC BUILDINGS

The built environment can have a fundamental effect on a person with dementia: probably greater than on people who are mentally fit. Generally speaking, the environment has the greatest effect on the person with the least capacity. Cohen and Day [77] have produced an influential book on the expertise of North America, and Judd *et al* [78] have produced another book on similar lines with Australian and Northern European examples.

Research on the impact of specific aspects of design is very rare [79,80]. Given this paucity of research, it is significant that there is an almost unanimous consensus about good design for dementia [81]. As far as design is concerned, it is helpful to see dementia as a disability: this approach provides clear pointers to the handicaps for which a building needs to compensate. Dementia as a handicap is characterized by: impaired memory, impaired reasoning, impaired ability to learn, high level of stress, and acute sensitivity to the social and the built environment. There are two ways of summarizing international consensus; one is agreement on principles, the other agreement on design features. The consensus on principles requires that design should: compensate for disability; maximize independence; enhance self-esteem and confidence; demonstrate care for staff; be orientating and understandable; reinforce personal identity; welcome relatives and the local community; allow control of stimuli. The consensus on design features includes: small size; familiar, domestic, homely in style; plenty of scope for ordinary activities (unit kitchens, washing lines, garden sheds); unobtrusive concern for safety; different rooms for different functions; age-appropriate furniture and fittings; safe outside space; single rooms big enough for lots of personal belongings; good signage and multiple cues where possible (e.g. light, smell, sound); use of objects rather than colour for orientation; enhancement of visual access; controlled stimuli, especially noise. However, a great range of issues make designing for dementia a challenge [81]. These include cost, regulations and cultural appropriateness.

There are numerous aspects to the cost issue. For example, small scale is at the top of the list of key design features, but what it actually means is widely divergent, primarily because of the staffing implications. Staff is the major expense consideration. A second aspect is that of designing for groups with different needs: people with dementia are far from a homogeneous group; people with challenging behaviours, for example, may need a great deal more visual access, in the sense that they need to be able to see the staff and the staff need to be able to see them; a cheap standard building will not be helpful.

There are numerous difficulties with fire and environmental health regulations. Fireproof doors and walls may divide the unit in such a way that concepts of domesticity and orientation are severely compromised. There is a growing recognition that small shared dwellings are houses, not institutions, and that technological changes such as sprinkler systems and smoke alarms may provide safety.

If people with dementia retain their past memories longer than their present, it must help to use familiar design and furniture. Again there is a challenge to this: the units have a mixed population in terms of class, ethnic background, occupational history. The great cultural diversity within Australia exemplifies this challenge [78,82].

On the one hand it is very stressful for people with dementia to move, but on the other hand they thrive in the new environment if it suits their needs better. Units for people with some social competence and low levels of physical dependence may be more like an ordinary house, but space for wheelchairs, hoists, challenging behaviour, etc. may need to be provided, so that people with dementia can increase their chances of remaining in a familiar environment. The social advantage of the group homes in Sweden, for example, is obvious, but aggression is the most frequent reason for leaving the group home for another institution [83]; the country still lacks an institution designed for elderly people with dementia where a medical-psychiatric approach can work side by side with the social one [84].

What is achieved will always be a compromise, mainly because of the difficulties inherent in the complex, interrelated issues. Such a compromise is illustrated by the design of the Ten Kerselaere Centre in Belgium [85]. This centre has to provide services at all stages of progressive geriatric and psychogeriatric disorders (long-term hospital care, nursing home care, ambulatory/day care, and sheltered housing) and at the same time suit the well-being and comfort of its elderly residents. All facilities, including living quarters, are at ground level, laid out to resemble a small, dynamic village, where all normal daily activities take place. Rather than long narrow corridors, there are wide streets, squares and street corners, a cafe, beauty parlour, chapel, shops, exhibits and events, attracting residents to a more social life style. Strolls are encouraged via sensory stimulation in the form of children's playgrounds, small livestock, birds, flowers, greenery. Therapeutic and rehabilitation activities are discretely open for all to see, avoiding apprehension and suspicion about the unknown among the residents. Integrated into daily living, they give a positive view of their potential benefits to residents, family and visitors alike.

Changing the physical environment *per se* may have a positive impact on people with dementia and their carers, but these changes have to be embedded in changes in the ways care is offered. In this context, clearly too little attention has been given as yet to adaptations to the person's own home. This is, no doubt, a top priority.

## CARER SUPPORT

For elderly individuals with primary caregivers, formal care is inextricably tied to informal care [86,87]. Care programmes and services need to target all caregivers if they are to be successful in reaching their goals. A principal caregiver who receives support at early stages, may benefit greatly from formal services and premature institutionalization may well be avoided. On the other hand, receiving support at too late a stage may do little to relieve stress and other negative outcomes.

In the near future, with more elderly people, there will be more disabled, eventually demented individuals in need of care. The present system in most countries consists of the overwhelming amount of caregiving being provided by informal caregivers in the community, while formal (professional and paid) support is responsible for a small amount. It is clear that neither formal services nor informal family caregivers can meet the needs of a growing population [88]. The need for coordination may be especially acute in cases of dementia, which places high amounts of stress on informal and formal carers alike. A book, *Profiles in Caregiving: The Unexpected Career* [89] gives a comprehensive overview of the caregiving burden.

Lyons and Zarit [86] explore the link between formal and informal care and discuss several models of such an interface. The mix of informal and formal help varies from country to country and is a matter of custom (e.g. filial responsibility), policy (e.g. reimbursement systems) and other factors. For instance, demented elders with an adult child caregiver were 4.8 times as likely to be institutionalized as those elders with spousal caregivers [90]. However, the risk of being placed in an institution was less for elders who lived with an informal caregiver: relationship between the two was less important than co-residence. Gender is also important: female caregivers tend to assist with more personal care and housekeeping tasks that are relevant to surviving in the community [91].

There is a need to assess the dynamic nature of caregiving, the relationship between formal and informal caregiving, the predictors of use and both positive and negative outcomes. An example of a common outcome in caregiving research is the amount of time that informal caregivers must provide care. Berry *et al* [92] compared caregivers of elders with dementia who received in-home help with those who used day care, and found that caregivers who used day care still had to provide assistance with activities of daily living (ADLs) such as toileting and dressing, whereas those care-givers who received in-home help were more continuously assisted with such tasks. Although both groups of caregivers expressed satisfaction with the respite they received, in-home help appeared to be more successful in alleviating stressful time-demands than day care. In this particular sample, it was concluded that a supplementary interface (as followed in in-home care) has a more positive outcome than a dual-specialization model (as followed in day care).

In general, those elderly persons who are older, suffer greater disability and are demented, are more likely to be placed in institutions than their younger, less disabled and cognitively intact counterparts. Also, those care-givers who experience personal burden are more likely to institutionalize their relative. Formal health care was found to have a strong moderating effect on physical disability for three important caregiver outcomes (depression, health deterioration and social isolation); it was also found to buffer the impact of the patient's dementia on caregiver depression [93]. Formal personal care, on the other hand, was found to have a strong moderating effect on the problem behaviours in demented elderly for all three caregiver outcomes; household services did buffer the effect of problem behaviour on caregiver depression only.

Personal care tasks involve daily routines such as eating and toileting, and the use of formal personal care may provide a much-needed respite to the informal caregiver, as well as allowing a trained helper to monitor the sources of behaviour problems and offer emotional support. Problem beha-viours in a demented elder can be extremely stressful to a principal care-giver and have in fact been associated with greater negative outcomes than physical disability [94,95]. The relationship between the carer's burden and negative outcomes has been extensively studied according to pathogenic stress models.

Antonovsky [96] has proposed a "salutogenic" (health-promoting) stress model, with the "sense of coherence"—a person's view that his or her world is comprehensible, manageable and meaningful—as a core mechanism. In the face of stressful life situations, persons with a strong sense of coherence are protected against negative stress outcomes, whereas persons with a low sense of coherence suffer distress and breakdown. Studying the impact of high burden of dementia caregiving, Baro et al [97] found that principal caregivers with a strong sense of coherence are not only significantly less likely to manifest negative outcomes, but also more likely to develop adaptive coping and to improve their use of adequate social support. On the contrary, principal caregivers with a high burden but a low sense of coherence are very likely to manifest distress and breakdown. Surprisingly, the study also found that the sense of coherence makes no significant difference in conditions of low burden. These findings join the evidence by such researchers as Pearlman and Crown [98], who concluded that the more social support is needed, the greater effect it has.

Advocacy means making the case for someone, or a group of people, or helping them to represent their views, to define their rights and to promote their interests. The concept has special relevance to people who are less able to speak for themselves and as a consequence have largely been overlooked, such as older people with dementia and their principal carers [99].

There are many types of advocacy [100]. Legal advocacy is perhaps the most widely known form of advocacy and is undertaken by professionally qualified lawyers on behalf of their clients. Self-advocacy, on the contrary, means speaking up for yourself. Self-advocacy with a specific focus upon dementia is at the origin of the worldwide "Alzheimer movement", a growing body of collective advocacy, mutual support, better information and communication, skill development and a common call for research and change. Organizationally, this movement includes many small local groups as well as national and international networks (e.g. Alzheimer's Disease International, Alzheimer Europe).

## QUALITY OF LIFE

Age-related dementia has an obvious impact on the quality of life of those impaired, their families, and the community.

Quality of life may be defined as a person's perception of his or her position in life in the context of the culture and value systems in which he or she lives, and in relation to his or her goals, expectations, standards and concerns [101]. The World Health Organization (WHO) has a commitment to holistic views of health, which includes the health-related quality of life. It refers not only to health in its narrow sense of the absence of disease and impairment, but also to health as a state of physical, mental and social well-being. The primary aim of any health intervention is to maximize health and minimize disease, thereby enhancing the person's quality of life.

Three components of quality of life should be distinguished: subjective well-being, objective functioning, and environmental living conditions [102]. Different life domains should be assessed separately, since a person's quality of life might be excellent in one (e.g. family) and inferior in another life area (e.g. work); also, helping actions have to address those segments of life which are most in need of assistance. Assessment should be carried out by the patient, a family member or friend, and a professional. The three components are highly related to cognitive status and thus interrelated, but cannot be accurately predicted from knowledge of the cognitive status and therefore should be independently assessed.

Subjective evidence of impaired quality of life due to dementia is given by strong feelings of difficulty, anxiety, frustration, etc. Denial, depression, "fight or flight" as emotional responses to the advent of cognitive impairment or to an increasingly dependent position are often prominently evident, as well as feeling handicapped by errors or inability in everyday tasks.

Secondly, objective evidence of impaired quality of life due to dementia is found whenever the person cannot meet adaptive challenges independently, such as going out and returning home, recognizing family and friends, dressing in the right order. Intact quality of life is regarded as emanating from adaptive responses, while impaired quality of life emanates from maladaptive functioning.

Thirdly, the failure in adaptation, especially under challenging conditions, will inevitably lead to stand-by supervision, a sheltered environment, and demand for personal care services. Also, the environment modifies adaptation. Distressed or burdened caregivers may be motivated to intrude into the patient's life, because it may be easier and quicker for the caregiver to take over the task than to fit into the patient's limits of competence. In other cases, restructuring the home or provision of assistance can extend or restore the patient's adaptation and quality of life [103].

Falls and fear of falling offer a good example of the interplay of the three quality of life components (subjective well-being, objective functioning, and environmental living conditions). Studying risk factors for falling among elderly persons living in the community, Tinetti et al [104,105] concluded that cognitive impairment, second only to sedative use, is associated with a very high risk of falling. Older persons with dementia may be at particular risk of serious sequelae when they fall, either because cognitive impairment may be associated with compromised protective responses or because impaired judgement may predispose cognitively impaired persons to engage in more hazardous activities. Prevention of falls in these elderly remains a challenge [106]. Those who survive falls may have soft-tissue injuries, or fractures requiring hospitalization or immobilization. Fear of falling, with consequent restriction of activities and social isolation, are among the sequelae of falls in older people. It is known that cognitively impaired elderly who experience loneliness tend to show greatest dependence on help in ADLs [107].

The quality of life approach in the area of age-related dementia is very relevant and innovative, but only meaningful if its assessment is carried out in a comprehensive and individual way.

A good example of the importance of assessment in quality of life issues is related to driving. Cognitive impairment may imperil the driver, passengers and others on the road. How to balance the need for public safety with the preservation of personal independence for the person with suspected or mild dementia? In the 1994 International Consensus Conference on Dementia and Driving, there was agreement that persons with moderate and severe dementia should not drive [108]. Consensus was reached that diagnosed mildly demented individuals with functional deterioration should be considered for specialized assessment of driving competence.

For older drivers, the car is often a vital link in maintaining independence, acquiring goods and socializing. Hu and Young [109] have reported that 88% of older Americans rely on a private automobile for most of their transportation needs. Clearly, for an older person, loss of driving may represent a loss of a vital function as well as a loss of autonomy. It may have an added dimension in that it may be the first time that the person is confronted with a loss of function associated with cognitive impairment. Discussion of driving cessation should take place with the patient alone in the first instance, then with family involvement if this is unsuccessful.

Two complementary sets of factors need to be considered: those associated with reluctance or refusal to stop driving and those associated with problems for the patient and the family after eventually stopping driving. Certain factors, such as anosognosia, living alone, poor access to public transport, continued driving after a crash, and male sex may be expected to produce resistance to advice about cessation of driving [110]. Difficulties as a result of stopping driving may be anticipated in terms of coping with the change in lifestyle and mobility status. For example, many ex-drivers like to have their automobile in the driveway or retain their driver's licenses to maintain a sense of belonging to the community.

In fact, the whole issue of dealing with driving limitations parallels how one succeeds or fails in helping the person deal with the reality of the cognitive impairment [111]. Patients with early or mild dementia should be given the opportunity to demonstrate the capacity to drive through a re-examination process. A periodic follow-up is always advised; the time interval depends on the rate of progression of the disease.

The above-mentioned salutogenic model, proposed by Antonovski [96], presents opportunities for improving quality of life of both patients and carers [112]. Posing research questions salutogenically allows us to broaden the perspective of psychosocial interventions and look to ways in which people adapt to a most challenging life situation with healthy responses as opposed to pathogenic ones. This is a vital issue for elderly persons with dementia, principal carers and professionals alike. Offering and evaluating a sense of coherence-based support program, well integrated within the framework of a problem-oriented approach, is suggested as one of the key elements to consider [113].

The problem-oriented approach aims at directing the carer's response towards problem-solving activities and away from maladaptive reactions, by identifying and emphasizing those aspects of the problem that lend themselves to meaningful action. The program includes 120 specific problems, from patient's night-time confusion and wandering, to carer's guilt feelings and anticipatory bereavement. At the same time, the salutogenic approach offers a fundamental contribution to learning about the habitual life goals and ways of understanding and managing stressful situations. In order to maintain "meaningfulness", it is helpful for the patient to be oriented towards those aims in life that they do not have to give up yet, and for the carer to be encouraged to talk about the meaning of being a principal carer. In order to maintain "manageability", it is important to convey a feeling of security to bear the painful reality and commitment to offer continuing help. Maintaining "comprehensibility" implies handling misinterpretations completely and helping both patient and carer to understand the problem and its consequences. In fact, the salutogenic model requires that the professional abandons unilateral decision-making, exchanging it for a partnership with the carer in an atmosphere of mutual trust.

## SUMMARY

The psychosocial component of dementia care is a very dynamic and rapidly developing field. Various studies have shown that good practices are successful in maintaining a person with dementia at a particular level of functioning without further loss, and in improving the quality of life of both patient and carer. There is a great choice of methods and approaches, from changing the individual to changing the environment, but in practice there are many difficulties and complex ethical issues. Dementia care is hard and demanding work; principal carers as well as professional staff need advice and assistance. Research evidence is still scarce.

## Consistent Evidence

Consistent evidence has been published concerning the positive impact of a variety of psychosocial interventions. According to the available evidence, the positive changes directly related to psychosocial interventions include:

- A reassuring foundation in reality provided by reality orientation therapy.
- The many meaningful activities linked to reminiscence work with individuals and groups.
- The surprising ability of demented members of validation groups to share feelings and problems.
- The reduction of challenging behaviour and improvement of adapted behaviour, offered by the use of behaviour modification based on reward techniques tailored to individual preferences.

- The same positive responses following sensory stimulation approaches, such as music therapy, presence of pets, meetings with school-age children, and relaxation sessions.
- The optimal use of remaining adaptive capabilities, induced by cognitive-motor exercise.
- The temporarily stabilizing and comforting effects of group living and environmental adaptations.

Moreover, the support needs of the principal carers are well known, as well as the salutogenic importance of the carer's sense of coherence. Improvements in staff morale and job satisfaction have also been demonstrated.

## Incomplete Evidence

Theories and practices seem to have developed in an unconnected way, and there has been little concern with systematically monitoring the impact of psychosocial approaches on people with dementia. Also, many anecdotal reports discuss psychosocial interventions that seem to be a practical coming-together of methods and ideas, rather than having, from the start, a firm, reliable, conceptual base. Finally, regardless of the specific psychosocial approach used, the outcome for the person with dementia will always be co-determined by the interaction with environmental conditions and with the carer who uses the psychosocial tool, as well as with the positive or negative impact of concomitant biomedical interventions (e.g. medication).

Mood changes, for instance, are often the focus of reports. However, there are strong difficulties in assessing mood in people with dementia. The reliability of existing self-report measures or carer's feelings of well-being is open to doubt. Are the mood changes appropriately described as, for example, "depressive"? How important are anxiety and fear, neglect and understimulation? How determinant are the effects and side effects of medication? Many elderly persons with a diagnosis of early dementia may, in fact, enter depression, whereas others may have depression plus early dementia. Clearly, these psychosocial concepts, processes and research methodology need systematic exploration.

## Areas Still Open to Research

Despite promising research findings about older people and the conditions causing dementia, research on psychosocial interventions faces obstacles at every step (subject selection, design, measurement, etc.). Therefore, as a first research priority, it is recommended to focus on the methodological issues involved in conducting psychosocial intervention research, in the hope of stimulating more and better studies of innovative treatment programmes.

The second research priority is related to the advances in biomedical interventions. One has to re-define a set of methodological guidelines specifically applied to psychosocial interventions in interaction with biomedical interventions and taking into account the complex and interdisciplinary nature of research in this field. Such research is critical in order to ensure a more efficient evaluation and comparison of the numerous projects currently undertaken and to find the optimal interactions.

The third research priority concerns a most important psychosocial issue: to what extent can families assume long-term responsibility for the care of patients without harming their own health and well-being? One has to develop action research projects, which include both a problem-oriented dimension and a salutogenic dimension. Such projects could even be designed in such a way as to emphasize the fundamental aspects of human behaviour, thereby promoting their use in multicultural situations.

There needs to be a continued effort to evaluate the effectiveness of psychosocial interventions in enabling man to adapt with minimal trauma to a most severe challenge and in positively interacting with more and more effective biomedical interventions.

## REFERENCES

1. Taulbee L.R., Folsom J.C. (1966)   Reality orientation for geriatric patients. *Hosp. Commun. Psychiatry*, **17**: 234–239.
2. Holden U.P., Woods R.T. (1995)   *Positive Approaches to Dementia Care*, Churchill Livingstone, Edinburgh.
3. William R., Reeve W., Ivison D., Kavanagh D. (1987)   Use of environmental manipulation and modified informal reality orientation with institutionalized, confused elderly subjects: a replication. *Age Ageing*, **16**: 315–318.
4. Breuil V., de Rotrou J., Forette F., Tortrat D., Ganansia-Ganem A., Frambourt A., Moulin F., Boller F. (1994)   Cognitive stimulation of patients with dementia: preliminary results. *Int. J. Geriatr. Psychiatry*, **9**: 211–217.
5. Bowlby M.C. (1991)   Reality orientation thirty years later: are we still confused? *Can. J. Occup. Ther.*, **58**: 114–122.
6. Butler R.N. (1963)   The life review: an interpretation of reminiscence in the aged. *Psychiatry*, **26**: 65–76.
7. Garland J. (1994)   What splendour, it all coheres: life-review therapy with older people. In *Reminiscence Reviewed* (Ed. J. Bornat), pp. 21–31, Open University Press, Buckingham.
8. Tabourne C.E. (1995)   The effects of a life review program on disorientation, social interaction and self-esteem of nursing home residents. *Int. J. Aging Hum. Develop.*, **41**: 251–266.
9. Norris A. (1986)   *Reminiscence*, Winslow Press, London.

10. Schweitzer P. (Ed.) (1998)  *Reminiscence in Dementia Care*, Age Exchange, London.
11. Gibson F. (1997)   Owning the past in dementia care: creative engagement with others in the present. In *State of the Art in Dementia Care* (Ed. M. Marshall), pp. 134–139, Centre for Policy on Ageing, London.
12. Murphy C., Moyes M. (1997)   Life story work. In *State of the Art in Dementia Care* (Ed. M. Marshall), pp. 149–153, Centre for Policy on Ageing, London.
13. Rentz C. (1995)   Reminiscence: a supportive intervention for the person with Alzheimer's disease. *Psychosoc. Nursing Ment. Health Serv.*, **33**: 15–20.
14. Woodrow P. (1998)   Interventions for confusion and dementia: 3. Reminiscence. *Br. J. Nursing*, **7**: 1145–1149.
15. Haight B.K. (1991)   Reminiscing: the state of the art as a basis for practice. *Int. J. Aging Hum. Develop.*, **33**: 1–32.
16. Woods R.T., McKiernan F. (1995)   Evaluating the impact of reminiscence on older people with dementia. In *The Art and Science of Reminiscence: Theory, Research, Methods and Applications* (Eds B.K. Haight, J. D. Webster), pp. 233–242, Taylor and Francis, Washington, DC.
17. Gibson F. (1994)   What can reminiscence contribute to people with dementia? In *Reminiscence Reviewed* (Ed. J. Bornat), pp. 46–60, Open University Press, Buckingham.
18. Coleman P. (1986)   *Aging and Reminiscence Processes. Social and Clinical Implications*, Wiley, New York.
19. Osborne C. (1989)   Reminiscence: when the past eases the present. *J. Gerontol. Nursing*, **15**: 6–12.
20. Berghorn F.J., Schäfer D.E. (1987)   Reminiscence intervention in nursing homes: what and who changes? *Int. J. Aging Hum. Develop.*, **25**: 113–127.
21. Crisp J. (1995)   Making sense of the stories that people with Alzheimer's tell: a journey with my mother. *Nursing Inquiry*, **2**: 133–140.
22. Feil N. (1982)   *V/F Validation: The Feil Method*, Feil Productions, Cleveland.
23. Miesen B.M.L. (1993)   Alzheimer's disease, the phenomenon of parent fixation and Bowlby's attachment therapy. *Int. J. Geriatr. Psychiatry*, **8**: 147–153.
24. Feil N. (1993)   *The Validation Breakthrough: Simple Techniques for Communicating with People with Alzheimer's Type Dementia*, Health Professions Press, Baltimore.
25. Bleathman C., Morton I. (1992)   Validation therapy: extracts from 20 groups with dementia sufferers. *J. Adv. Nursing*, **17**: 658–666.
26. Kitwood T. (1992)   How valid is validation therapy? *Geriatr. Med.* (April): 23.
27. Van Amelsvoort Jones G.M.M. (1985)   Validation therapy: a companion to reality orientation. *Can. Nurse*, **81**: 20–23.
28. Stokes G., Goudie F. (Eds) (1990)   *Working with Dementia*, Winslow Press, Bicester.
29. Miller E., Morris R. (1993)   *The Psychology of Dementia*, Wiley, Chichester.
30. Baltes M.M. (1988)   The etiology and maintenance of dependence in the elderly: three phases of operant research. *Behav. Ther.*, **19**: 301–319.
31. Sandman C.A. (1993)   Memory rehabilitation in Alzheimer's disease: preliminary findings. *Clin. Gerontol.*, **13**: 19–33.
32. Doyle C., Zapparoni T., O'Connor D., Runci S. (1997)   Efficacy of psychosocial treatments for noisemaking in severe dementia. *Int. Psychogeriatrics*, **9**: 405–422.
33. Kim E.J., Buschmann M.T. (1999)   The effect of expressive physical touch on patients with dementia. *Int. J. Nursing Studies*, **36**: 235–243.
34. Woods R.T., Britton P.G. (1977)   Psychological approaches to the treatment of the elderly. *Age Ageing*, **6**: 104–112.

35. Norberg A., Melin E., Asplund K. (1986)  Reactions to music, touch and object presentation in the final stage of dementia: an exploratory study. *Int. J. Nursing Studies*, **23**: 315–323.
36. Lord T.R., Gardner J.E. (1993)  Effects of music on Alzheimer patients. *Percept. Motor Skills*, **76**: 451–455.
37. Bright R. (1992)  Music therapy in the management of dementia. In *Care-Giving in Dementia* (Eds G. Jones, B.M.L. Miesen), pp. 162–180, Routledge, London.
38. Clark M.E., Lipe A.W., Bilbrey M. (1998)  Use of music to decrease aggressive behaviours in people with dementia. *J. Gerontol. Nursing*, **24**: 10–17.
39. Langford S. (1993)  A shared vision. *Nursing Times*, **98**: 86–89.
40. Elliott V., Milne D. (1991)  Patient's best friend? *Nursing Times*, **87**: 34–35.
41. Haughie E., Milne D., Elliott V. (1992)  An evaluation of companion dogs with elderly psychiatric patients. *Behav. Psychother.*, **20**: 367–372.
42. Benson S. (1994)  Sniff and doze therapy. *J. Dementia Care*, **2**: 12–14.
43. Molloy D.W., Richardson L.D., Grilly R.G. (1988)  The effects of a three-month exercise programme on neuropsychological function in elderly institutionalized women: a randomised controlled trial. *Age Ageing*, **17**: 303–310.
44. Morgan K. (1991)  Trial and error: evaluating the psychological benefits of physical activity. *Int. J. Geriatr. Psychiatry*, **4**: 125–127.
45. Dvorak R.V., Poehlman E.T. (1998)  Appendicular skeletal muscle mass, physical activity, and cognitive status in patients with Alzheimer's disease. *Neurology*, **51**: 1386–1390.
46. Dick-Muehlke C., Cotman C.W., Kean M.L. (1996)  Acquisition and long term retention of a gross motor skill in Alzheimer's disease patients under constant and varied practice conditions. *J. Gerontol. Psychol. Sci.*, **51B**: 103–111.
47. Jacobs D.H., Adair J.C., Williamson D.J., Na D.L., Gold M., Foundas A.L., Shuren J.E., Cibula J.E., Heilman K.M. (1999)  Apraxia and motor-skill acquisition in Alzheimer's disease are dissociable. *Neuropsychologia*, **37**: 875–880.
48. Burgio L.D., Burgio K., Engel B.T., Tice L.M. (1986)  Increasing distance and independence of ambulation in elderly nursing home residents. *J. Appl. Behav. Analysis*, **19**: 357–366.
49. Welden S., Yesavage J.A. (1982)  Behavioural improvement with relocation training in senile dementia. *Clin. Gerontol.*, **1**: 45–49.
50. West B., Brockman S. (1994)  The calming power of aromatherapy. *J. Dementia Care*, **2**: 20–22.
51. Snyder M., Egan E.C., Burns K.R. (1995)  Interventions for decreasing agitation behaviours in persons with dementia. *J. Gerontol. Nursing*, **21**: 34–40.
52. Droës R.M., Van Tilburg W. (1992)  Effects of psychomotor therapy in demented patients. Presented at the 8th International Meeting on Alzheimer's Disease, Bierbeek, Belgium, September 25–27.
53. Hendrickx F., De Lausnay L. (1992)  Cognitive interpretation of the motor behaviour of demented elderly. Presented at the 8th International Meeting on Alzheimer's Disease, Bierbeek, Belgium, September 25–27.
54. Reisberg B., Kenowsky S., Franssen E.H., Auer S.R., Souren L.E. (1999)  Towards a science of Alzheimer's disease management: a model based upon current knowledge of retrogenesis. *Int. Psychogeriatrics*, **11**: 7–23.
55. Asplund K., Jansson L., Norberg A. (1995)  Facial expressions of patients with dementia: a comparison of two methods of interpretation. *Int. Psychogeriatrics*, **7**: 527–534.

56. Tappen R.M., Williams C., Edelstein J., Touhy T., Fishman S. (1997) Communicating with individuals with Alzheimer's disease: examination of recommended strategies. *Arch. Psychiatr. Nursing*, **11**: 249–256.
57. Ikeda M., Mori E., Hirono N., Imamura T., Shimomura T., Ikeijri Y., Yamashita H. (1998) Amnestic people with Alzheimer's disease who remembered the Kobe earthquake. *Br. J. Psychiatry*, **172**: 425–428.
58. Fairbarn A. (1997) Insight and dementia. In *State of the Art in Dementia Care* (Ed. M. Marshall), pp. 13–18, Centre for Policy on Ageing, London.
59. McDaniel K.D., Edland S.D., Heyman A. (1995) Relationship between level of insight and severity of dementia in Alzheimer disease. CERAD Clinical Investigators. Consortium to Establish a Registry for Alzheimer's Disease. *Alz. Dis. Assoc. Disord.*, **9**: 101–104.
60. Vasterling J.J., Seltzer B., Watrous W.E. (1997) Longitudinal assessment of deficit unawareness in Alzheimer's disease. *Neuropsychiatry Neuropsychol. Behav. Neurol.*, **10**: 197–202.
61. Starkstein S.E., Chemerinski E., Sabe L., Kuzis G., Petracca G., Teson A., Leiguarda R. (1997) Prospective longitudinal study of depression and anosognosia in Alzheimer's disease. *Br. J. Psychiatry*, **171**: 47–52.
62. Wagner M.T., Spangenberg K.B., Bachman O.L., O'Connell P. (1997) Unawareness of cognitive deficit in Alzheimer disease and related dementias. *Alz. Dis. Assoc. Disord.*, **11**: 121–122.
63. Sinason V. (1992) The man who was losing his brain. In *Mental Handicap and the Human Condition: New Approaches from the Tavistock* (Ed. V. Sinason), pp. 87–110, Free Associations Books, London.
64. Killick J. (1997) Confidences: the experience of writing with people with dementia. In *State of the Art in Dementia Care* (Ed. M. Marshall), pp. 32–36, Centre for Policy on Ageing, London.
65. Hausman C. (1992) Dynamic psychotherapy with elderly demented patients. In *Caregiving in Dementia: Research and Applications* (Eds G. Jones, B.M.L. Miesen), pp. 181–189, Routledge, London.
66. Thompson L. W., Wagner B., Zeiss A., Gallagher D. (1990) Cognitive/behavioural therapy with early stage Alzheimer's patients: an exploratory view of the utility of this approach. In *Alzheimer's Disease: Treatment and Family Stress* (Eds E. Light, B.D. Lebowitz), pp. 383–397, Hemisphere, New York.
67. Sutton L.J., Cheston R. (1997) Rewriting the story of dementia: a narrative approach to psychotherapy with people with dementia. In *State of the Art in Dementia Care* (Ed. M. Marshall), pp. 159–163, Centre for Policy on Ageing, London.
68. King's Fund (1986) *Living Well into Old Age: Applying Principles of Good Practice in Services for Elderly People with Severe Mental Disabilities*, King's Fund, London.
69. Kitwood T. (1993) Towards a theory of dementia care: the interpersonal process. *Ageing Society*, **13**: 51–67.
70. Goldwasser A.N., Auerbach S.M., Harkins S.W. (1987) Cognitive, affective and behavioural effects of reminiscence group therapy in demented elderly. *Int. J. Aging Hum. Develop.*, **25**: 209–222.
71. Heron J. (1991) *The Facilitator's Handbook*, Kogan Page, London.
72. Bender M., Norris A. (1987) *An Introduction to Group Work with the Elderly*, Winslow Press, London.
73. Foster K. (1997) Pragmatic groups: interactions and relationships between people with dementia. In *State of the Art in Dementia Care* (Ed. M. Marshall), pp. 164–169, Center for Policy on Ageing, London.

74. Booth T., Phillips D. (1987) Group living in homes for the elderly: a comparative study of the outcomes of care. *Br. J. Soc. Work*, **17**: 1–20.
75. Wimo A., Wallin J.O., Lundgren K., Ronnback E., Asplund K., Mattsson B., Krakau I., (1991) Group living, an alternative for dementia patients: a cost analysis. *Int. J. Geriatr. Psychiatry*, **6**: 21–29.
76. Annerstedt I., Gustafson L., Nilsson K. (1993) Medical outcome of psychosocial intervention in demented patients: one-year clinical follow-up after relocation into group living units. *Int. J. Geriatr. Psychiatry*, **8**: 833–841.
77. Cohen U., Day K. (1993) *Contemporary Environments for People with Dementia*, Johns Hopkins University Press, Baltimore.
78. Judd S., Marshall M., Phippen P. (1998) *Design for Dementia*, Hawker, London.
79. Netten A. (1993) *A Positive Environment? Physical and Social Influences on People with Senile Dementia in Residential Care*, Asgate, Aldershot.
80. Wilkinson T.J., Henschke P.J., Handscombe K. (1995) How should toilets be labelled for people with dementia? *Aust. J. Ageing*, **13**: 163–165.
81. Marshall M. (Ed.) (1997) *State of the Art in Dementia Care*, Centre for Policy on Ageing, London.
82. Kidd B.J. (1997) A journey with Alice. In *State of the Art in Dementia Care* (Ed. M. Marshall), pp. 169–174, Centre for Policy on Ageing, London.
83. Wimo A., Asplund K., Mattsson B., Adolfsson R., Lundgren K. (1995) Patients with dementia in group livings: experiences 4 years after admission. *Int. Psychogeriatrics*, **7**: 123–127.
84. Malmberg B. (1997) Group homes, an alternative for older people with dementia. In *State of the Art in Dementia Care* (Ed. M. Marshall), pp. 78–82, Centre for Policy on Ageing, London.
85. Baro F., Dom R. (1993) Ten Kerselaere, a contemporary approach to geriatric care in Belgium. In *Life-Span Design of Residential Environments for an Aging Population. Proceedings of an International Conference* (Eds R. Haroetyan, E. Stern), pp. 95–98, American Association of Retired Persons, Washington, DC.
86. Lyons K.S., Zarit S.H. (1999) Formal and informal support: the great divide. *Int. J. Geriatr. Psychiatry*, **14**: 183–196.
87. Clarke C. (1999) Commentary. *Int. J. Geriatr. Psychiatry*, **14**: 194–196.
88. Zarit S.H., Pearlin L.I. (Eds) (1993) *Caregivers Systems: Formal and Informal Helpers*, Erlbaum, Hillsdale.
89. Aneshensel C., Pearlin L., Mullan J., Zarit S., Whitlatch C. (Eds) (1995) *Profiles in Caregiving: the Unexpected Career*, Academic Press, San Diego.
90. Scott W.K., Adwards K.B., Davis D.R., Cornman C.B., Macera C.A. (1997) Risk of institutionalization among community long-term care clients with dementia. *Gerontologist*, **37**: 46–51.
91. Jette A.M., Tennstedt S., Crawford S. (1995) How does formal and informal community care affect nursing home use? *J. Gerontol.*, **50**: 4–12.
92. Berry G.L., Zarit S.H., Rabatin V.X. (1991) Caregiver activity on respite and non-respite days: a comparison of two service approaches. *Gerontologist*, **31**: 830–835.
93. Bass D.M., Noelker L.S., Rechlin L.R. (1996) The moderating influence of service use on negative caregiving consequences. *J. Gerontol.*, **51**: 121–131.
94. Bass D.M., McClendon M., Deimling G.T., Mukherjee S. (1994) The influence of a diagnosed mental impairment on family caregiver strain. *J. Gerontol.*, **49**: 146–155.
95. Gallagher T., Wagenfeld M.O., Baro F., Haepers K. (1994) Sense of coherence, coping and caregiver role overload. *Soc. Sci. Med.*, **39**: 1615–1622.

96. Antonovsky A. (1982) *Unraveling the Mystery of Health*, Jossey-Bass, San Francisco.
97. Baro F., Haepers K., Wagenfeld M., Gallagher T. (1996) Sense of coherence in demented elderly persons in Belgium. In *Neuropsychiatry in Old Age: an Update* (Eds C. Stagagnis, H. Hippius), pp. 145–156, Hogrefe & Huber, Seattle.
98. Pearlman D.N., Crown W.H. (1991) Alternative sources of social support and their impacts on institutional risk. *Gerontologist*, **32**: 527–535.
99. Killeen J. (1996) *Advocacy and Dementia*, Alzheimer Scotland Action on Dementia, Edinburgh.
100. Dunning A. (1997) Advocacy and older people with dementia. In *State of the Art in Dementia Care* (Ed. M. Marshall), pp. 95–101, Centre for Policy on Ageing, London.
101. Orley J., Kuyken W. (Eds) (1993) *Quality of Life Assessment: International Perspectives*, Springer, Berlin.
102. Katschnig H. (1998) How useful is the concept of quality of life in psychiatry? In *Quality of Life in Mental Disorders* (Eds H. Katschnig, H. Freeman, N., Sartorius), pp. 3–16, Wiley, Chichester.
103. Gurland B., Katz S. (1998) Quality of life and mental disorders of elders. In Quality of Life in Mental Disorders (Eds H. Katschnig, H. Freeman, N. Sartorius), pp. 193–211, Wiley, Chichester.
104. Tinetti M.E., Doucette J., Claus E., Marottoli R. (1995) Risk factors for serious injury during falls by older persons in the community. *J. Am. Geriatr. Soc.*, **43**: 1214–1221.
105. Tinetti M.E., Speechley M., Ginter S.F. (1988) Risk factors for falls among elderly persons living in the community. *N. Engl. J. Med.*, **319**: 1701–1707.
106. Myers A.H., Young Y., Langlois J.A. (1996) Prevention of falls in the elderly. *Bone*, **18** (Suppl. 1): 875–1015.
107. Holmen K., Ericsson K., Andersson L., Winblad B. (1993) ADL capacity and loneliness among elderly persons with cognitive impairment. *Scand. J. Prim. Health Care*, **11**: 56–60.
108. Johansson K., Lundberg C. (1997) The 1994 international consensus conference on dementia and driving: a brief report. *Alz. Dis. Relat. Disord.*, **11** (Suppl. 1): 62–69.
109. Hu P.H., Young J. (1994) *Nation-wide Personal Transportation Survey: Demographic Special Reports*, Oak Ridge National Laboratories Report FHWA-PL-94–019.
110. Kington R., Reuben D., Rogowski J., Lillard L. (1994) Socio-demographic and health factors in driving patterns after 50 years of age. *Am. J. Publ. Health*, **84**: 1327–1329.
111. O'Neill D. (1997) Predicting and coping with the consequences of stopping driving. *Alz. Dis. Relat. Disord.*, **11** (Suppl. 1): 70–72.
112. Wagenfeld M., Baro F., Gallagher T., Haepers K. (1994) The correlates of coherence in caregivers to demented and nondemented elderly in Belgium. In *Sense of Coherence and Resiliency* (Eds H. McCubbin, E. Thompson, A. Thompson, J. Fromer), pp. 21–40, The University of Wisconsin System, Wisconsin.
113. Baro F., Meulenbergs L. (1998) *The European Alzheimer Clearing House*, Ministry of Health, Brussels.

# Commentaries

## 5.1
## Psychosocial Dimensions of Dementia Care
### Kathleen C. Buckwalter[1]

Caring for persons with dementia is a challenge, whether they are in home, community-based or institutional settings. As noted by Hall [1], "The desired outcomes at all levels of care are to maximize the potential for safe function by controlling for excess disability and providing appropriate levels of assistance; encourage participation in activities as desired by the client; minimize discomfort caused from physical and emotional stressors; and maximize expressions of comfort". Certain therapeutic principles underlie all therapeutic goals [2], including: (a) the goal of treatment should depend on the severity of the disease; (b) therapeutic goals belong to no single scientific or health care discipline; and (c) patient and family-valued outcomes are key considerations. Weiner [3] has also set forth several general psychological principles that facilitate management and effective psychosocial intervention with this population: correcting sensory impairment; non-confrontation; finding optimal level of autonomy; simplification, structuring; multiple cuing; repetition; guiding and demonstration; positive and negative reinforcement; reducing choices; distraction; avoiding new learning; determining and using overlearned skills; coupling learning with emotional arousal; minimizing anxiety; and optimal stimulation. Although the psychosocial interventions discussed in Prof. Baro's review aim to promote quality of life for both caregivers and care recipients, some do so far better than others.

*Environment.* The concepts of person–environment fit and interaction [4] are logical frameworks for understanding and managing behavioural and functional changes in persons with dementia, in that sensory, perceptual and cognitive processes affect the individual's ability to interact successfully with the environment. Thus, repetitive, catastrophic and situationally inappropriate behaviours may be viewed as disordered person–environment interaction. Successful interventions are aimed at restructuring (simplification/modification) the environment to compensate for deficits, and redu-

---

[1] *University of Iowa, 234 Medicine Administration Building, Iowa City, IA 52242-1101, USA*

cing internal and external stressors. One of the biggest challenges in developing effective interventions that include modification of the environment, is to create strategies that reduce stimuli (e.g. television, mirrors) that appear to cause dysfunctional behaviour, while at the same time maintaining sufficient stimulation to prevent sensory deprivation [5].

*Communication.* There are many communication-related issues that effect both individual and group psychotherapy and psychosocial interventions with this population. As noted by Prof. Baro, it is not always possible to understand what patients with dementia are attempting to communicate. In many cases it will be necessary to deduce needs from past behaviour or to have family members help staff understand names or phrases that patients call out, in order to facilitate understanding of the expressed meaning. It is also useful to avoid asking questions that begin with "why" because this often requires a response that demented patients are unable to provide [6]. General principles for communicating with cognitively impaired persons, set forth by Bartol [7], include: identifying oneself and addressing the person by name; using short words and simple sentences; asking one question at a time; giving adequate time for a response; repeating when necessary; using nouns vs. pronouns; speaking slowly and enunciating clearly; and accompanying speech with clarifying or reinforcing gestures. Nonverbal communication becomes increasingly important as verbal language deteriorates.

*Reality orientation and validation therapy.* Although there has been little empirical support for validation therapy [8], most practitioners believe it is preferable to confrontation or to reality orientation, especially in cognitively impaired patients who are hallucinating or delusional. In addition to accepting the patient's feelings, clinicians often find distraction and redirection into some reality-based activity most helpful. Reality orientation may irritate, embarrass, or agitate patients with dementia, reminding them of their deficits [9]. The most appropriate role for reality orientation with dementia patients is in helping to deal with the acute confusion that may occur when they are admitted to a health care facility. In this situation, staff and visitors should always identify themselves to the patients and continuously indicate where they are and that they have not been abandoned by their families. Of course it is always appropriate to respond succinctly to patients' requests for orienting information, recognizing that the information will likely not be retained, and may be requested again in a short period of time [3].

*Reminiscence/reassurance techniques/Sensory stimulation.* Encouraging persons with dementia to reminisce and tell stories about themselves helps to increase socialization and quality of life, in that activities that elicit pleasant memories such as review of photo albums, personal memorabilia, or listening to favourite music may help them to feel comfortable. In addition to the research cited by Prof. Baro in this area, Gerdner [10] found that preferred music reduced agitated behaviours in confused nursing home residents. Bailey *et al* [11] used dolls and stuffed animals to provide companionship and comfort to demented residents. This intervention was particularly effective for a woman who incessantly tried to elope and talked about the need to go home and care for her family.

*Behavioural approaches.*   Behavioural interventions are often targeted to persons with dementia who are agitated or aggressive or who exhibit behaviours that are troubling to staff, other patients and family members. The goal of care in this situation is to identify those components, whether social, personal or environmental, that contribute to aggressive behaviour and to act to reduce the risk that violence occurs in the first place. As noted in Prof. Baro's review, appropriate management of these residents depends upon accurate assessment and preventative care. The A–B–C approach (Antecedents/Behaviours/Consequences) to behavioural management (as opposed to modification which relies on the person's ability to learn new ways to behave) has been shown to reduce patient discomfort as well as the potential for aggression [12]. This model requires that, before behavioural goals are set, practitioners must describe the behaviour in detail, review all possible internal and external conditions that may precipitate aggression, and describe consequences of the behaviour from the perspective of the patient and staff. With this information at hand, antecedents and consequences of the disturbing behaviours can be changed and replaced by more positive ones, which are consistently reinforced. Because of cognitive impairment and diminished ability to learn new behaviours, persons with dementia cannot be expected to perform in the absence of a stimulus or cut to prompt the desired behaviour.

*Intervention frameworks.*   It is heartening to note that quality of life has emerged as a dominant concept in the evaluation of psychosocial interventions for persons with dementia, and that preservation of life without quality and function is viewed as a tragedy [13]. Similarly, Burgener and Chiverton [14] have argued for psychological well-being as an appropriate framework for guiding knowledge development in the care of cognitively impaired elders. A number of conceptual frameworks other than Antonovsky's, as described in the Baro review, have also been used to guide psychosocial intervention research, including Meddaugh's [15] theory of reactance; Norberg *et al*'s [16] use of Piagetian concepts; Hurley and colleagues' [17] work on resistance and Boettcher's [18] basic need model.

Although the theoretical frameworks and interventions used to assist cognitively impaired elders are diverse, they do share some commonalities, including: (a) finding ways to introduce choice and participation, thus maximizing personal freedom and choice; (b) increasing comfort levels; and (c) enabling persons with dementia to function at their maximum potential.

# REFERENCES

1. Hall G.R. (1991)   Altered thought processes: dementia. In *Nursing Diagnoses and Interventions for the Elderly* (Eds M. Maas, K.C. Buckwalter, M. Hardy), pp. 332–347, Addison-Wesley, Redwood City.
2. Whitehouse P. (1996)   Conceptual framework of therapeutic goals in Alzheimer's disease. Presented at the Meeting of the Department of Health and Human Services Advisory Panel on Alzheimer's Disease, Washington, DC, February 17.
3. Weiner M.F. (1991)   Psychological and behavioural management. In *The Dementias: Diagnosis, Management and Research* (Ed. M.F. Weiner), pp. 107–133, American Psychiatric Press, Washington, DC.
4. Lawton M.P. (1975)   Competence, environmental press and the adaptation of older people. In *Theory Development in Environment and Aging* (Eds P. Windley, T. Byerts, F. Ernst), pp. 13–83, Gerontological Society, Washington, DC.
5. Gerdner L.A., Stolley J.M., Hall G.R., Garand L., Buckwalter K.C. (1996)   Nursing management of persons with dementia. In *The Dementias: Diagnosis, Management and Research* (Ed. M.F. Weiner), pp. 281–329, American Psychiatric Press, Washington, DC.
6. Feil N. (1992)   Validation therapy. *Geriat. Nursing*, **13**: 129–133.
7. Bartol M.A. (1979)   Nonverbal communication in patients with Alzheimer's disease. *J. Gerontol. Nursing*, **5**: 23–31.
8. Robb S., Stegman C., Wolanin M.O. (1986)   No research versus research with compromised results: a study of validation therapy. *Nursing Res.*, **35**: 113–118.
9. Dietch J.T., Hewett L.J., Jones S. (1989)   The adverse effects of reality orientation. *J. Am. Geriatr. Soc.*, **37**: 974–976.
10. Gerdner L. (1997)   An individualized music intervention for agitation. *J. Am. Psychiatr. Nurses Assoc.*, **3**: 117–184.
11. Bailey J., Gilbert E., Herweyer S. (1992)   To find a soul. *Nursing*, **22**: 63–64.
12. Cohn M.D., Horgas A.L., Marisiske M. (1990)   Behaviour management training for nurse aides: is it effective? *J. Gerontol. Nursing*, **16**: 21–25.
13. Buckwalter K.C., Stolley J.M., Farran D. (1999)   Managing cognitive impairment in the elderly: conceptual, intervention and methodological issues. *Online Journal of Knowledge Synthesis for Nursing*, **6**: Document 10.
14. Burgener S.C., Chiverton P. (1992)   Conceptualizing psychological well-being in cognitively impaired older persons. *Image*, **24**: 209–214.
15. Meddaugh D.I. (1990)   Reactance: understanding aggressive behaviour in long-term care. *J. Psychosoc. Nursing Ment. Health Services*, **28**: 28–33.
16. Norberg A., Melin E., Asplund K. (1986)   Reactions to music, touch, and object presentation in the final stage of dementia: an exploratory study. *Int. J. Nursing Studies*, **23**: 315–323.

17. Hurley A.C., Volicer B.J., Hanrahan P.A., Houde S., Volicer L. (1992) Assessment of discomfort in advanced Alzheimer's patients. *Res. Nursing Health*, **15**: 369–377.
18. Boettcher E.G. (1983) Preventing violent behaviour: an integrated theoretical model for nursing. *Perspect. Psychiatr. Care*, **21**: 54–58.

5.2
## First Experience, then Evidence, then Possibly New Criteria

M. Powell Lawton[1]

In few areas is the contrast between evidence and experience better illustrated than in the topic of Prof. Baro's review, psychosocial interventions with dementia. Although dementia has been studied for well over a century, we are still in our first generation of recognizing that people with dementia could be studied as people rather than as sites for pathology of nervous tissue. Even more recently has there been serious effort to apply psychosocial interventive procedures to people with dementia. We are thus still collecting first bodies of literature in both the evidence and the experience categories.

In the human intervention sciences it is usual for clinical experience to accumulate over some extended period before evidence becomes a developed focus of interest. Put bluntly, innovative clinical procedures do not commonly arise from the work of positivist behavioural scientists. Virtually all of the great systems of intervention have been created by artist–clinicians. Although their practice is clearly based on evidence, the evidence is clinical and very likely to be holistic in nature. Clinical practice is thus a first testing ground for the validity of a good idea. A quarter of a century does not seem too long to give a good clinical idea to be tried by enough practitioners to provide a first reading on whether that technique has a future.

Evidence of a more formal sort (as exemplified, for example, in experimental design or a randomized clinical trial) is a necessary next step, in which theory becomes better articulated, the processes are specified, and the critical hypotheses tested, usually resulting in various mixes of iconoclastic rejection of the original idea, revisionist operations, and, if we are fortunate, enshrinement of the core idea in a modified setting.

The review of psychosocial interventions is necessarily based on only a partial growth period for creative interventions. A next step will be appro-

[1] *Polisher Research Institute, Philadelphia Geriatric Center, Temple Continuing Care Center, 5301 Old York Road, Philadelphia, PA 19141-2996, USA*

priate and badly needed in just a few more years. The fact is that dementia is such a daunting illness that creative clinicians have been loath to risk entering such a treatment-recalcitrant area. When a new idea is proffered, its rarity sometimes precipitates its premature adoption. Most of our current approaches to the psychosocial treatment of dementia are still in the clinical tryout phase. But the hunger for something, *anything*, to try to help the desperate situation of a person with dementia is so great that such candidate treatments seem to gain lives of their own, even after the early search for evidence proves fruitless.

Some of the treatments covered in Prof. Baro's review fall into this category. Reality orientation, life review, the several planned reminiscence therapies and validation therapy fall into a group of interventions that have had their time for clinical use and sharpening. They are clearly ready for the evidence phase to be applied in a rigorous manner. Although some reports on attempts to validate their efficacy have appeared, their results are not terribly encouraging at this point. The next critical review may be able to provide a definitive "stop" vs. "proceed" message for some of these interventions, but that review needs to be merciless in its assessment of the evidence. Sensory stimulation and motor activity display a slightly better state of encouraging validation research. Behaviour modification is clearly in the best position as far as outcomes of research-based assessment is concerned.

Individual and group therapy in their different forms, although not new in application to dementia, are still in great need of purely clinical use with differing types of patients. Environmental design in its physical and social forms is flourishing as an approach to the care of people with dementia. The type of research best suited to the global nature of these interventions, however, may well not be the traditional experiment. The coalition of behavioural and environmental scientists who have been so active in creating this technology owe us now a new research paradigm that accounts for the global and non-linear character of the dynamics of well-being when many people behave in such complex environments.

Finally, Prof. Baro's sage comments on quality of life lead to a basic question about the goals of intervention on behalf of people with irreversible brain damage: why do we have to apply our usual scientific evidential criteria of permanence of effect or generalization beyond the trained response in order to conclude that a treatment has a positive effect? A preferred criterion is offered here: an acceptable goal of an intervention is any increment in time where pleasure is experienced, time when interest is evoked, or occasion when personal control or autonomous behaviour occurs. Thus we will do well in our future research to focus on microprocesses and cumulative time rather than global and permanent change as the basic evidence in our efforts to intervene in dementing illness. Such a perspective on the nature of evidence may also lead us to return to some of the experiential trials that have not fared well in formal validation. Have we tried hard enough to assess the pleasure, the distress, the autonomy of the moment, as these therapies, such as reality orientation or validation therapy, are applied? How about occupational therapy or recreational therapy? Psychotherapy or an attractive living environment may be liked (i.e. evoke pleasure, interest, or a sense of control) even if they do not reconstruct the whole person. The moral: seize the moment.

5.3
## The Development of Cognitive Neurorehabilitation for Alzheimer's Disease
Takashi Asada[1]

Prof. Baro's sophisticated review provides us with a guide to the most promising strategies of psychosocial intervention currently available for dementia. Roughly speaking, many of these interventions seem to be effective for psychiatric and behavioural symptoms. However, it remains an open question whether they are effective for cognitive impairment and able to delay the progression of dementing illnesses. As there are few empirical data relating to this issue, I would like to discuss some recent findings pertaining to human neurogenesis and related areas from the viewpoint of Alzheimer's disease (AD) prevention.

Recently, neurogenesis in the adult human brain, especially the hippo-campus, has been demonstrated. Eriksson *et al* [1] indicated that the human hippocampus retains its ability to generate neurons throughout life. A series of animal experiments have demonstrated that an enriched environment [2], running [3] and learning [4] enhance adult neurogenesis in the hippocampus. In contrast, prolonged stress can cause damage in the rat brain. It is well known that characteristic neuronal loss is evident in the hippocampus even at early stage of AD, and this neuronal loss impairs memory retention [5]. Thus, these recent findings concerning neurogenesis seem to favour the possible AD-protective effect of psychosocial factors. It is now necessary to clarify which factors have the potential to facilitate neurogenesis in humans.

From this viewpoint, it is perhaps appropriate to refer first to the prefrontal cortex. Very recently, it was revealed that the prefrontal cortex plays

[1] *Department of Rehabilitation, National Center of Neurology and Psychiatry, Ogawahigashicho 4-1-1, Kodaira City, Tokyo, 187–8551 Japan*

major roles in memory retrieval [6], complex problem-solving and planning [7]. In addition, Kramer *et al* [8] reported that aerobic exercise can improve executive control processes supported by the prefrontal and frontal regions of the brain.

Second, it may be worthwhile re-evaluating music as a brain activator. For many years, correlations between intelligence scores and musical ability tests have been examined. Magnetic resonance imaging (MRI) has shown that the left planum temporale region is larger in musicians than in non-musicians [9]. In connection with this finding, it is known that verbal memory is mediated mainly by the left temporal lobe, and in fact Chan *et al* [10] have proved that adults with music training should have better verbal memory than adults without such training. Although the "Mozart effect" on the cognitive function of the normal individuals is controversial, Rauscher [11] reported that the effect is limited to spatial–temporal tasks involving mental imagery and temporal ordering. These two reports appear to indicate that music has potential to improving the cognitive functions of both normal and demented individuals.

It is generally agreed that preventive measures are not always able to delay the progression of AD. However, whether psychosocial intervention or brain activation might prevent further decline and neuronal loss even after the onset of AD is a line of research worth pursuing. In this connection, a recent study by Johnson *et al* [12] demonstrated enhancement of spatial–temporal reasoning after a Mozart listening condition in a patient with AD.

As a basis for developing effective intervention measures, knowledge about the pathological process of AD is indispensable. On gross inspection, the brains of AD patients are most atrophic in the temporoparietal and anterior frontal regions, with sparing of the primary motor, somatosensory and occipital cortices [13]. A positron emission tomography (PET) study [14] in the early phase of the illness revealed that parietal hypometabolism is most marked; as the disease progresses, premotor metabolic reduction also becomes severe. From these findings, it would appear that the prefrontal cortex and planum temporale are the regions which are relatively being spared in AD brain.

Researchers and clinical staff who are attempting to develop effective psychosocial interventions for AD should bear the following issues in mind: (a) whether certain types of brain activation are able to ameliorate the impaired functions corresponding to regions of the brain that are affected by the disease; (b) whether activation of one brain region is able to compensate for impaired functions in another affected brain region. Taking these issues into consideration, we should re-evaluate the promising strategies of intervention reviewed by Prof. Baro. For such studies, neuroimaging techniques, including magnetoencephalogram, may bring fruitful results.

## REFERENCES

1. Eriksson P.S., Perfilieva E., Bjork-Eriksson T., Alborn A.M., Nordborg C., Peterson D.A., Gage F.H. (1998)   Neurogenesis in the adult human hippocampus. *Nature Med.*, **4**: 1313–1317.
2. Kempermann G., Kuhn H.G., Gage F.H. (1997)   More hippocampal neurons in adult mice living in an enriched environment. *Nature*, **386**: 493–495.
3. van Praag H., Kemperman G., Gage F.H. (1999)   Running increases cell proliferation and neurogenesis in the adult mouse dentate gyrus. *Nature Neurosci.*, **2**: 266–270.
4. Gould E., Beylin A., Tanapat P., Reeves A., Shors T.J. (1999)   Learning enhances adult neurogenesis in the hippocampal formation. *Nature Neurosci.*, **2**: 260–265.
5. Hyman B.T., Arriagada P.V., van Hoesen G.W., Damasio A.R. (1993)   Memory impairment in Alzheimer's disease: an anatomical perspective. In *Neuropsychology of Alzheimer's Disease and Other Dementias* (Eds R.W. Parks, R.F. Zec, R.S. Wilson), pp. 138–150, Oxford University Press, New York.
6. Tomita H., Ohbayashi M., Nakahara K., Hasegawa I., Mitashita Y. (1999)   Top-down signal from prefrontal cortex in executive control of memory retrieval. *Nature*, **401**: 699–703.
7. Koechlin E., Basso G., Pietrini P., Panzer S., Grafman J. (1999)   The role of the anterior prefrontal cortex in human cognition. *Nature*, **399**: 148–151.
8. Kramer A.F., Hahn S., Cohen N.J., Banich M.T., McAuley E., Harrison C.R., Chason J., Vakil E., Bardell L., Boileau R.A. *et al* (1999)   Ageing, fitness and neurocognitive function. *Nature*, **400**: 418–419.
9. Schlaug G., Jancke L., Huang Y., Steinmetz H. (1995)   *In vivo* evidence of structural brain asymmetry in musicians. *Science*, **267**: 699–701.
10. Chan A.S., Ho Y.C., Cheung M.C. (1998)   Music training improves verbal memory. *Nature*, **396**: 128.
11. Rauscher F.H. (1999)   Prelude or requiem for the "Mozart effect"? *Nature*, **400**: 827–828.
12. Johnson J.K., Cotman C.W., Tasaki C.S., Shaw G.L. (1998)   Enhancement of spatial–temporal reasoning after Mozart listening condition in Alzheimer's disease: a case study. *Neurol. Res.*, **20**: 666–672.
13. Cummings J.L., Benson D.F. (1992)   *Dementia*, 2nd edn, Butterworth-Heinemann, Stoneham.
14. Haxby J.V., Grady C.L., Koss E., Horwitz B., Schapiro M., Friedand R.P., Rapoport S.I. (1988)   Heterogeneous anterior–posterior metabolic patterns in dementia of the Alzheimer type. *Neurology*, **38**: 1853–1863.

## Psychosocial Interventions and Behavioural Treatments for Dementia
### Linda Teri[1]

Psychosocial interventions for dementia patients often have an intuitive appeal. Oftentimes consisting of providing support, education and advice to caregivers, and simple environmental changes and suggestions for patients, these interventions are sometimes mistakenly seen as simplistic or unscientific. Prof. Baro has done an exceptional job of showing how psychosocial interventions often draw upon a diverse literature of scholarly work. The connections he makes between various psychosocial interventions and different areas of scientific inquiry offer intriguing avenues for future conceptual and empirical research.

One form of psychosocial treatment, as Prof. Baro discusses, is training for family and staff caregivers. Training families to provide care to dementia patients has a long clinical history. In recent years, the amount and popularity of this kind of information has grown exponentially, as is evident in the proliferation of books, training programs and self-help groups. Numerous programs have focused on caregivers themselves seeking to reduce caregiver burden, cope with disease, improve well-being, and enhance social support (as reviewed in [1]). Many of these have shown that caregivers enjoy participation in supportive and psycho-educational groups, but overall treatment effects have been modest and short-term.

Another form of psychosocial treatment is, as Prof. Baro indicates, behaviour modification. It is a misnomer, however, to suggest that such treatments are solely based on cognitive learning. If this were the case, dementias might be least amenable to this treatment given the deficits in learning that characterize them. Rather, such treatments are more often based upon social-learning, operant and classical conditioning theories and research—i.e. individuals respond to social and environmental stimuli and, by changing the stimuli, one can change the response. This paradigm has been successful in altering the behaviour in even severely brain-impaired patients.

Similar to caregiver education programs, behavioural treatment incorporates providing basic education about Alzheimer's dementia, information about community and family resources to assist with caregiving responsibilities, and developing short- and long-term care plans. More uniquely, behavioural treatment involves teaching methods of behaviour observation and change, identifying and developing strategies to maximize patient

---

[1] *Department of Psychosocial and Community Health, University of Washington School of Nursing, Seattle, WA 98195–7263, USA*

function, and teaching effective problem-solving skills for day-to-day difficulties in patient care. Studies using this approach have focused on patient outcomes and have demonstrated impressive success. One series of investigations by Mittleman and colleagues [2] points to maintenance of gains 8 years following treatment; another by Teri and colleagues [3–5] indicates that a structured systematic approach can successfully reduce depression in dementia patients and in their caregivers. Others have shown that family caregivers were able to learn specific behavioural techniques to successfully reduce problematic patient behaviours (e.g. [6–9]) and that staff training programs can be similarly effective in decreasing patient problems and increasing staff skills [10–12]. Thus, diverse programs, focusing on both institutional and family caregivers, have been successful in achieving short- and long-term success.

The growth of randomized controlled clinical trials in the area of psychosocial interventions represents a significant advance in the field. I could not agree more with Prof. Baro's conclusion that more research is needed in this field. Thus far, the majority of published studies focus on pharmacological approaches to care. It is time for psychosocial approaches to be subjected to comparable rigor. Support is needed for the development and investigation of psychosocial approaches on their own and in conjunction with pharmacotherapy. Only by merging the best of what we learn can we hope to optimize care for our dementia patients.

## REFERENCES

1. Zarit S.H., Teri L. (1991)   Interventions and services for family caregivers. *Ann. Rev. Gerontol. Geriatrics*, **11**: 241–265.
2. Mittelman M., Ferris S., Steinberg G., Shulman E., Mackell J., Ambinder A., Cohen J. (1993)   An intervention that delays institutionalization of Alzheimer's disease patients: treatment of spouse-caregivers. *Gerontologist*, **33**: 730–740.
3. Teri L., Uomoto J. (1991)   Reducing excess disability in dementia patients: training caregivers to manage patient depression. *Clin. Gerontol.*, **31**: 49–63.
4. Teri L. (1994)   Behavioural treatment of depression in patients with dementia. *Alz. Dis. Assoc. Disord.*, **8**: 66–74.
5. Teri L., Logsdon R.G., Uomoto J., McCurry S. (1997)   Behavioural treatment of depression in dementia patients: a controlled clinical trial. *J. Gerontol. B: Psychol. Sci. Soc. Sci.*, **52B**: P159–P166.
6. Pinkston E.M., Linsk N. (1984)   Behavioural family intervention with the impaired elderly. *Gerontologist*, **24**: 576–583.
7. Aronson M.K., Levin G., Lipkowitz R. (1984)   A community based family/patient group program for Alzheimer's disease. *Gerontologist*, **24**: 339–342.
8. Haley W.E., Brown S.L., Levine E.G. (1987)   Family caregiver appraisals of patient behavioural disturbance in senile dementia. *Clin. Gerontol.*, **6**: 25–37.
9. Pinkston E.M., Linsk N., Young R.N. (1988)   Home based behavioural family treatment of the impaired elderly. *Behav. Ther.*, **19**: 331–344.

10. Burgio L., Scilley K., Hardin J.M., Hsu C., Yancey J. (1996) Environmental "white noise": an intervention for verbally agitated nursing home residents. *J. Gerontol. B: Psychol. Sci. Soc. Sci.*, **51B**: P364–P373.
11. Burgio L.D. (1997) Behavioural assessment and treatment of disruptive vocalization. *Semin. Clin. Neuropsychiatry*, **2**: 123–131.
12. Beck C.K. 91998) Psychosocial and behavioural interventions for Alzhemer's disease patients and their families. *Am. J. Geriatr. Psychiatry*, 6 (Suppl. 1): 541–548.

5.5
# The Need for Greater Specificity in Psychosocial Interventions
## Cornelia Beck[1]

The paper by Franz Baro provides an excellent overview of common psychosocial interventions used with persons with dementia, as well as addressing the needs of caregivers. What stands out from this review is that while a few interventions have been shown to be effective through the rigor of scientific evaluation, many more are still supported primarily by anecdotal evidence.

Reality orientation, while having demonstrated some positive benefits, as Baro indicates, can also serve as a trigger for problem behaviours and even more confusion. It seems more appropriate for those with reversible memory loss. Dietch *et al* [1] reported three case studies of demented elderly people who experienced negative effects when caregivers used reality orientation with them. The authors then tried validation therapy and found it more effective. They concluded that: (a) caregivers must employ reality orientation carefully and observe its results, and (b) researchers must test the efficacy of validation therapy in controlled studies.

Prof. Baro makes a useful distinction between life review, simple reminiscence, life history, and life story. Additional research on reminiscence includes work by the European reminiscence project, which includes 11 European countries [2]. They have concluded from observations that it is therapeutic for persons with dementia, as have Mills and Coleman [3] and Woods and McKiernan [4]. Schweitzer's book [5] provides an excellent overview, although primarily not research-based.

In the discussion of behaviour modification, Prof. Baro makes an important point about the areas of learning which are preserved in dementia. These include implicit memory and verbal learning and retention. While not discussed specifically, these retained abilities have implications for memory

[1] *Departments of Psychiatry and Geriatrics, University of Arkansas for Medical Sciences, 4301 W. Markham, Slot 748, Little Rock, AR 72205, USA*

interventions. For example, Camp *et al* [6] distinguish between interventions which use internal vs. external mnemonics and explicit (effortful or conscious) vs. implicit (automatic or unconscious) learning. Neuropsychological literature suggests that some memory systems (implicit, indirect, procedural memory) operate unconsciously or automatically, or both. Persons with dementia seem to retain motor and verbal priming (implicit or procedural memory). Therefore, they often benefit from interventions that use external mnemonics and capitalize on implicit learning, especially in the early and middle stages.

Although these preserved areas of memory have provided direction for interventions that capitalize on and support remaining cognitive abilities, the heterogeneity of cognitive losses means that interventions must be individualized to specific cognitive disabilities. Also, studies are needed which combine pharmacotherapy with the new cholinergic agents and cognitive enhancement interventions.

The retrogenesis model does suggest that the motor-cognitive stages of dementia can be translated into developmental age equivalents. Matteson *et al* have both proposed [7] and tested [8] a retrogenesis model using Piaget's cognitive developmental levels. They have found it helpful in matching the interventions used with dementia patients to their remaining cognitive abilities.

Studies of sensory stimulation interventions have, for the most part, demonstrated fairly immediate positive effects, such as decreases in anxiety, improvements in mood and social interaction, and decreased agitation. Baro notes, in relation to the Benson [9] study, that there was little carry-over effect beyond the session. This same finding emerges also from the other studies reviewed, as well as those not discussed. Such a finding seems realistic, given the cognitive deficits of the subjects. Perhaps investigators do not need to continue to measure for these carry-over effects and consider that increasing the quality of life during the time that the intervention occurs is sufficient.

Baro's discussion of the use of individual psychotherapy is important, particularly given the trend toward earlier diagnosis and the availability of cholinergic therapies which may delay cognitive decline. The work of the Bradford Dementia Group has highlighted the importance of understanding the personal experience of the disease [10,11]. Assisting individuals with dealing with the losses brought on by the disease is an important component of individual therapy. It would be interesting to document the effect of psychotherapy early in the disease process on later behavioural outcomes, such as problem behaviours. Baro makes the important point that people with dementia are able to express their views and feelings to a much greater degree and for a longer period of time than has generally thought to be possible. For example, Simmons' and Schnelle's work with nursing home residents shows that persons with moderate cognitive impairment are still able to report accurately on the quality of care they are receiving [12].

Baro is accurate in his observation that there seems to be a consensus on environmental designs for dementia care despite a paucity of research in this area. Perhaps this points to a need to develop a science that underlies the recommendations that designers are currently making. Formal educational programs for interior designers and architects that are focused on the needs of persons with dementia could then be developed.

# REFERENCE

1. Dietch J.T., Hewett L.J., Jones S. (1989) Adverse effects of reality orientation. *J. Am. Geriatr. Soc.*, **37**: 974–976.
2. Rasmussen L. (1999) A response to the Pan-European project: remembering yesterday, caring today. *Reminiscence*, **18**: 10–11.
3. Mills M.A., Coleman P.G. (1994) Nostalgic memories in dementia: a case study. *Int. J. Aging Hum. Develop.*, **38**: 181–202.
4. Woods B., McKiernan F. (1994) Evaluating the impact of reminiscence on older people with dementia. In *The Art and Science of Reminiscing: Theory, Research, Methods, and Applications* (Eds B.K. Haight, J.D. Webster), pp. 233–242, Taylor and Francis, Washington, DC.
5. Schweitzer P. (Ed.) (1998) *Reminiscence in Dementia Care*, Age Exchange, London.
6. Camp C.J., Foss J.W., Stevens A.B., Reichard C.C., McKitrick L.A., O'Hanlon A.M. (1993) Memory training in normal and demented elderly populations: the E–I–E–I–O model. *Exp. Aging Res.*, **19**: 277–290.
7. Matteson M.A., Linton A.D., Barnes S.J. (1996) Cognitive developmental approach to dementia. *Image*, **28**: 233–240.
8. Matteson M.A., Linton A.D., Cleary B.L., Barnes S.J., Lichtenstein M.J. (1997) Management of problematic behavioural symptoms associated with dementia: a cognitive developmental approach. *Aging Clin. Exp. Res.*, **9**: 342–355.
9. Benson S. (1994) Sniff and doze therapy. *J. Dementia Care*, **2**: 12–14.
10. Kitwood T. (1997) The experience of dementia. *Aging Ment. Health*, **1**: 13–22.
11. Kitwood T. (1998) Toward a theory of dementia care: ethics and interaction. *J. Clin. Ethics*, **9**: 23–34.
12. Simmons S.F., Schnelle J.F., Uman G.C., Kulvicki A.D., Lee K.H., Ouslander J.G. (1997) Selecting nursing home residents for satisfaction surveys. *Gerontologist*, **37**: 543–550.

### 5.6
### Psychosocial Interventions in Dementia: the Nature and Focus of Intervention, Outcome Measurement and Quality of Life

Sube Banerjee[1]

Prof. Baro's elegant review of psychosocial interventions for people with dementia focuses on management strategies at the level of the individual with dementia. However, such a consideration of psychosocial interventions raises important basic questions concerning the goal and the focus of such interventions. These issues are of interest because there is a complex web of potential outcomes (and therefore outcome measures) and there are interventions which may be of benefit to the person with dementia (PWD) but which are not necessarily individually focused upon that person. This brief commentary cannot cover these issues in detail, but will instead consider some of the active debates in definitions and measurement of outcome and in the focus of intervention which are of particular salience in dementia care.

When considering intervention in a disorder, we need to ask what we are trying to achieve. The answer to this question is usually self-evident in most disorders where there is an understanding of aetiology and the focus of the disease process, and there are interventions of proven effectiveness. The intention of intervention will generally be to prevent the occurrence of disease (primary prevention), to cure the disease (secondary prevention), or to stabilize or palliate the disease (tertiary prevention). However, the state of the art in dementia is such that, despite increasingly compelling biological research and development, we have no clear understanding of the aetiology of the vast majority of dementias, and no treatments available which can reverse or stabilize disease progression. Added to this, the nature of the syndrome of dementia is that it is a chronic relentlessly progressive neurodegenerative disorder in which there is a massive impact not only on the PWD but also on informal (family/friends) carers and health and social welfare services.

What we want to achieve depends on the focus of our intervention. Interventions can be focused anywhere along an axis which includes the PWD, informal carers, formal carers (including care settings), the community, and nationally or internationally. At each of these levels there are interventions that have been suggested to address the needs of the PWD, but these interventions necessarily vary.

At the individual PWD level, interventions may be focused on the cognitive features of dementia (this is the primary focus of much pharmacological intervention following from the requirements of national drug licensing

[1] Institute of Psychiatry, King's College, De Crespigny Park, London SE5 8AF, UK

agencies) or on non-cognitive features, as discussed in Prof. Baro's review. The role of informal carers in maintaining PWD in the community and in maximizing quality of life is well recognized, and such carers have been identified as an important resource for the delivery of psychosocial interventions for the PWD. Equally, it is clear that the caring role is strongly associated with carer burden and carer mental ill-health, both of which can be detrimental to the PWD under their care. Thus, interventions at the level of informal care can be directly provided through the carer (as with much formal behaviour modification) or can be focused on the carer her- or himself. Primary and secondary preventative strategies (to prevent burden of mental disorder) include psychoeducational approaches, respite care, support groups, and carer-specific counselling or psychotherapy. These seek to be of direct help to the carer and also of indirect help to the PWD on the basis that a more informed, supported and a healthier carer will look after and interact better with the PWD.

The interventions in the preceding paragraph can be categorized as individually focused interventions (either on the PWD or the carer). However, there is another potentially beneficial set of approaches that might be called integrative interventions. In these, the carer/PWD dyad is treated as a system whose individual parts need joint as well as separate assessment and intervention. The rationale for such an approach is that an analysis of the system as a whole, and the development, delivery and review of a package of care individualized to the particular situation, will be more likely to be effective than a plan which narrowly construes the problems and the intervention. Examples of this include some more or less intensive models of case/care management and other multidimensional approaches. This idea of producing a holistic and individually tailored management plan for each referral is in accord with the general practice of old age psychiatry.

Formal carers, for example those social service, health or welfare staff providing home care and institutional care in nursing homes, have also been the subjects of interventions designed to improve the management and quality of life of the PWD under their care. In common with the interventions for informal carers discussed above, the psychoeducational, training and support packages that have been advocated, have a dual focus: first, to be of direct help to the PWD, by improving the care delivered, and also to be of indirect help by improving the quality of care by decreasing unwanted staff outcomes, such as burnout, stress and high staff turnover.

At the community level, interventions will generally concern the formation of health and social policy and the delivery of health and social services. Few psychosocial interventions have no cost; therefore, if interventions are to be provided to a community, those who purchase and provide services, including the private sector, local government and the voluntary sector, need to recognize, prioritize and facilitate the delivery of services for PWD and their carers. This population level facilitation of interventions by the formulation of health and social policy is also the main conduit for positive action for PWD on a national and international basis. However, it is not only narrow health and social policy which is of importance here, but also population level health education and promotion, transport provision and employment law, as well as targeted financial benefits which can be used to help PWD and their carers. At this national level, the motors for intervention are likely to be financial as well as humanitarian. Dementia costs health and social services and families a very large amount, with institutionalization a major source of financial outlay in many countries. The primary objective of intervention at a national level may therefore be to minimize the spend on PWD.

This multiplicity of levels and foci for intervention means that, in dementia, outcome measurement can be particularly challenging. The conundrum of how best to evaluate and compare the clinical and cost-effectiveness of interventions at an individual and service level, when outcomes may be as diverse as cognition, behavioural disturbance, carer burden, staff turnover or national spend, is one that engages those who purchase, provide, plan and receive services as well as researchers. This is one of the major reasons for the growing interest in developing a methodology for measuring health-related quality of life in dementia. The paradox in dementia care is that supposedly hard outcome measures, such as cognition, may deteriorate while an intervention that is of major benefit to the PWD and carers is delivered. A quality of life measure that is able to distinguish systematically and empirically between degrees of good and poor quality of life and is psychometrically responsive to change would enable this paradox to be resolved.

However, this requires a development of the scientific base in the measurement of quality of life. Many purists would hold that this is a purely subjective construct, and that without self-report quality of life cannot be ascertained. This standpoint may be tenable for the majority of disorders, where it is very unlikely that a significant proportion of those affected will be unable to provide a valid self-assessment. However, while there is increasing evidence that a substantial proportion of PWDs of mild to moderate severity can provide such data, there are many who cannot. Also, those who cannot complete these assessments, such as those with severe dementia in residential care and those with active or passive behavioural disturbance, may be just the groups who require intervention. If we accept that the inability to provide a valid self-report of quality of life means that quality of life cannot be assessed, then this is tantamount to denying that there is variation in quality of life in dementia (which is patently untrue) and that interventions designed to improve quality of life are untestable. In our increasingly evidence-based health care systems, untestability equates with unfundability. What is needed are innovative approaches to the measurement of quality of life in dementia which are based on the soundest of psychometrics. These might integrate self-report, proxy carer data and potentially external observer ratings into a valid and reliable measure that can be used in clinical and research settings.

With such a measure, studies of the clinical and cost effectiveness and of the cost utility of interventions for PWD and their carers could be conducted. Without them, it is far less likely that a successful case can be made for the provision of such interventions in the real world, because other disorders and client groups will be able to present a more coherent evidence base than is possible for dementia care. Equally, where there is competition for research funding, trials in disorders where there are clear and clinically relevant outcome measures are more likely to be funded that those where there are not. Dementia care is complex, as is the measurement of outcome in dementia, but our best chance of improving the lot of PWDs and their carers will come from intervention at multiple levels that is based on sound outcome data.

5.7

### General Comments on Psychosocial Interventions for Dementia

Edgar Miller[1]

Franz Baro has provided an extensive review of psychosocial interventions for dementia. This commentary will not attempt to add further detailed information. Instead it will deal with some general and fundamental issues that complement the information provided in the review.

The first point is to emphasize (or re-emphasize) that elderly patients with dementia are sensitive to environmental influences. Discussions of the psychosocial aspects of dementia often focus on impairments, and it is certainly true that dementia does lead to profound psychological and functional deficits [1,2]. Despite this, it is important to remember that there are also many findings indicating that patients with dementia can show appreciable learning, under at least some circumstances [3,4]. These experimental investigations, considerably reinforced by the positive outcomes obtained by many of the therapeutic studies described in the review by Franz Baro, attest to the very real ability of even quite markedly afflicted patients to respond to environmental manipulations. This responsiveness is an essential prerequisite for work on psychosocial interventions and offers a major justification for further research and development.

[1] *Department of Psychology, University of Leicester, Leicester LE1 7RH, UK*

Many of the methods of interventions described in the review, such as reality orientation and reminiscence, are general in nature and based on assumptions about the nature of the problems revealed by those with dementia as a whole. For example, that problems in maintaining orientation for time, place and person are a central issue in dementia was a fundamental assumption in the development of reality orientation. Similarly, reminiscence as a therapy is based on notions about the importance of life review for older people. Although these approaches can be adapted to the needs of individuals, as in using individual background experience in reminiscence sessions, they fail to take into account the wide range of difficulties and impairments that arise in dementia. This contrasts with the major approaches to psychological treatment in other contexts, that depend on carefully analysing the nature of the particular individual's problems and what maintains them, and devising therapeutic investigations accordingly. Of the approaches to intervention described in the review, behaviour modification and individual psychotherapy are different in this respect and are directed at the problems of individual clients.

Possibly the different nature of many interventions for older people with dementia, like reality orientation, is because of a tendency to see their problems as being very different from those of other patient groups and thus requiring their own particular forms of intervention. In fact, problems such as difficulty in maintaining activities of everyday living, failing memory, disordered speech and personality change, are far from unique to those with dementia. This suggests that the types of therapy used to deal with similar problems in other patient groups could effectively be exploited to deal with the problems of those with dementia.

Although positive changes have been shown to follow from many of the interventions described in the review, these typically show two features. First, the gains are hard won and considerable therapeutic effort goes into achieving quite modest gains [5]. The fact that dementia is a progressive, deteriorating condition may be one reason for this. The second feature is that where follow-up data has been collected, any gains tend to be lost quite quickly after any special intervention is discontinued [6]. An implication that follows from this is that psychosocial interventions for dementia should typically not be viewed as "treatments", in the sense that a "treatment" is designed to put right or reverse a pathological situation [7]. Having dealt with that situation, the treatment can then be withdrawn. Rather, greater emphasis should be placed on what Lindsley [8] originally described as "prosthetic environments". Psychosocial environments should be designed so as to maximize the functioning of individuals, with many of the interventions involved being regarded as more-or-less permanent features of the environment, rather than something which is put in place to achieve a therapeutic goal and then withdrawn when that goal appears to have been achieved.

Finally, it is important to emphasize the point, made in the Franz Baro's review, that much dementia care is, and will remain, informal care, usually provided by spouses and other relatives. Abundant evidence now attests to the strains placed on informal carers who look after someone with dementia [1,9]. An important facet of developing effective psychosocial interventions is the requirement to consider not only the sufferer but also to take into account the difficulties faced by the carer.

## REFERENCES

1. Miller E., Morris R.G. (1993) *The Psychology of Dementia*, Wiley, Chichester.
2. Morris R.G. (Ed.) (1996) *The Cognitive Neuropsychology of Alzheimer-type Dementia*, Oxford University Press, Oxford.
3. Eslinger P., Damasio A.R. (1986) Preserved motor learning in Alzheimer's disease: implications for anatomy and behaviour. *J. Neurosci.*, **6**: 3006–3009.
4. Morris R.G. (1987) Matching and oddity learning in moderate to severe dementia. *Quart. J. Exp. Psychol.*, **39**: 215–227.
5. Miller E. (1994) Psychological strategies. In *Principles and Practice of Geriatric Psychiatry* (Eds J.R.M. Copeland, M.T. Abou-Saleh, D.G. Blazer), pp. 427–430, Wiley, Chichester.
6. Powell-Proctor I., Miller E. (1982) Reality orientation: critical appraisal. *Br. J. Psychiatry*, **140**: 457–463.
7. Lindsley O.R. (1964) Geriatric behavioural prosthesis. In *New Thoughts on Old Age* (Ed. R. Kastenbaum), pp. 126–143, Springer, New York.
8. Woods R., Bird M. (1999) Non-pharmacological approaches to treatment. In *Diagnosis and Management of Dementia* (Eds G.K. Wilcock, R.S. Bucks, K. Rockwood), pp. 311–331, Oxford University Press, Oxford.
9. Morris R.G., Morris L.W., Britton P.G. (1988) Factors affecting the emotional wellbeing of caregivers of dementia sufferers. *Br. J. Psychiatry*, **153**: 147–156.

5.8
## Changing Therapeutic Paradigms
Bernard Groulx[1]

What is remarkable in Prof. Baro's review on psychosocial interventions in dementia should be that it is thorough, covers literally all forms of psychosocial interventions in dementia and addresses the needs of patients and their families. But, in a sense, it is what is not written or is between the lines that surprises, i.e. how far our vision, our attitudes regarding patients suffering from dementia, have come in perhaps 10–15 years.

[1] *Ste. Anne's Veterans Hospital, 305 Anciens Combattants Blvd., Ste.-Anne-de-Bellevue, Quebec H9X 1Y9, Canada*

It does not seem that long ago that interest in the field was almost restricted to neuropathological features, such as neuritic plaques and neurofibrillary tangles. Now, by contrast, Reisberg *et al* show us that the functional stages in Alzheimer's disease (AD) can be translated into developmental age equivalents that can be utilized to understand and react to observed changes in the disease [1]. It is a complete change in thinking, a focus that has moved from a narrow observation of the brain to a real interest in what the patient is living, is feeling; a focus that has gone from studying the illness from the greatest distance possible (autopsies) to a genuine attempt at putting oneself, empathically, in the patient's place.

In the presence of agitation or any behavioural problems, the clinicians of not long ago were mainly interested, in absolute good faith, in helping the family and professional caregivers. The interest has now shifted to understanding why the patient is behaving in such a way and what are the needs he is trying to express.

It is not that the needs of caregivers are no longer important, it is that instead of putting the highest value on their quality of life, it is now put on the patient's quality of life, on the patient's well-being and capacity for pleasure. That is, indeed, another remarkable change in paradigm.

Of course, recognizing these changes does not mean that we are there yet. It is still estimated that, in nursing homes, over 90% of treatment for mental illnesses, agitated or aggressive behaviour, etc. is by medication. And indeed, there are reasons for this. It is easier and certainly cheaper when compared with hiring clinical personnel. When applicable, the reimbursement is easier. Mostly, however, it is simply because many professional caregivers do not know how to conduct non-pharmacological psychosocial interventions or are too entrenched in their routines.

We have always known that, with these patients and their difficult behaviour, medications sometimes do not work and can actually harm them. In fact, medication can certainly mask the expression of a distress and its communication, therefore decreasing our ability to help the individual. However, it is with the more recent growing body of evidence for the efficacy of non-pharmacological psychosocial interventions, so well documented in Prof. Baro's paper, that, again, focus was redirected from unmet needs of others to unmet needs of dementia patients.

These needs, of course, are not mysterious or abnormal. They are normal physiological needs: health, control of pain, of physical discomfort. They are needs for safety and comfortable environmental conditions; needs for love and belonging, for social contacts, for self-actualization and stimulation. It is the life conditions of the patient that are mysterious and abnormal: inability to communicate needs, inability to use prior coping mechanisms or obtaining means for meeting the needs; being in an environment that does not comprehend the needs or satisfy them; actual unawareness of the needs [2].

At the risk of sounding minimalist, it is perhaps in the area of interpersonal communication that these changes in paradigms have been most dramatic. We certainly do not have to go very far back in time to acknowledge that, in the face of verbal expressions of distress by dementia patients, the accepted clinical approaches, again practiced in all good faith, were basically to suppress them. Orthodox psychotherapies found little value in exploring the psyche of elderly people, let alone ones afflicted with dementia, and the belief, in caregivers, was that a happy or serene patient was a quiet one, a silent one. That Prof. Baro is able to document the interesting results of individual as well as group psychotherapies with these patients, is a tremendous leap forward.

And if this is true in a professional setting, it is equally true in a familial one. In the past few years, psychologists, linguists, psychoeducators, etc. have developed and, most importantly, have applied better and better communication strategies that families can use with their loved one suffering from dementia, even in the more severe stages. In contrast with times when families were instructed to diminish stimulation, even verbal ones and, in doing so, create unwittingly a devastating solitude, they now have the possibility of taking training programs in functional communications with AD patients (e.g. [3]).

It would be naive to believe, at this point in time, that the psychosocial interventions described in Prof. Baro's review are the norm in the management and treatment of dementia patients worldwide. Contacts with psychogeriatric institutions in North America, Europe and Japan have shown me that we still have a long way to go. But the attribution of a full chapter to issues of not only psychosocial interventions but the psychotherapeutic needs and, most importantly, the quality of life of patients suffering from dementia, should be a great incitement to change ways of thinking and philosophies on clinical approaches. It will also certainly act as a guideline for education, for training of family and professional caregivers and, hopefully, an impetus for further research.

## REFERENCES

1. Reisberg B., Kenowsky S., Franssen E.H., Huer S.R., Souren L.E. (1999) Towards a science of Alzheimer's disease management: a model based upon current knowledge of retrogenesis. *Int. Psychogeriatrics*, **11**: 7–23.
2. Cohen-Mansfield J., Billig N. (1986) Agitated behaviours in the elderly. A conceptual review. *J. Am. Geriatr. Soc.*, **34**: 711–721.
3. Ripich B.N. (1994) Functional communication with AD patients: a care giver training program. *Alz. Dis. Assoc. Disord.*, **8**: 95–109.

5.9
## Psychosocial Interventions in Dementia: Attitudes, Approaches, Therapies and Quality of Life

Edmond Chiu[1]

Working with persons with dementia invites the immediate response of having to "do something" for these persons. From the perspective of the traditional medical and scientific stand, the response is to make a diagnosis, identify etiologies and provide the most appropriate and efficacious treatment or therapy. Until an effective, specific and safe treatment is available, management of the person with dementia rests with individual carers (formal and informal) using pragmatic strategies derived from their experience and personality. Psychosocial interventions are, thus, the pragmatic, non-scientific, intuitive responses to such a stressful and stress-inducing condition.

Prof. Baro's review presents studies and comments on a list of the most common psychosocial interventions, citing evidence where it exists in a sparse literature. This parallels a similar systematic review of research findings by Opie *et al* [1], which identified 43 studies meeting the authors' criteria for review. They pointed out that areas of scientific weakness include a small number of subjects, inadequate description of study participants, imprecise data collection methods, high attrition rates and inadequate statistical analysis. Despite these flaws, the authors concluded that there is evidence to support the efficacy of activity programmes, music, behavioural therapy, light therapy, carer education and changes to the physical environment. Evidence in favour of multi-disciplinary teams, massage and aromatherapy is inconclusive.

Herein lies a fundamental difficulty. Scientific methods to measure efficacy require a clear definition of improved outcomes. This focuses one's mind on narrowly but clearly defined objectives, which within the framework of scientific methods are laudable and necessary.

In dementia care, however, concentration on scientific method may lead to a blinkering of vision regarding the person who has dementia. Tom Kitwood [2], in his masterly text, advocated for the personhood to be central and pre-eminent. Holden and Woods [3] supported the development of integrated approaches able to satisfy the diversity of individual needs, responses and preferences of people with dementia. Antonovsky's [4] "salutogenic" (health-promoting) approach argued for the person's "sense of coherence", with a view of the world that is comprehensive, manageable and meaningful. The WHO commitment to holistic views of health and

[1] *Academic Unit for Psychiatry of Old Age, University of Melbourne, St. George's Health Service, 283 Cotham Road, Kew, Victoria 3101, Australia*

quality of life also provided a basis for re-valuing the person as the centre and object of our attention. Whilst scientific method is necessary to evaluate all interventions, it may be wise, at this time, to see all psychosocial interventions as "approaches" to developing and maintaining a better relationship with persons with dementia, in valuing them as genuine human beings and seeing them not as objects for "treatment", but as people for caring.

Baro's review, whilst presenting as much "evidence" as available in a world of "evidence-based medicine", should also remind readers not to discard "narrative-based medicine" [5], which is the context of psychosocial intervention for people with dementia and has equal, if not more valid, foundation for the building of appropriate attitudes in caring. Not using the word "therapy" after the name of each psychosocial intervention has the potential to de-mystify such valuable humane and positive approaches to care, eschewing mistakenly grandiose expectations that "therapy" and "treatment" may be provided for the subjects of such interventions. It may be argued that all psychosocial interventions in dementia care should be founded on the development of genuine caring and positively valuing attitudes on the part of formal and informal carers. The dictum *primum non nocere* (first do not harm) and the principle of "unconditional positive regard" should constantly underpin the development, practice and evaluation of all psychosocial interventions in dementia, as in all aspects of practice of medicine and psychiatry.

## REFERENCES

1. Opie J., Rosewarne R., O'Connor D.W. (1999) The efficacy of psychosocial approach to behaviour disorders in dementia—a systemic review. *Austr. N.Zeal. J. Psychiatry*, **33**: 789–799.
2. Kitwood T. (1997) *Dementia Reconsidered—The Person Comes First*, Open University Press, Buckingham.
3. Holden U.P., Woods R.T. (1995) *Positive Approach to Dementia Care*, Churchill Livingstone, Edinburgh.
4. Antonovsky A. (1982) *Unravelling the Mystery of Health*, Jossey-Bass, San Francisco.
5. Greenhaugh T., Hurwitz B. (1998) *Narrative Based Medicine*, British Medical Journal Books, London.

### 5.10
### The Importance of Touch and Contact
Yoram Barak[1]

Prof. Baro's review on the psychosocial interventions in dementia highlights the large body of knowledge that has accumulated over the last decade in this important area of treatment. The traditional pharmacologically-focused treatments offered to patients suffering from dementia do not address the psychological needs of either patients or their principal caregivers. However, one must acknowledge the lack of well-designed and methodologically sound studies in this area. Allen-Burge et al [1] have recently evaluated the methodology of research in the area of behavioural interventions for decreasing dementia-related challenging behaviour and conclude that both increasing patients' engagement and patients' social interactions hold promise of benefit.

The two avenues for the improvement of patients' social interaction, engagement and quality of life, are touch and contact. "A longing for touch is no doubt common to many ill and elderly persons...", writes Connelly in the recent supplement to the *Lancet* devoted to "Literature and Ageing" [2]. Touch is unique among the senses in that it not only provides information essential for survival, but is a reminder that one is alive. Therapeutic massage is being practised regularly in many nursing homes and has been incorporated in our centre as part of enhancing structured touch between staff and patients. Additional strategies to enhance touch are undertaken in group settings in which grooming, fashion and sport activities are performed. Lack of touch is the "rule" in many hospitals and nursing homes and patients over time become uncommunicative concerning their need for it [3]. In patients suffering from dementia, the pleasure of being touched may be forgotten and rekindled only after the initial massage or other form of therapeutic touch. It is not only the patient but also the caregiver who enjoys and benefits from touching. Humane touch offers the possibility of establishing new mutual experiences, especially for patients who suffer from progressive aphasia or impairment of sight and hearing.

Animals serve as the symbol of contact in many cultures and are the second approach to be mentioned in this commentary. Since the observation in the 1970s that an elderly patient who is progressing well may have a pet, more than 1000 references have been published focusing on the use of a variety of animals in therapeutic settings. However, animal-assisted therapy (AAT) has both suffered and benefited from the enthusiastic public attention.

[1] *Psychogeriatric Department, Abarbanel Mental Health Center, 15 KKL Street, Bat-Yam, 59100 Israel*

The scope of "indications" for AAT is wide, ranging from hypertension to depression and Alzheimer's disease. The functions of animals within therapy are thought to be as a companion, a social facilitator or as a substitute for close interpersonal relationships. Animals are also thought to enhance health status, increase sensory stimulation, provide emotional support, reinforce feelings of independence, and affect behaviour modification. We have recently completed a 1-year study evaluating by a controlled design the effects of AAT on a group of patients suffering from dementia. The primary outcome measure for the study was a change in the Social-Adaptive Functioning Evaluation (SAFE) scores. The items in the scale measure social-interpersonal, instrumental and life skills functioning and are designed to be rated by observation and interaction with the subject. Patients were rated on the SAFE before the study, after 6 months of treatment, and upon completion (12 months). AAT was undertaken once weekly. The therapists and assisting animals came to the ward at 10.30 a.m. and the group session was of 3 hours. Three AAT counsellors were regularly accompanied by a psychiatric nurse, providing a ratio of 1:2.5 caretakers to patients. Each patient was provided with his own dog or cat, according to personal preference.

Sessions included petting, feeding, grooming, bathing and teaching the animals to walk on a lead for greater mobility. Another major component of the treatment plan was to increase mobility and socialization through walking the animals outside the hospital grounds. These excursions facilitated interaction with people of all ages outside, who were inevitably drawn to these very special animals. Each session was concluded in the ward with a summation of the day's activities and a special time allocated for a "parting between friends"—between the patients, staff members and their animal assistants.

Statistical analysis demonstrated that the AAT groups' SAFE total score improved significantly as compared with the control group. Impulse control did not change in either group; instrumental and self-care improved in both groups, but this change did not attain statistical significance, and social functions improved significantly in the AAT group. The social functioning dimension of the SAFE scale consists of the following items: conversational skills, instrumental social skills, social appropriateness/politeness, social engagement, friendships, recreation/leisure, and participation in hospital programmes. This approach further validates the results of the comprehensive study by Raina et al [4], demonstrating enhancement of activities of daily living (ADL) functioning levels of older people.

In summary, it can be seen that the addition of touch and contact to the evolving field of psychosocial interventions in dementia adds a creative and humane aspect in the treatment of these demanding diseases.

## REFERENCES

1. Allen-Burge R., Stevens A.B., Burgio L.D. (1999)  Effective behavioural interventions for decreasing dementia related challenging behaviour in nursing
   homes. *Int. J. Geriatr. Psychiatry*, **14**: 213–232.
2. Connelly J.E. (1999)  "Back rub": reflections on touch. *Lancet*, **354** (Suppl.): 2–4.
3. Montagu A. (1986)  Touch and age. In *Touching, the Human Significance of the
   Skin* (Ed. A. Montagu), pp. 393–400, Harper & Row, New York.
4. Raina P., Waltner-Toews D., Bonnett B., Woodward C., Abernathy T.
   (1999)  Influence of companion animals on the physical health of older
   people: an analysis of a one-year longitudinal study. *J. Am. Geriatr. Soc.*, **47**:
   323–329.

**5.11**
**The Need to Improvise and Look for Evidence**

Abdel Moneim Ashour[1]

Besides the systematic review by Prof. Baro on the techniques and strategies, I would like to highlight some rules about psychosocial interventions
in dementia. These "general rules" may be the only technology available to
a worker in a less developed country, and hopefully can guide his or her
practice and research:

1. Cognitive—particularly memory—impairment, which is globally present in all cases of dementia, limits sustainability and generalization in
   rehabilitation. Yet, there is evidence that new learning is still possible in
   demented people.
2. Cognitive management covers cognitive deficits other than memory and
   learning. It utilizes the techniques of reducing cognitive load, providing
   external memory aids, enhancing new learning, and enhancing implicit
   and procedural memory.
3. Behaviouural disturbances, including challenging behaviour, have
   wider aetiology than cognitive defect. Besides roots in the organic
   brain pathology of the patient, there is the impact of reactions of the
   carers to the needs of the patient, which are confounded by their degree
   of stress and communication state. Kitwood [1] has coined a "malignant
   social psychology" model for that: "In many ways dementia is a time of
   feeling rather than knowing—feelings that are essentially inborn and
   develop without any special opportunities for learning".

[1] *Department of Neurology and Psychiatry, Faculty of Medicine, Ain Shams University, 1, Gawad
Hossny St., Abdeen, Cairo, Egypt*

4. The behaviour of confused people denotes some form of coded but meaningful communication. Confusion is rooted in social and environmental background, besides organic mental impairment. The counsellor of a confused demented person should deal effectively with the social and emotional problems within the counselling process. Confusion can be mental withdrawal from a complex modern life that taxes the person's diminished coping abilities.

5. Adopting more positive attitudes, like value and worth of the patient, individualization and the contention that learning is possible, is more important than using techniques of proven efficacy. This includes careful and creative selection of targets, addressing first the key issues that make real difference to the person concerned.

6. Prevention is an intervention. For example, positive experiences distract patients from problematic behaviour. Also, identifying the triggers of catastrophic behaviour allows avoiding them [2]. Anticipation and planning are the secrets.

7. Intervention-based neuropsychological assessment allows a caregiver of any degree of sophistication to produce interventions after gaining understanding of objectives, targets and methods. Improvising all the time and all the way allows creative thinking inherent in most carers to surface. Widening the base of applicants of psychological techniques to include informal caregivers compensates for the shortage of "therapists".

8. Evaluative research should be intensified. Some of the methodological problems should be solved, e.g. definition of the problematic behaviour and measurement of the outcome. Sophisticated theoretical models should be worked out to supply the notions for more rational interventions.

9. The environmental approach to dealing with mood and behaviour problems involves adapting the physical and social surroundings to provide safety, reduce distractions, increase non-verbal cues, etc. In familiar environments and with familiar routines, patients are less likely to become confused and disoriented and thus less likely to become frightened, agitated and restless.

10. In home settings and in most nursing homes, limitations of resources preclude the creation of an ideal environment, but patients benefit from even simple interventions.

11. Interventions that change the physical or psychosocial environment include: concrete advice, general guidelines, problem solving, support of caregivers, creation of prosthetic environment and milieu therapy.

12. Carer's needs and expectations include information concerning dementia and existing support systems. There is also a severe need

for psychological support, including opportunities to discuss the oppressive matters with the nursing staff.

13. Sense of competence, that is decreased in carers by long duration of illness and agitated behaviours of the patient cared for, rises if the carer receives professional supportive intervention.

14. Dementia, even in mild degree, is notorious for instigating stress and depression in spouses and children of patients [3]. This explains the importance of caregiver support programs in care strategies of dementia.

15. Carer support should be considered more in the light of the trend to manage dementia patients within their families. Family members are thus "partners" in the cornerstone formal care system.

16. Indicators of mental health of the carer will not be improved by moving the patient to an institution [4].

To sum up, Bere Miesen [5] wrote: "Persons with dementia are not crazy. They behave like all persons do in strange situations, and in unsafe conditions. When they cannot find safety and attachment in their environment, they become difficult and demand our attention...". A new psychology of dementia is born.

## REFERENCES

1. Kitwood T. (1993) Person and process in dementia. *Int. J. Geriatr. Psychiatry*, **8**: 541–545.
2. Mace N.L. (Ed.) (1990) *Dementia Care*, Johns Hopkins, Baltimore.
3. Braekhus A., Oksengard A.R., Engedal K., Laake K. (1998) Social and depressive strain suffered by spouses of patients with mild dementia. *Scand. J. Prim. Health Care*, **16**: 242–246.
4. Matsuda O., Hasebe N., Ikehara K., Futatsuya M., Akahane N. (1997) Longitudinal study of the mental health of caregivers caring for elderly patients with dementia: effect of institutional placement on mental health. *Psychiatry Clin. Neurosci.*, **51**: 289–293.
5. Bere Miesen M.L. (1999) *Dementia in Close-up*, Routledge, London.

5.12
## The Need for Psychosocial Interventions in Dementia
Manuel Suárez Richards[1]

The psychiatric management of dementia involves a broad range of psycho-social interventions for the patient and his or her family. The different types of interventions described by Prof. Baro are intended to replace lost functions by the available ones or to enhance those impaired.

Psychosocial interventions have two ultimate specific goals, closely related: the preservation or restoration of the greatest possible autonomy and the patient's mobilization. Psychosocial resources must be used to keep the patient ambulant: the demented should not be in bed when there is no physical reason for it.

One of the most important factors affecting quality of life in a demented old person is immobilization, which, in turn, leads to social isolation, a destabilizing factor.

Psychosocial interventions are intended to slow or avoid disintegration and avoid or modify immobilization. Measures are directed to the patient and the physical and human environment surrounding him or her. Beyond cognitive impairment, human and physical environment directly affects the evolution of dementia [1].

Specific psychosocial interventions may be effective in reducing behavioural symptoms such as agitation, apathy and depression. Psychoeducational strategies in the support of caregivers may be effective in reducing behavioural symptoms of demented patients in daily living [2].

A solid alliance is critical among the demented patient, family and other caregivers. Family members and other caregivers are a critical source of information, as the patient is frequently unable to give a reliable history. They are generally responsible for implementing and monitoring treatment plans. Their own attitudes and behaviours may have a profound effect on the patient, and they often need the treating psychiatrist's compassion and concern.

It is also helpful to educate the family regarding basic principles of care. These include keeping requests and demands relatively simple and avoiding overly complex tasks that might lead to frustration; avoiding confrontation and deferring requests if the patient becomes angry; remaining calm, firm and supportive if the patient becomes upset; being consistent and avoiding unnecessary change; providing frequent reminders, explanations and orientation cues; recognizing declines in capacity and adjusting expectations appropriately; bringing sudden declines in function and the emergence of new symptoms to professional attention. In addition, the

[1] *Department of Psychiatry, School of Medicine, University of La Plata, Argentina*

psychiatrist can offer more specific behaviourally or psychodynamically informed suggestions for techniques that caregivers can use to avoid or deal with difficult behaviours.

While these interventions differ in philosophy, focus and methods, they have the broadly overlapping goals of improving quality of life and maximizing function in the context of existing deficits. Many have, as an additional goal, the improvement of cognitive skills, mood or behaviour.

These interventions are necessary to keep quality of life, not merely to keep the patient alive, and they are essentially oriented to preserve the human right to live worthily.

## REFERENCES

1. Maheu S., Cohen C. (1996)   Support of families. In *Clinical Diagnosis and Management of Alzheimer's Disease* (Ed. D. Gautier), pp. 293–304, Dunitz, London.
2. Haupt M. (1999)   The course of behavioural symptoms and their psychosocial treatment in dementia sufferers. *J. Gerontol. Geriatr.*, **32**: 159–166.

5.13
### Sharing and Supporting Families with Dementia
R. Srinivasa Murthy[1]

Recognition of the needs of the elderly and organization of services for elderly individuals is a recent development in India and other developing countries. Community-based services are rare or non-existent. There are three aspects on which to comment: the understanding of dementia, the use of psychosocial interventions and the needs of carers.

During the last decade, there has been a growing interest in understanding the magnitude of the needs and developing methods to address them. Initial epidemiological studies in the community [1,2] used largely clinical criteria. More recent studies have utilized standarized tools and multistage screening for dementia [3–8]. The development of simple instruments for use in the rural and illiterate population [9,10] has provided new avenues for multicentre research in India. The studies have provided norms for categorizing cognitive deficits in the elderly [11] and shown important cross-cultural differences in US–India comparisons. There are series of studies utilizing the same methodology in Delhi, India and Pittsburgh, USA. The findings show that the prevalence of dementia is low in India—

[1] *National Institute of Mental Health and Neurosciences, Bangalore 560029, India*

0.84% in the population aged 55 years and older and 1.36% in the population aged 65 years and older. A major benefit of this collaborative study was the functional ability scale for use in the rural general population [10]. Availability of such instruments can be expected to result in a large number of studies in different regions and population groups.

The majority of the dementia patients in India are living in the community and with the families. Alternative institutions are still the exception. There are also differences in care perceptions between rural and urban populations and between different social classes [12].

The real challenge for the psychiatrists is sharing and supporting families with a person suffering from dementia. The advances made in psychosocial interventions need to be simplified and shared with carers. There are a number of innovations in developing countries. One example is the programme DIGNITY Dialogue in Bombay city. As part of this programme, there is a linking of elderly with youth, use of a monthly magazine as a network, the starting of regional enrichment centres, organization of workshops on living skills, etc.

The psychosocial interventions reviewed in Baro's paper provide an excellent knowledge base for community care. Different methods, such as reality orientation therapy, reminiscence, validation therapy, behaviour modification, sensory stimulation, reorganization of motor activity, individual psychotherapy, are relevant and applicable. There is scope for integrating culturally relevant practices in these methods. An example is the use of yoga in India, which is part of the larger understanding of the community. Group therapy has had difficulties in India, as sharing highly personal details is limited in the general population.

With regard to quality of life, the role of religion in understanding old age as a natural transition, as well as a period of decreased activity and a stage of preparation for future life, could be an advantage for those working in traditional societies. This is an area that has not been adequately explored and exploited.

Carer support is the biggest challenge for psychiatrists. This situation offers an opportunity to develop innovative methods, as professional barriers are outdone in thinking of new ways of addressing the needs. Some examples are the use of the extended/joint family network, including community members, as supporters in rural areas. Support to carers will have to be more substantive than occasional help. In India and other developing countries, there is very little formal mental health care. As a result, the carer has to meet multiple needs. The carers need more knowledge about the condition, course, various physical and psychosocial treatments, and guidance about levels and limits of care. A useful method of support to carers is to think of nine components: (1) information to patients/general public; (2) medical and psychosocial care; (3) strengthening family life; (4) coping

skills; (5) networking of families; (6) respite care/support; (7) day care—
rehabilitation; (8) stigma/discrimination; and (9) empowerment. The
psychosocial interventions are at an early stage of development. There are
enormous challenges and new opportunities for sharing and supporting
families.

## REFERENCES

1. Ramchandran V., Sarada Menon M., Ramamurthy B. (1979)  Psychiatric disorders in subjects aged over fifty. *Indian J. Psychiatry*, **22**: 193–198.
2. Venkoba Rao A., Madhavan T. (1982)  Geropsychiatric morbidity survey in a semi-urban area near Madurai. *Indian J. Psychiatry*, **23**: 256–267.
3. Rajkumar S., Kumar S. (1996)  Prevalence of dementia in the community: a rural–urban comparison from Madras, India. *Austral. J. Ageing*, **15**: 9–13.
4. Rajkumar S., Kumar S., Thara R. (1997)  Prevalence of dementia in a rural setting: a report from India. *Int. J. Geriatr. Psychiatry*, **12**: 702–707.
5. Shaji S., Promodu K., Abraham T., Roy K.J., Verghese A. (1996)  An epidemiological study of dementia in a rural community in Kerala, India. *Br. J. Psychiatry*, **168**: 745–749.
6. Chandra V., Ganguli M., Ratcliff G., Pandav R., Sharma S., Gilby J., Belle S., Ryan C., Baker C., Seaberg E. *et al* (1994)  Studies of the epidemiology of dementia: comparisons between developed and developing countries. General conceptual and methodological issues. *Aging Clin. Exp. Res.*, **6**: 307–321.
7. Chandra V., Ganguli M., Ratcliff G., Pandav R., Sharma S., Belle S., Ryan C., Baker C., DeKosky S., Nath L. (1998)  Practical issues in cognitive screening of elderly illiterate populations in developing countries. *Aging Clin. Exp. Res.*, **10**: 349–357.
8. Chandra V., Ganguli M., Pandav R., Johnston J., Belle S., DeKosky S.T. (1998)  Prevalence of Alzheimer's and other dementias in rural India: the Indo-US study. *Neurology*, **51**: 1000–1008.
9. Ganguli M., Ratcliff G., Chandra V., Sharma S., Gilby J., Pandav R., Belle S., Ryan C., Baker C., Seaberg E. *et al* (1995)  A Hindi version of the MMSE: the development of a cognitive screening instrument for a largely illiterate rural elderly population in India. *Int. J. Geriatr. Psychiatry*, **10**: 367–377.
10. Fillenbaum G.G., Chandra V., Ganguli M., Pandav R., Gilby J.E., Seaberg E.C., Belle S., Baker C., Echement D.A., Nath L.M. (1999)  Development of an activities of daily living scale to screen for dementia in an illiterate rural older population in India. *Age Ageing*, **28**: 161–168.
11. Ganguli M., Chandra V., Gilby J.E., Ratcliff G., Sharma S.D., Pandav R., Seaberg E.C., Belle S. (1996)  Cognitive test performance in a community-based non-demented elderly sample in rural India: the Indo-US Cross-National Dementia Epidemiology Study. *Int. Psychogeriatrics*, **8**: 507–524.
12. Irudaya Rajan S., Mishra U.S., Sarma P.S. (1999)  Indian elderly: some views of populace. *Indian J. Social Work*, **60**: 488–506.

# 6

# Costs of Dementia: A Review

**Bengt Jönsson[1], Linus Jönsson[2] and Anders Wimo[2]**

[1]*Stockholm School of Economics, Box 6501, S-113 83 Stockholm, Sweden;*
[2]*Division of Geriatric Medicine, Neurotec, Karolinska Institute, S-171 76
Stockholm, Sweden*

## INTRODUCTION

This paper reviews the evidence on the costs of dementia. In the first section
we summarize and compare most of the published cost of illness (COI)
studies of dementia. These studies reveal that most costs of care are found
outside traditional health care. They also show that indirect costs in terms
of lost productivity are a small part of the total costs, since most of the
victims of the disease are retired. However, these costs are not negligible in
absolute terms.

In the following section we discuss some specific issues related to costing
of dementia. The first relates to the direct costs of care. Only a small share of
costs is found in traditional hospitals. Most formal care is delivered as day
care, nursing home care and home care. A second important problem in
costing dementia is how to identify, quantify and value informal care. The
different methods available are presented and discussed.

Subsequently we present the evidence on the relation between the severity of dementia and costs. Different measures of severity are discussed, but
the main empirical results presented are from the relation between costs and
Mini-Mental State Examination (MMSE) scores.

This review focuses on costs. But an important use of costing data is as a
basis for economic evaluations comparing costs and outcome for different
treatment alternatives. Particularly with the introduction of new drugs,
there has been a rapidly growing number of economic evaluations of therapies. The difficulties in defining relevant outcome measures for economic
evaluations in dementia has the consequence that most of these evaluations
only compare costs for different interventions. In particular, these studies
are investigating whether the cost of new drugs is totally or partially offset

*Dementia, Second Edition.* Edited by Mario Maj and Norman Sartorius.
© 2002 John Wiley & Sons Ltd.

by reductions in costs from progression of patients to more severe and costly states of the disease. The review ends with some conclusions and suggestions for further research.

## COST OF ILLNESS (COI) STUDIES IN DEMENTIA—A REVIEW OF PUBLISHED STUDIES IN DIFFERENT COUNTRIES

This review is an update and a complete revision of an earlier review article by Wimo et al [1]. The first COI study in dementia was published for the USA in the late 1980s. In the last decade, similar studies have been published for Canada and a number of European countries. The overall results from these studies are presented in Table 6.1.

There is a great range in the share for different cost categories in the various COI studies, mainly depending on how many cost categories are included. This aspect is clearly illustrated in the paper by Huang et al [4]. Hay and Ernst [3] analysed Alzheimer's disease (AD) alone. In an update, the same authors [6] found higher figures than in their previous study. The study by Manton et al [7] is the only one regarding COI of dementia where comorbidity has been systematically analysed; they estimated the costs of medical care for the total population of 65 and older (with different states of interacting comorbidity, including dementia) to US$ 388 billion. In a simulation, a total elimination of dementia would decrease the costs by US$ 32.2 billion, which could be regarded as the net cost of dementia.

The estimated costs of dementia in the USA can be compared to an estimation of the total costs of illness in the USA, US$ 805 billion, where US$ 374 billion were direct costs [18] (updated to 1996 prices). The American studies mainly focus on net costs (i.e. the extra costs that are caused by dementia). Schneider and Guralnik's figures [5] also give the opportunity to compare the costs of dementia with those of hip fractures. At 1996 prices, the cost of hip fractures was US$ 2.4 billion for 220 000 fractures or US$ 11 000 annually per fracture (US$ 10 per citizen), to be compared to US$ 63.4 billion for 2.4 million demented or US$ 26 400 annually per demented (US$ 270 per citizen).

Plausible explanations for the rather low costs in England found by Gray and Fenn [9] are the amount of volunteers, the low daily cost of residential care or nursing home care, the low estimated proportion of demented people in residential care/nursing homes, the fact that only AD was included, and the fact that only paid family efforts were included. The English cost figures presented by Smith et al [8] and Livingston et al [19] are at the same level as those of Gray and Fenn [9], while the figures by Kavanagh et al [10], Schneider et al [20] and Holmes et al [11] are more in line

**TABLE 6.1** Cost of illness studies of dementia: distribution in different cost categories*

| Country | Year | Estimated dementia cases | Currency | Cost (billions) | Cost (billions US$ 1996) | Direct costs (%) | Out-of-pocket (%) | Indirect costs (%) | Informal care (%) | Note | Source |
|---|---|---|---|---|---|---|---|---|---|---|---|
| USA | 1983 | | US$ | 38 | 75.3 | 49 | | | 51 | Net costs | OTA [2] |
| USA | 1983 | 1 535 000 | US$ | 27.1 | 53.6 | | | | 36 | Net AD costs | Hay and Ernst [3] |
| USA | 1985 | 4 280 000 | US$ | 87.9 | 155.6 | 7.5 | 7.5 | 49 | | | Huang et al [4] |
| USA | 1985 | 2 400 000 | US$ | 35.8 | 63.4 | 100 | | | | Gross costs | Schneider and Guralnik [5] |
| USA | 1991 | 1 595 000 | US$ | 67.3 | 83.9 | 31 | | 20 | 49 | | Ernst and Hay [6] |
| USA | 1991 | | US$ | 25.8 | 32.2 | | | | | | Manton et al [7] |
| England | 1995 | 370 000 | £ | 0.9 | 2.5 | 94 | 6 | | | | Smith et al [8] |
| England | 1991 | | £ | 1.03 | 1.9 | 94 | | | 6 | Paid informal care | Gray and Fenn [9] |
| England | 1991 | 320 000 | £ | 5.04 | 9.4 | 87 | | | 13 | Advanced cognitive impairment | Kavanagh et al [10] |
| UK | 1996 | 650 000 | £ | 16.1 | 24.3 | 67 | | | 33 | | Holmes et al [11] |
| Canada | 1991 | 281 000 | Can$ | 3.9 | 3.4 | 84 | | | 16 | | Østbye and Crosse [12] |
| Sweden | 1991 | 153 000 | SEK | 30.7 | 3.6 | 100 | | | | Gross costs | Wimo et al [13] |
| Sweden | 1991 | | SEK | 20 | 2.4 | 100 | | | | Net costs | Wimo et al [13] |
| Italy | 1995 | 735 000 | US$ | 38.8 | 40.6 | 16 | | | 84 | | Cavallo et al [14] |
| Germany | | 932 500 | US$ | 7.2 | 7.7 | 100 | | | | Low alternative | Schulenburg et al [15] |
| Germany | | 1 260 000 | US$ | 15.5 | 16.6 | 100 | | | | High alternative | Schulenburg et al [15] |
| Denmark | 1996 | 58 000 | DK | 4.5 | 0.5 | 100 | | | | | Kronborg Andersen et al [16] |
| Holland | 1994 | 180 000 | HFL | 3.31 | 1.6 | 100 | | | | | Koopmanschap et al [17] |

*Some cost figures have been extrapolated from individual costs to national costs by national prevalence figures.
AD, Alzheimer's disease; OTA, Office of Technology Assessment, Philadelphia

**TABLE 6.2** Cost of illness studies of dementia: comparison of cost per patient and cost per inhabitant*

| Country | Estimated dementia cases | Cost (billions US$ 1996) | Annual cost per patient (US$ 1996) | Annual cost per citizen (US$ 1996) | Cost categories included | Source |
|---|---|---|---|---|---|---|
| USA | 1 595 000 | 83.9 | 52 600 | 335 | D, IC | Ernst and Hay [6] |
| England | 370 000 | 2.5 | 6 720 | 53 | D | Smith et al [8] |
| Canada | 252 600 | 3.4 | 12 060 | 125 | D, IC | Østbye and Crosse [12] |
| Sweden | 153 000 | 3.6 | 23 600 | 420 | D | Wimo et al [13] (gross costs) |
| Sweden | 153 000 | 2.4 | 15 400 | 274 | D | Wimo et al [13] (net costs) |
| Germany | 932 500–1 260 000 | 7.7–16.6 | 8 300–13 200 | 115–250 | D | Schulenburg et al [15] (low-high) |
| Denmark | 58 000 | 0.52 | 9 100 | 100 | D | |
| Italy | 735 000 | 6.3–40.6 | 8 600–55 300 | 110–710 | D, IC | Cavallo et al [14] |
| Holland | 180 000 | 1.6 | 9 000 | 105 | D | Koopmanschap et al [17] |

*Figures are rounded and expressed as US$; currency conversions by PPPs (purchasing power parities); time transformations by national price index of health. Source: OECD (Organization for Economic Cooperation and Development). D, directs costs; IC, costs of informal care with the other studies. In the cost calculations by Livingston *et al* [19], no costs for accommodation were included.

Østbye and Crosse [12] from Canada have estimated the net Canadian costs of dementia as US$ 3.4 billion, based on a dementia population of 281 000 individuals. The high Italian costs [14] depend on a high estimate of informal care.

The costs of dementia care in Sweden were estimated to be US$ 3.6 billion in 1996 [13], where 93% were gross direct costs of moderate and severe dementia. The net cost of dementia care in this study was estimated to be about 65% of the gross costs. Figures from the Netherlands [17] and Denmark [16] show a rather low cost per demented person, which can at least partly be explained by the fact that costs of informal care are not included.

It is very difficult to compare the results of the different studies. In an attempt to make a rough comparison, we have recalculated the figures of a number of studies to make them comparable. Results are presented as cost per demented patient and cost per inhabitant in 1996 US$ (see Table 6.2).

Cost per person with dementia varies from US$ 6720 in one study for England to US$ 55 300 in Italy. Moreover, two different studies from the USA give estimates which differ more than two-fold. The variation in cost per inhabitant varies even more. To some extent the high figure for Sweden reflects the high share of the population in the older age groups. But the major explanation for the difference between the studies is probably related to differences in methodology, particularly which costs to include, and in the data sources used.

## METHODOLOGICAL ASPECTS OF COSTING DEMENTIA

The general methodology for costing in COI studies is well developed, although there is some controversy over the most appropriate method for costing different types of resources. For each specific disease, some types of resources are more important for the total cost of the disease. For example, for diseases that mainly affect the working population, the identification, quantification and valuation of loss of production (indirect costs) is very important. For dementia, which mainly affects the elderly, indirect cost is not the key resource item. Neither is the traditional health care cost component, including hospitalization, ambulatory care and drugs, the most important cost item in dementia.

What poses a particular problem in estimating the costs of dementia is that the majority of the costs of care are found outside the health care sector. We can label these "non-medical" direct costs. A distinction can be made between two types of non-medical direct costs. The first is formal care, which is undertaken by paid professionals, either in special institutions, such as nursing homes, or in the patients' homes. The second is informal care, which is undertaken by the patients' relatives or an unpaid voluntary worker. We will examine the specific problems involved in costing these categories.

## Institutional Care

### Nursing Home Care

Nursing home care costs are often referred to as "reference costs" when other care alternatives are evaluated. However, to be valid, such comparisons must assume that institutional care is the only alternative, otherwise comparisons are misleading. Costs can be dementia-specific and include a detailed analysis of the costs of all activities linked to dementia patients, while the other and most common way is to provide the average costs of nursing home patients. The gross cost per day per demented person (1996 prices) varies between US$ 78 and US$ 233, with an average cost of about US$ 135 (see Table 6.3).

According to Hu et al [22] the costs of care for demented nursing home patients was 36% higher than the costs of care for non-demented patients. Hay and Ernst [3] and Ernst and Hay [6] also present net costs due to dementia of approximately US$ 26–29 per day. However, this issue is complicated and controversial. Coughlin and Liu [21] found only slight differences between the cognitively impaired and cognitively unimpaired. Rovner et al [26] found, in a randomized study, that even if an intervention program reduced behavioural disturbances, costs were not significantly lower during a 6-month follow-up. In the UK, the concept of Domus care comprises registered mental health nursing homes where residents live in a purpose-built facility with their own rooms. The costs of a Domus care unit with demented residents were much higher than the costs of private or voluntary nursing homes in the UK [28].

### Intermediate Care Alternatives

Care and living arrangements between home and nursing homes are under development in many countries. These settings are staffed around the clock and the number of residents is smaller than in nursinghome wards. The main purpose is to offer community, supervision/surveillance and a natural life situation. There are few published costing studies, and all cover short periods, 12 months or fewer (see Table 6.4).

A comparison with nursing home care may be appropriate if demented patients must stay at nursing homes because intermediate care options are

**TABLE 6.3** Costs per patient of nursing home care[*]

| Country | Year | Costs/day (total) | Costs/day (US$ 1996) | Out-of-pocket (%) | Cost categories included | Note | Source |
|---|---|---|---|---|---|---|---|
| USA | 1982 | US$ 61.10 | 130 | | D | | Coughlin and Liu [21] |
| USA | 1983 | US$ 61.53 | 122 | | D | | Hu et al [22] |
| USA | 1983 | US$ 50.68 | 100 | | D | Low alternative | Hay and Ernst [3] |
| USA | 1983 | US$ 61.64 | 122 | | D | High alternative | Hay and Ernst [3] |
| USA | 1983 | US$ 14.59 | 29 | | D | Net costs | Hay and Ernst [3] |
| USA | 1985 | US$ 64.38 | 114 | | D? | | Schneider and Guralnik [5] |
| USA | 1990 | US$ 115.20 | 152 | 60 | D | | Rice et al [23] |
| USA | 1990 | US$ 130.38 | 172 | 53 | D, IC | | Rice et al [23] |
| USA | 1991 | US$ 37.95 | 47 | | D | Low alternative, net costs | Welch et al [24] |
| USA | 1991 | US$ 48.02 | 60 | | D | High alternative, net costs | Welch et al [24] |
| USA | 1990 | US$ 101.37 | 134 | | D | | Weinberger et al [25] |
| USA | 1991 | US$ 105.48 | 131 | | D | Low alternative | Ernst and Hay [6] |
| USA | 1991 | US$ 113.15 | 125 | | D | High alternative | Ernst and Hay [6] |
| USA | 1991 | US$ 20.74 | 26 | | D | Net costs | Ernst and Hay [6] |
| USA | 1991 | US$ 77 | 95 | | D | | Rovner et al [26] |
| UK | 1992 | £ 135.86 | 233 | | D | Domus care | Beecham et al [27] |
| UK | 1993 | £ 48.29 | 78 | | D | Private or voluntary nursing home | Knapp [28]; Kavanagh et al [10] |
| Sweden | 1985 | SEK 837 | 147 | 5 | D | | Annerstedt [29] |
| Sweden | 1987 | SEK 900 | 143 | 6 | D | | Wimo et al [30] |
| Sweden | 1993 | SEK 1 150 | 112 | 12 | D | | NBHW (Sweden) [31] |
| Netherlands | 1990? | US$ 115 | 132 | 20 | D | | Ribbe [32] |

[*] All costs are gross costs if nothing else is noted.
D, direct costs; IC, costs of informal care

**TABLE 6.4** Costs per patient of intermediate care alternatives

| Country | Year | Costs/day | Costs/day (US$ 1996) | Out-of-pocket (%) | Nursing home costs (US$ 1996) | Out-of-pocket (%) | Group living (% of nursing home costs) | Cost categories included | Source |
|---------|------|-----------|----------------------|-------------------|-------------------------------|-------------------|----------------------------------------|--------------------------|--------|
| Sweden | 1985 | SEK 472 | 83 | | 106 | | 78 | D | Wimo et al [33] |
| Sweden | 1985 | SEK 338 | 59 | 18 | 147 | 5 | 40 | D | Annerstedt [29] |
| Sweden | 1987 | SEK 612 | 97 | 13 | 143 | 6 | 68 | D | Wimo et al [30] |
| Sweden | 1987 | SEK 541 | 86 | | 138 | | 69 | D | Wimo et al [34] |
| Sweden | 1992 | SEK 986 | 114 | | | | | | Svensson et al [35] |
| USA | 1985? | US$ 43 | 76 | | 126 | | 60 | ? | OTA [2]; Sands and Belman [36] |
| USA | 1985? | US$ 565 | 115 | | 126 | | 92 | ? | OTA [2]; Sands and Belman [36] |
| UK | 1993? | £ 34–51 | 55–83 | | 78 | | 70–106 | | Knapp [28]; Ka vanagh et al [10] |

D, direct costs

not available. A Swedish study [30] correlated the costs of dementia care in different care alternatives with the decline in cognitive function, activity of daily living (ADL) capacity and behavioural disturbances. The costs increased considerably in home care and in a day care group, parallel to the progression of dementia, but not in group living (GL). In another Swedish study [34], GL costs and three comparison alternatives were analysed. GL costs were 68% of nursing home costs, 91% of the costs of the home care group and 81% of a mixed comparison alternative; i.e. GL was cheaper than all alternatives. Johansson [37] and Wimo [38] have estimated the costs of GL to about 60–70% of nursing home costs.

In the UK, the cost of residential care for people with advanced cognitive impairment [28] was somewhat lower as compared to Sweden. Knapp *et al* [32] compared the costs of community care with those of hospital care of a population of mainly demented patients who were relocated from hospital to community care. They found that the costs of community care were considerably lower, about 40% of the nursing home costs. Some cost reports of "residential care for dementia patients", sometimes called "boarding home care" in the USA, indicate similar costs to GL in Sweden, from 60% (low nursing load) to 92% (high nursing load) of nursing home costs [36,40].

## Day Care

The health economic literature on dementia day care is limited (Table 6.5). Two different approaches of cost analysis have been used. The first is to analyse the cost of a day care unit, and the second approach is longitudinal. Day care can take place in different settings: in hospitals, apartments or special bungalows, and the number of staff per patient also vary, resulting in different costs. Comparisons are often made with nursing home costs, but such an approach may be questioned, since the study populations are often not comparable with respect to the degree of dementia. There are three US papers from the 1980s and one from the 1990s [41–44] presenting uncontrolled results, with great variability of costs. There are four Scandinavian papers with control groups [30,45–47], presenting cost data from the 1980s. In a Swedish study [45], in which the patients were their own controls during the period previous to day care the costs were higher during the period of day care. In two other Swedish studies [30,46], in which waiting list patients were used as controls, day care was cheaper. In a randomized Norwegian study [47], the costs were lower in absolute figures compared to the Swedish studies, but the relation between the day care group and the controls was the same, 86%. Reifler *et al* [48] studied the ratio between operating revenue (fee-for service payments from families or government) and non-operating revenue (donations, philanthropy, etc.) in a US dementia day care program. On average, 64% of the income was of the operating revenue type.

## Special Care Units and Other Types of Formal Care

The US special care unit (SCU) concept is broad, but care is provided in nursing homes or similar settings. Economic evaluations were sparse in 1988 [40], and the situation is still the same [49]. Some principles for cost evaluations have been presented [50], but no cost figures. In one study, which did not measure the basic costs of care, it was found that the annual costs for medication, radiology, laboratory service and treatment (catheterization, tracheal suctioning, etc.) were US$ 1477 lower in SCUs than in traditional nursing home care [51]. Costs of fever management [52] were studied in a small sample of SCU patients with dementia compared to nursing home patients. Maas *et al* [49] reported higher care costs for AD patients in SCUs as compared to traditional units.

Wray *et al* [53] studied the effects on costs of withholding medical treatment, and found that mortality was higher in the group where treatment was withheld, but there were no significant differences regarding costs.

Demented patients stay longer in acute care than non-demented patients [54], causing losses for New York hospitals paid through capitation according to diagnosis-related groups (DRG). Similar conclusions regarding Medicare capitation were drawn by Weiner *et al* [55].

In a decision model [56], surgery was estimated to be US$ 17000 more expensive per treatment episode than conservative intervention in the therapy of stage III pressure ulcers among demented patients. However, decision-makers preferred surgery if they did not have to consider costs.

## Home Care

Home care costs are often presented from two viewpoints. The first is to analyse costs for home care *per se* (a "typical" day of home care), implicitly assuming that institutionalization or other care options are avoided. The second approach is longitudinal and examines a wide range of resource utilization and costs of a "home care dementia population" during a specific period of time. With the longitudinal approach, patients who not are categorized as permanently institutionalized can be regarded as being in "home care", even if they also sometimes use different resources, such as institutional care. In some of the studies referred to, different cost categories were presented, making it possible to analyse both approaches. However, there may be difficulties in finding out whether longitudinal aspects were

**TABLE 6.5** Costs per patient of day care

| Country | Method | Year | Costs/day | Costs/day (US$ 1996) | Out-of-pocket (%) | Controls costs/day | Controls costs/day (US$ 1996) | Costs vs. controls (%) | Cost categories included | Source |
|---|---|---|---|---|---|---|---|---|---|---|
| USA | DC-unit | 1981 | US$ 23 | 56 | 70 | | | | D | Sands and Suzuki [41] |
| USA | DC-unit | 1983 | US$ 35 | 69 | 71 | | | | D | Kays and Szpak [42] |
| USA | DC-unit | 1984 | US$ 77 | 144 | 91 | | | | D? | Panella et al [43] |
| USA | DC-unit | 1992? | US$ 53 | 62 | 77 | | | | D? | Cox and Reifler [44] |
| Sweden | Long. | 1985 | SEK 269 | 47 | | SEK 199 | 35 | 135 | D | Wimo et al [45] |
| Sweden | Long. | 1987 | SEK 473 | 75 | | SEK 546 | 87 | 87 | D | Wimo et al [46] |
| Sweden | Long. | 1987 | SEK 619 | 98* | | SEK 661 | 105 | 94 | D, IC (paid) | Wimo et al [46] |
| Sweden | Long. | 1987 | SEK 466 | 74 | | SEK 534 | 85 | 87 | D, IC (unpaid) | Wimo et al [30] |
| Norway | Long. | 1989 | NOK 330 | 45 | | NOK 383 | 53 | 86 | D | Engedal [47] |

* "Hotel costs" also included.
DC-unit, costs of a day care unit; Long., longitudinal analysis; D, direct costs; IC, cost of informal care

TABLE 6.6  Costs per patient of home care

| Country | Method | Year | Costs/day | Costs/day (US$ PPP) | Costs/day (US$ 1996) | Cost categories | Out-of-pocket (%) | Family care (%) | Degree of dementia | Note | Source |
|---|---|---|---|---|---|---|---|---|---|---|---|
| USA | TD | 1982 | US$ 32.11 | 32 | 68 | D | | | Severe–moderate | | Coughlin and Liu [21] |
| USA | TD | 1983 | US$ 17.85 | 18 | 35 | D, IC | | 83 | Moderate | | Hu et al [22] |
| USA | TD | | US$ 40.59 | 41 | 80 | D, IC | | 93 | Severe | | Hu et al [22] |
| USA | TD | | US$ 32.15 | 32 | 64 | D, IC | | 91 | Moderate–severe | | Hu et al [22] |
| USA | TD | 1983 | US$ 28.76 | 29 | 57 | D, IC | | 81 | Moderate–severe | Net costs | Hay and Ernst [3] |
| USA | TD | 1990 | US$ 34.44 | 34 | 45 | D | 63 | | Mild–moderate (?) | | Rice et al [23] |
| USA | TD | | US$ 129 | 129 | 170 | D, IC | 17 | 73 | Mild–moderate (?) | | Rice et al [23] |
| USA | TD | 1989 | US$ 50 | 50 | 70 | IC | 29 | 71 | Mild–moderate (?) | | Stommel et al [57] |
| UK | TD | 1991 | £ 29.54 | 46 | 55 | D, IC | 35 | 23 | "Advanced" | Living alone | Kavanagh et al [10] |
| UK | TD | 1991 | £ 33.81 | 53 | 63 | D, IC | 32 | 28 | "Advanced" | Not living alone | Kavanagh et al [10] |
| Sweden | Long. | 1985 | SEK 199 | 25 | 35 | D, IC | | 1.5 | Mild–severe | | Wimo et al [45] |
| Sweden | Long. | 1987 | SEK 534 | 63 | 85 | D, IC | | 0.5 | Mild–severe | | Wimo et al [46] |
| Sweden | Long. | 1987 | SEK 562 | 67 | 90 | D, IC | | 20 | Mild–severe | | Wimo et al [30] |
| USA | Long. | 1990 | US$ 94.57 | 95 | 125 | IC | | | | | Max et al [58] |
| USA | Long. | 1990 | US$ 42.59 | 43 | 55 | D, IC | 48 | | Mild–moderate (?) | Net costs | Weinberger et al [25, 59] |
| USA | Long. | 1990 | US$ 144.11 | 144 | 190 | D, IC | 14 | 68 | Mild–moderate (?) | Net costs | Weinberger et al [25] |
| France | Long. | 1991 | US$ 23.08 | 23 | 29 | D, IC, ID | | 33 | MMSE < 15 | | Souêtre et al [60] |
| France | Long. | 1991 | US$ 14.16 | 14 | 17 | D, IC, ID | | 41 | MMSE > 15 | | Souêtre et al [60] |

PPP, purchasing power parities; TD, "typical day" analysis; Long., longitudinal analysis; D, direct costs; IC, costs of informal care; ID, indirect costs; MMSE, Mini-Mental State Examination included, even if the first approach is in the focus. In some studies, the costs of home care were used as a comparison alternative (e.g. with day care, see above). Studies presenting costs of home care must also be judged with four other aspects in mind: the degree of dementia; whether informal care is included; whether the value of the family efforts is based on paid or unpaid work; and whether gross or net costs are presented.

With the first approach, unpaid informal care makes up a large part of the total costs. There is also a wide range in the cost estimates (see Table 6.6).

Rice *et al* [23] showed that the out-of-pocket expenses for the families is approximately 63% of the health sector costs. Adding informal care increases costs considerably and the costs of home care are almost the same as for nursing home care, whereas the relative part of out-of-pocket expenses decreases to 17%. The family burden is double: out-of-pocket costs and informal unpaid care. Stommel *et al*'s [57] study on the costs for the families showed that the greatest part (71%) was unpaid (i.e. the same level as in Rice *et al*'s [23] study, 73%). The cost level in UK seems to be lower compared to USA when the same cost categories are included. Weinberger *et al* [25,59] presented net costs in a longitudinal study and also studied the effects of a social intervention program [59], where costs were not significantly lower than for the controls. The French study [60] illustrated that even if the value of informal care increases by the degree of the dementia, its relative part is higher (41%) among those with mild to moderate dementia than in moderate to severe dementia (33%), because more formal care is needed in severe dementia. The paid part of the family efforts is very low (0.5–1.5%) in comparison to unpaid efforts. In an English study, it was found that community-based services had lower total costs than long-term hospital stay, although the social service costs were higher [61,62]. In contrast, Donaldson and Gregson [63] found that the cost to maintain patients in home care could be very high. In Dellasega *et al*'s study [64], home care costs were lower for cognitively impaired than for intact persons if only the home care costs were analysed, but if informal care and hospitalization costs had been included, the total costs would have been greater for the impaired group.

When comparisons are made between home care and nursing home care (see Tables 6.3 and 6.6), it is notable that the costs may be higher in home care when all relevant cost categories are included.

## Informal Care

### Demand and Supply of Informal Care

Informal care is the unpaid care provided by family members, friends or voluntary workers to disabled and impaired individuals in the community

[65]. Most disabled elderly persons benefit from informal care to some degree, and many families choose informal care over formal, paid care [66,67]. Spouses form a major proportion of the informal care-giving network [2], but increasingly, elders reach their 70s without a spouse. Because of the greater than 7-year discrepancy between life-expectancy for men and women, this phenomenon is one which confronts women more often than men [68].

Most disabled individuals prefer to remain in their own homes, instead of moving into an institutional setting, to obtain the care they need. Values cited as important for describing the qualities of living at home include maintaining personal privacy, pleasant living environment, being at home and personal space. Informal caregivers often enable family members and friends to maintain their homes when otherwise they would be forced to accept institutional care. Even so, elders often favour paid assistance in their homes so that they can avoid burdening their families.

While the growing elderly population indicates that the demand for informal caregivers will be high, other socioeconomic and demographic trends indicate that the availability of informal caregivers is decreasing. However, supply of caregivers is difficult to measure, due to the obviously large variety of behavioural and cultural factors which determine the willingness of one adult to care for another.

## Measuring and Costing Informal Care

Different approaches for measuring informal care have been used, such as diaries/questionnaires, direct observation and interviews in retrospect. Support in ADLs and instrumental ADLs (IADLs) can be defined rather well. However, a great part of the caregiver's time is linked to supervision of the patient in various activities, to meet and treat behavioural disturbances and to watch over the patient to prevent dangerous events with hot water, fire, etc. The assessment of such supervision, in terms of minutes and hours, is difficult. Two other important factors are care productivity and joint production. A formal professional carer is probably more efficient and takes less time to support ADL tasks than an informal caregiver, which must be considered if a replacement costing approach is used (see below). Joint production means that the patient and the caregiver are doing things together, particularly in IADL tasks such as shopping or preparing meals.

The costing of informal care is controversial [69–71]. Whether informal care should be viewed as a direct (non-medical) cost or as an indirect cost is debatable. The ability to substitute informal caregivers for formal caregivers demonstrates similar resource qualities, which would argue for classifying it as a direct cost. Also, according to consumer theory, informal care giving can be viewed as a service product of a household or family [72]. Thus, it is reasonable to view the family members of a household producing informal care by using time, medical supplies, pharmaceutical and other goods in order to maximize their utility. Implicitly, this suggests that income and prices will contribute strongly to their decision to use formal vs. informal care. In most instances, the informal care produced by the household can be viewed as interchangeable with the home care provided by paid individuals and agencies.

Indirect costs compose a distinct type of foregone opportunity, that of production losses [73]. When a relative of a demented person takes time off from other activities to care for this person, it might be reasonable to interpret this as an indirect cost. However, if the household is viewed as a small production facility, then the time spent away from the formal labour market will not necessarily be considered an indirect cost. When a family member or friend foregoes employment time to provide informal care, his or her time becomes part of the household production function and, therefore, the time is not lost. In some cases this is the purpose for which such persons prefer to use their time and thus attempt to maximize their utility.

There are two frequently used methods for valuing informal care: the opportunity cost method and the replacement method, which both have drawbacks when applied in the field of dementia. The opportunity cost of a resource is the value of the resource (in this case the caregiver's time) put to its best alternative use. Whether or not the caregiver is paid for the care is not of interest; payment has impact on the distribution of the burden but not on the total societal cost. Thus, the question of interest is to find out what the alternative use of the caregiver's time actually is. If the caregiver is of working age and the alternative is working on the labour market, the cost for informal care should be valued to the production loss due to absence from work (with methods used in the estimation of labour cost).

More complicated is the costing of the caregiver's time regarding leisure and caregiver time produced by retired persons (such as spouses) since there are no market prices available. There is no consensus on how this should be performed [74]. Survey methods, such as the contingent valuation method, may be useful regarding caregiver's leisure time, but as far as we know no such empirical studies have been published yet regarding dementia.

The second option is to value time to the cost of professional formal care, e.g. the cost for professional home help (the replacement cost approach). It is assumed that a professional carer would replace the informal caregiver if this particular informal carer were not available. It is also assumed that the informal caregiver's time and the professional caregiver's time are perfect substitutes. The cost of informal care is, therefore, the corresponding cost for a formal carer. This approach also has several drawbacks. Firstly, we do not know if there actually would be a replacement with a professional carer if the informal carer were not available, at least not to the full corresponding time. Other complicated issues (which to some extent are also problematic with the opportunity cost approach) are, as mentioned above, the discussions about joint production and supervision time.

It has also been suggested that the loss of leisure time should be measured as a reduction of the caregiver's quality of life [71], as part of the "outcome side" in the evaluation. But it is unclear how a reduction in quality of life for the caregiver should be integrated in an economic evaluation.

Yet another approach is to give caregiver time a zero value. There are two reasons for this: the methodological problems described above and the fact that some caregivers to demented persons do not feel any burden or sacrifice in their situation; on the contrary, they sometimes describe their situation in very positive terms. These cases are, however, the exception rather than the rule; there is a large body of evidence in the literature that dementia has a heavy impact on the caregiver's situation in terms of burden, depression, quality of life, coping, stress, morbidity and social network [75].

To summarize, there are a number of issues that need to be resolved in the measurement and costing of informal care. We have argued for interpreting informal care as a direct cost, mainly by referring to issues of substitution and seeing the household as a production centre. Further, we recommend researchers to include all three costing options in the analysis, preferably with the opportunity cost approach as the main alternative and the replacement and zero approaches in the sensitivity analysis.

## COSTS IN RELATION TO SEVERITY OF DISEASE

### Disease Severity Scales in Dementia

Disease severity scales in dementia range from detailed, multidimensional descriptions of the different stages of dementia to unidimensional measures of, for example, cognitive functioning. The Clinical Dementia Rating (CDR) and the Global Deterioration Scale (GDS) are both widely used for classifying AD patients into a limited number of disease stages (four in the case of CDR and seven with the GDS) [76]. The advantage with these scales is that they incorporate several dimensions of the disease (memory impairment, ADL skills, etc.) into a single measure. Variables such as education, occupation and cultural factors have less influence than what is seen with scales only measuring cognitive function [76].

| Clinical diagnosis | Incipient/questionable AD | | Mild AD | Moderate AD Moderately severe AD | | | Severe AD |
|---|---|---|---|---|---|---|---|
| CDR stage | 0.5 | | | 1 | 2 | 3 | n/a |
| GDS stage | 3 | | 4 | 5 | 6 | | 7 |
| MMSE | 29 | 25 | 19 | 14 | 5 | 0 | |

Progression

FIGURE 6.1 Relationship between different severity scales in dementia. AD, Alzheimer's disease; CDR, Clinical Dementia Rating; GDS, Global Deterioration scale; MMSE, Mini-Mental State Examination
*Source*: adapted from Reisberg *et al* [76]

The MMSE is a test aimed at measuring the degree of cognitive impairment [77] with a score ranging from 30 (no cognitive impairment) to 0 (severe cognitive impairment). As mentioned above, the results are likely to be affected by the education of the subject and cultural factors. Also, results will be worse if the patient is tired or is having a "bad day." There may also be a "bottoming out" effect in subjects with very severe AD, who may score 0 on the MMSE before they have reached the final stage of progression. Advantages with the MMSE are that the test is easy to administer and has a more detailed scale than the staging scales.

Figure 6.1 shows the relationship between clinical diagnosis, CDR and GDS and the average MMSE score for patients in the different stages of dementia. The ideal severity scale for economic evaluation in AD should be easy to administer, reflect even small deterioration in health status and be highly correlated with costs. Of the available disease scales, the MMSE most closely matches these requirements. Whether the other scales also fulfil these criteria must be analysed further.

## Relation Between Costs and MMSE Score

The correlation between MMSE level and total costs has been investigated in several studies. Ernst *et al* [78] used a log-linear regression model to estimate the dollar savings from preventing or reversing cognitive decline in AD patients. For a patient with an initial MMSE score of 7, preventing a two-point decline would save $3700, while a two-point increase in MMSE score rather than a two-point decline would save $7100.

Jönsson *et al* [79] employed a linear regression model to analyse the relationship between MMSE and costs, including medical expenditures, costs of accommodation and home help. Data was taken from a population-based study (the Kungsholmen project [80]) including persons aged 75 and above, both with and without a diagnosis of dementia. A decrease in MMSE score by 1 point was associated with an increase in cost by $2000 (15 000 SEK).

Preliminary data from a further analysis of the Kungsholmen material [81] indicate a close correlation between costs and indicators of dementia severity. A change of CDR by one stage corresponds to a cost of about $12 500, a change of MMSE by one point to about $2000–2300 and a change by one step in the Katz index of ADL [82] to $6000.

In a Canadian study [83], MMSE was used to estimate stage-specific costs of AD. The annual costs were CAN$ 9451 for mild disease (MMSE 21–26), CAN$ 16 054 for mild–moderate disease (MMSE 15–20), CAN$ 25 714 for moderate disease (MMSE 10–14), and CAN$ 36 794 for severe disease (1996 prices).

It appears that even slight changes in MMSE score may be associated with significant changes in resource utilization and costs. However, studies have focused on the cross-sectional relationship between MMSE and costs, and the cost implications of changes in MMSE score still remain to be explored.

## ECONOMIC EVALUATION IN DEMENTIA

### Methods for Economic Evaluation

Economic evaluation means a comparative analysis of alternative treatments or other interventions in terms of cost and outcome. Depending on the outcome measure used, the different evaluation techniques are called cost-minimization analysis, cost–effectiveness analysis, cost–utility analysis and cost–benefit analysis [73].

### Cost-minimization Analysis

In cost-minimization analysis, only the costs of alternative treatments (or one treatment compared with doing nothing) are compared, whereas the health effects are assumed to be equal. The methodological difficulties associated with defining and measuring outcome in dementia have led to a frequent use of cost-minimization analysis in economic evaluation. If cost-minimization analysis is used in a case where the health effects of the comparators are not equal, it will provide guidance for decisions only if the alternative which is thought to give the best health effects is also the least costly. If a treatment has a positive health effect but is cost adding in relation to a comparator, cost-minimization analysis does not help the decision-maker on whether or not to use the treatment.

*Cost–effectiveness Analysis*

In cost–effectiveness analysis, health effects are expressed in some natural unit (most commonly life-years gained) and results are presented as the marginal (extra) cost per additional unit of effectiveness obtained (cost per life-year gained, for example). In dementia, there is a lack of good disease measures to be used for cost–effectiveness analysis. Using disease severity scales as an effectiveness measure leads to difficulties in interpreting the results. For example, what is the willingness to pay per MMSE point gained? Another possibility is to use the time spent in non-severe states of the disease as an outcome measure. Effectiveness is defined as 1 if the patient avoids reaching the state and 0 if he reaches it. The cost–effectiveness ratio will be the cost to avoid that a patient reach the defined severe state, for example MMSE below 10, or the cost per additional year spent out of that state. Here, also the results become difficult to interpret. Another weakness with cost–effectiveness analysis is that cost–effectiveness ratios cannot be compared between different therapeutic areas. This limitation has led to the development of cost–utility analysis.

*Cost–utility Analysis*

In cost–utility analysis, the most common outcome measure is the number of quality-adjusted life-years (QALYs) gained. Using this method requires that we can estimate the quality of life for patients with different levels of dementia. These estimations are difficult to obtain, particularly among patients with severe dementia. A way around this problem is to let someone else (the patients' spouse, the physician or the general population) assign quality of life weights to different states of dementia. However, these weights could potentially differ a lot from the quality of life perceived by the patients themselves. A special problem is how to include potential quality of life losses for relatives or other caregivers. It is common to measure the impact of dementia on the quality of life of caregivers, while this is seldom included for other diseases. This makes it problematic to compare between different diseases. There is also a risk of double counting, since estimates of the cost of informal care include a valuation of the opportunity cost of time.

## Modelling Issues

Since dementia is a chronic, progressive disease, treatments aimed at altering the course of the disease might have consequences as far ahead in time as decades after the initiation of treatment. Clinical trials typically have a duration of less than a year up to a few years. To capture all the relevant consequences of the intervention, it is therefore necessary to predict the occurrence of events beyond the end of the clinical trial. Different modelling techniques have been developed for this purpose. The most commonly used technique is Markov modelling, where an imaginary cohort of patients is divided into a number of "states" defined according to the severity of the disease [84]. Having the patients move from less severe to more severe states simulates progression over time. For each cycle, the distribution of patients over the different states is estimated, and this information is used to calculate expected costs and outcomes. Another modelling technique is decision-tree analysis. This method requires the researcher to specify all sequences of events that are possible over the time period for the simulation and the costs and outcomes associated with each of these sequences. This method has several drawbacks compared with the Markov model. The most important weakness of decision-tree models in modelling progressive diseases is that the number of different chains of events that can occur increases rapidly with the length of the simulation period, so that the decision tree quickly becomes very large and difficult to handle.

## Cost-effectiveness of Tacrine

The first drug approved for the treatment of mild or moderate AD, the anticholinergic tacrine, was also the first anti-dementia drug to undergo an economic evaluation. Lubeck *et al* [85] created an economic model which linked cognitive changes observed in a 30-week clinical trial of tacrine [86] with estimates of the cost of AD, drug therapy, monitoring, time in a nursing home, and survival from diagnosis. Two patient groups were evaluated: one group consisting of 367 patients receiving varying doses of tacrine, including treatment failures, and a second group of 67 patients able to tolerate the high dose of 160 mg/day. Based on a literature review, a patient with AD survives a mean of 4.4 years from diagnosis and incurs lifetime treatment costs of $57 169 (1993 dollars). Patients taking doses of 80–160 mg/day showed an average improvement in MMSE of 1.0 point, which resulted in 9.5 months of predicted community and institutional care avoided, for annual savings of $2243/patient (range, $109–3342). Patients able to tolerate the 160 mg dose improved 2.0 points on the MMSE, resulting in a prediction of 12.1 months of reduced community and nursing home care, for annual savings of $4052/patient.

There are several methodological problems involved in this analysis. The most important difficulty lies in assessing the efficacy of tacrine and quantifying the benefits of treatment. In a review of clinical trials of tacrine

[87], three trials showed small but clinically unimportant improvements in patients treated with the drug, while the remaining 10 trials demonstrated no difference in the outcome measures related to cognition. Lubeck *et al*'s [85] results stem from a difference in MMSE score between treated and untreated patients of 1.0 (2.0 for the high-dose group). This is a very small difference but, since costs are so highly dependent on cognitive functioning, the treatment turns out to be cost saving in both groups.

Knopman *et al* [88] studied the effect of tacrine on nursing home placement (NHP) and mortality with efficacy data taken from the same 30-week clinical study as Lubeck *et al*. In a logistic regression model, it was shown that the likelihood of NHP was reduced by tacrine treatment in various doses (odds ratio 2.7 for doses > 80 mg/day and 2.8 for doses > 120 mg/day) over the 2-year unblinded follow-up period of the trial. Tacrine treatment had no statistically significant effect on mortality, although there was a trend towards lower mortality in high-dose groups. This data supports the notion that treatment has a beneficial effect on resource utilization and costs. However, it is difficult to quantify these possible cost savings and to put them in relation to the cost of intervention. Also, since the follow-up phase of the study was neither randomized nor blinded, the results are open to bias.

In conclusion, the cost–effectiveness of tacrine is difficult to judge, due to the very small therapeutic effect of the drug. Also, due to problems with poor tolerability, many patients will not be able to receive the full dosage required to reach optimal therapeutic effect. However, if the drug can be shown to have a significant effect on cognitive functioning in a selected patient material, it can very well be cost–effective when used in these patients.

## Cost-effectiveness of Donepezil

Donepezil is a specific acetylcholinesterase inhibitor that has been shown to maintain cognitive function above baseline levels for up to 1 year and slow the expected decline [89]. Donepezil is generally well tolerated and the frequency of side effects was similar to that of placebo in the clinical trials. Five Markov models analysing the economic effect of donepezil have recently been developed [90] for USA [91], UK [92], Canada [93,94] and Sweden [95]. Lanctôt *et al* [94] took the government payer perspective and included only direct medical costs, while all others adopted a societal perspective and included direct medical and non-medical costs, as well as costs for informal care (except for the Swedish study, which did not include unpaid caregiver costs). QALYs were used as outcome measure in two of the studies [91,94], while the other studies used the expected number of years with non-severe AD.

The results of these models suggest that donepezil is effectively cost-neutral (treatment causes either a slight decrease or a slight increase in total costs), while giving a better outcome than the no-treatment option, in terms of both time in less severe states and of QALYs. Donepezil was the dominant strategy (better outcome and lower costs in the base-case scenario) in three of the five studies. In the two other studies donepezil was slightly cost adding, but the incremental cost–effectiveness ratios were favourable under certain scenarios. In all studies, the increased drug costs were offset to a large extent by savings due to less utilization of other resources, particularly nursing home care and other types of institutionalization.

Donepezil is most likely a cost–effective treatment if prescribed to the right patients at the right time. Not all patients will respond to treatment, and at this time there is no way of identifying in advance those who will respond. The response to the drug should be evaluated after three months, and treatment should be discontinued if there is no perceived benefit. The indication for treatment with donepezil is mild to moderate disease, which implies that once the progression has reached a certain level, further treatment is of no benefit to the patient and certainly not a cost–effective use of resources.

## Cost-effectiveness of Rivastigmine

Rivastigmine is the third cholinesterase inhibitor that has been launched for treatment of AD. So far, one pharmacoeconomical evaluation is available [96]. This study used a different modelling approach to the donepezil studies, making comparisons difficult, but the presented benefits are of the same size as in the donepezil studies.

## SUMMARY

### Consistent Evidence

Dementia is a costly disease and causes considerable suffering to patients and caregivers. Inpatient care stands for a large share of direct medical expenditure, while drug costs and costs for physician visits are small by comparison. However, the majority of direct cost of care is found outside the traditional health care system. Indirect costs for patients with dementia are relatively small due to the age distribution of the patients.

## Incomplete Evidence

The great variety of care alternatives for patients with dementia makes it difficult to undertake relevant assessments and comparisons of costs. Although many studies have compared the cost for different treatment alternatives, there is no clear picture on their relative cost.

Another important aspect of costing dementia is the identification, quantification and valuation of the costs of informal care. These costs are difficult to measure, but the opportunity cost for these services is likely to be high. Many studies have included these costs, but limitations in both data and methods make it difficult to assess the precise importance of these costs.

Few treatment options are available that have an impact on the course of the disease. Cholinesterase inhibitors have been shown to delay the progression of the disease when used in patients with mild-to-moderate AD. Due to the strong impact of cognitive decline on costs, mainly through increased institutionalization, treatments that have a significant effect on the progression of AD will also lead to savings in costs. However, the evidence on cost–effectiveness of drug interventions as well as alternative arrangements for care is scarce.

## Areas Still Open to Research

There have been a number of costing studies published in dementia but, in relation to the size of the costs involved, the amount of research is small. The published studies are from a small number of countries, making international comparisons limited. There is also a need to standardize the methods for costing. The great variations shown between studies from different countries, as well as for a specific country, are probably mainly explained by differences in methods and data sources. In particular, there is a need for studies with individual costing data. Such studies are necessary to answer questions about the relationship between costs for people with dementia vs. the cost of dementia. This distinction is sometimes referred to as gross vs. net costs. Only the former can be observed, while the latter have to be estimated by comparisons with patients without dementia. Such studies are also important to answer questions about the cost related to different severities of the disease.

Further development of methods for costing informal care is important. These costs are important to include in the analysis to make comparisons between different alternatives of caring for dementia patients relevant.

Quality of life aspects are important both for patients and caregivers. There is a need for development and testing of methods for quality of life measurements in dementia, particularly of instruments that can be used for outcome measurement in economic evaluations. Further theoretical and empirical studies are also needed to find out how quality of life aspects should be included in economic evaluations. Is cost per QALY a relevant cost-effectiveness measure in dementia, and how should costs and QALY then be defined to avoid double counting and to make comparisons with other diseases relevant?

Research is needed to further investigate the link between measures of cognitive functioning (e.g. the MMSE) and resource utilization and costs.

There is also a need for developing the models used for the evaluation of the cost-effectiveness of treatments in dementia by combining results from clinical trials with data from long-term follow-up studies. In addition, it is necessary to undertake economic evaluations alongside clinical trials of sufficient length comparing relevant treatment strategies, in order to verify the results predicted by models based on efficacy data from short trials.

## REFERENCES

1. Wimo A., Ljunggren G., Winblad B. (1997) Costs of dementia and dementia care—a review. *Int. J. Geriatr. Psychiatry*, **12**: 841–856.
2. Office of Technology Assesment (OTA) (1988) Confronting Alzheimer's Disease and other Dementias, Chapter 1, pp. 3–55, Office of Technology Assessment, Philadelphia.
3. Hay J. Ernst R. (1987) The economic costs of Alzheimer's disease. *Am. J. Public Health*, **77**: 1169–1175.
4. Huang L., Cartwright W., Hu T. (1988) The economic cost of senile dementia in the United States, 1985. *Public Health Reports*, **103**: 3–7.
5. Schneider E., Guralnik J. (1990) The aging of America. Impact on health care costs. *JAMA*, **263**: 2335–2340.
6. Ernst R. Hay J. (1994) The US economic and social costs of Alzheimer's disease revisited. *Am. J. Public Health*, **84**: 1–4.
7. Manton K., Corder L., Clark R. (1993) Estimates and projections of dementia-related service expenditures. In *Forecasting the Health of the Oldest Old*. (Eds R. Suzman, B. Singer, K. Manton), pp. 207–238, Springer, New York.
8. Smith K., Shah A., Wright K., Lewis G. (1995) The prevalence and costs of psychiatric disorders and learning disabilities. *Br. J. Psychiatry*, **166**: 9–18.
9. Gray A., Fenn P. (1993) Alzheimer's disease: the burden of illness in England. *Health Trends*, **25**: 31–37.
10. Kavanagh S., Schneider J., Knapp M., Beecham J., Netten A. (1993) Elderly people with cognitive impairment: costing possible changes in the balance of care. *Health Soc. Care Commun.*, **2**: 69–80.
11. Holmes J., Pugner K., Philips R. (1998) Managing Alzheimer's disease: the cost of care per patient. *Br. J. Care Manag.*, **4**: 332–337.
12. Østbye T., Crosse E. (1994) Net economic costs of dementia in Canada. *J. Can. Med. Assoc.*, **151**: 1457–1464.
13. Wimo A., Karlsson G., Sandman P., Corder L., Winblad B. (1997) Cost of illness due to dementia in Sweden. *Int. J. Geriatr. Psychiatry*, **12**: 857–861.

14. Cavallo M.C., Fattore G. (1997)   The economic and social burden of Alzheimer disease on families in the Lombardy region of Italy. *Alz. Dis. Assoc. Disord.*, **11**: 184–190.

15. Schulenburg J., Schulenburg I., Horn R. (1998)   Cost of treatment and cost of care for Alzheimer's disease in Germany. In *The Health Economics of Dementia* (Eds A. Wimo, G. Karlsson, B. Jönsson, B. Winblad), pp. 217–230, Wiley, Chichester.

16. Kronborg Andersen C., Sogaard J., Hansen E., Kragh-Sørensen A., Hastrup L., Andersen J., Andersen K., Lolk A., Nielsen H., Kragh-Sørensen P. (1999)   The cost of dementia in Denmark: the Odense Study. *Dement. Geriatr. Cogn. Disord.*, **10**: 295–304.

17. Koopmanschap M., Poulder J., Meerding W. (1998)   Cost of dementia in the Netherlands. In *The Health Economics of Dementia* (Eds A. Wimo, G. Karlsson, B. Jönsson, B. Winblad), pp. 207–215, Wiley, Chichester.

18. Rice D., Hodgson T., Kopstein A. (1985)   The economic costs of illness: a replication and update. *Health Financing Rev.*, **7**: 61–80.

19. Livingston G., Manela M., Katona C. (1997)   Cost of community care for older people. *Br. J. Psychiatry*, **171**: 56–59.

20. Schneider J., Kavanagh S., Knapp M., Beecham J., Netten A. (1993)   Elderly people with advanced cognitive impairment in England: resource use and costs. *Ageing Soc.*, **13**: 27–50.

21. Coughlin T., Liu K. (1989)   Health care costs of older persons with cognitive impairments. *Gerontologist*, **29**: 173–182.

22. Hu T., Lien-Fu H., Cartwright W. (1986)   Evaluation of the costs of caring for the senile demented elderly: a pilot study. *Gerontologist*, **26**: 158–163.

23. Rice D., Fox P., Max W., Webber P., Lindeman D.A., Hauck W., Segura E. (1993)   The economic burden of Alzheimer's disease care. *Health Affairs*, **12**: 164–176.

24. Welch G., Walsh J., Larson E. (1992)   The cost of institutional care in Alzheimer's disease: nursing home and hospital use in a prospective cohort. *J. Am. Geriatr. Soc.*, **40**: 221–224.

25. Weinberger M., Gold D., Divine G., Cowper P., Hodgson L., Schreiner P., George L. (1993)   Expenditures in caring for patients with dementia who live at home. *Am. J. Publ. Health*, **83**: 338–341.

26. Rovner B., Steele C., Shmuely Y., Folstein M. (1996)   A randomized trial of dementia care in nursing homes. *J. Am. Geriatr. Soc.*, **44**: 7–13.

27. Beecham J., Cambridge P., Hallam A., Knapp M. (1993)   The cost of domus care. *Int. J. Geriatr. Psychiatry*, **8**: 827–831.

28. Knapp M. (1995)   Resource scarcity chasing scarce resources: health economics and geriatric psychiatry. *Int. J. Geriatr. Psychiatry*, **10**: 821–829.

29. Annerstedt L. (1993)   Development and consequences of group living in Sweden. A new model of care for the demented elderly. *Soc. Sci. Med.*, **37**: 1529–1538.

30. Wimo A., Mattsson B., Krakau I., Eriksson T., Nelvig A. (1994)   The impact of different levels of cognitive decline and work load on costs of dementia care at different caring levels. *Int. J. Geriatr. Psychiatry*, **9**: 479–489.

31. Sweden National Board of Health and Welfare (1994) *De Nya Avgifterna för Äldre och Handikappomsorg*, National Board of Health and Welfare Stockholm.

32. Ribbe M. (1993)   Care for the elderly: the role of the nursing home in the Dutch health care system. *Int. Psychogeriatrics*, **5**: 213–222.

33. Wimo A., Wallin J., Lundgren K., Rönnbäck E., Asplund K., Mattsson B., Krakau I. (1991) Group Living, an alternative for dementia patients. A cost analysis. *Int. J. Geriatr. Psychiatry*, **6**: 21–29.

34. Wimo A., Eriksson T., Mattsson B., Krakau I., Nelvig A., Karlsson G. (1995) Cost–utility analysis of group living in dementia care. *Int. J. Technol. Assess. Health Care*, **11**: 49–65.

35. Svensson M., Edebalk P., Persson U. (1996) Group Living for elderly patients with dementia—a cost analysis. *Health Policy*, **38**: 83–100.

36. Sands D., Belman J. (1986) *Evaluation of a 24-Hour Care System for Alzheimer's and Related Disorders*. Contract Report Prepared for the Office of Technology Assessment, US Congress, Office of Technology Assessment, Philadelphia.

37. Johansson L. (1990) Group dwellings for dementia patients: a new care alternative. *Ageing Int.*, **17**: 35–37.

38. Wimo A. (1997) Are costs of dementia care reduced by the introduction of group living? In *Research and Practice in Alzheimer's Disease* (Eds B. Vellas, J. Fitten, G. Frisoni), pp. 447–458, Springer, New York.

39. Knapp M., Cambridge P., Thomason C., Beecham J., Allen C., Darton R. (1994) Residential care as an alternative to long-stay hospital: a cost-effectiveness evaluation of two pilot projects. *Int. J. Geriatr. Psychiatry*, **9**: 297–304.

40. Office of Technology Assessment (OTA) (1988) *Confronting Alzheimer's Disease and Other Dementias*, Chapter 7, pp. 240–270 Office of Technology Assessment, Philadelphia.

41. Sands D., Suzuki T. (1983) Adult day care for Alzheimer's patients and their families. *Gerontologist*, **23**: 21–23.

42. Keys B., Szpak G. (1983) Day care for Alzheimer's disease, profile of one program. *Postgrad. Med.*, **73**: 245–250.

43. Panella J., Lilliston B., Brush D., McDowell F. (1984) Day care for dementia patients: an analysis of a four-year program. *J. Am. Geriatr. Soc.*, **32**: 883–886.

44. Cox N., Reifler B. (1994) Dementia care and respite services program. *Alz. Dis. Assoc. Disord.*, **8**: 113–121.

45. Wimo A., Wallin J., Lundgren K. (1990) Impact of day care on dementia patients costs, well-being and relatives views. *Fam. Pract.*, **4**: 279–287.

46. Wimo A., Mattsson B., Krakau I., Eriksson I., Nelvig A. (1994) Cost-effectiveness analysis of dementia in day care for patients with dementia disorders. *Health Economics*, **3**: 395–404.

47. Engedal K. (1989) Day care for demented patients in general nursing homes. Effects on admission to institutions and mental capacity. *Scand. J. Prim. Health Care*, **7**: 161–166.

48. Reifler B., Henry R., Rusching J. (1997) Financial performance among adult day centers: results of a national demonstrating program. *J. Am. Geriatr. Soc.*, **45**: 146–153.

49. Maas M., Specht J., Weiler K., Buckwalter K., Turner B. (1997) Special care units for people with Alzheimer's disease. Only for the privileged few? *J. Gerontol. Nursing*, **24**: 28–37.

50. Holmes D., Ory M., Teresi J. (1994) Special dementia care: research, policy, and practice issues. *Alz. Dis. Assoc. Disord.*, **8** (Suppl. 1): S5–S13.

51. Volicer L., Collard A., Hurley A., Bishop C., Kern D., Karon S. (1994) Impact of special care unit for patients with advanced Alzheimer's disease on patient's discomfort and costs. *J. Am. Geriatr. Soc.*, **42**: 597–603.

52. Hurley A., Volicer B., Mahoney M., Volicer L. (1993)   Palliative fever management in Alzheimer patients: quality plus fiscal responsibility. *Adv. Nursing Sci.*, **16**: 21–32.
53. Wray N., Brody B., Bayer I., Boisaubin E. (1988)   Withholding medical treatment from the severely demented patient. *Arch. Intern. Med.*, **148**: 1980–1984.
54. Torian L., Davidson E., Fulop G., Sell L., Fillit H. (1992)   The effect of dementia on acute care in a geriatric medical unit. *Int. Psychogeriatrics*, **4**: 231–239.
55. Weiner M., Powe N., Weller W. (1998)   Alzheimer's disease under managed care: implications from Medicare utilization and expenditure patterns. *J. Am. Geriatr. Soc.*, **46**: 762–770.
56. Siegler E., Lavizzo-Mourey R. (1991)   Management of stage III pressure ulcers in moderately demented nursing home residents. *J. Intern. Med.*, **6**: 507–513.
57. Stommel M., Collins C., Given B. (1994)   The costs of family contribution to the care of persons with dementia. *Gerontologist*, **34**: 199–205.
58. Max W., Webber P., Fox P. (1995)   Alzheimer's disease. The unpaid burden of caring. *J. Aging Health*, **7**: 179–199.
59. Weinberger M., Gold D., Divine G., Cowper P., Hodgson L., Schreiner P., George L. (1993)   Social interventions for caregivers of patients with dementia: impact on health care utilization and expenditures. *J. Am. Geriatr. Soc.*, **41**: 153–156.
60. Souêtre E., Qing W., Vigoureux I. (1995)   Economic analysis of Alzheimer's disease in outpatients: impact of symptom severity. *Int. Psychogeriatrics*, **7**: 115–122.
61. Keen J. (1993)   Dementia: questions of cost and value. *Int. J. Geriatr. Psychiatry*, **8**: 369–378.
62. Challis D., Darton R.A., Johnson L., Stone M., Traske K. (1991)   An evaluation of an alternative to long-stay hospital care for frail elderly patients: II. Costs and effectiveness. *Age Ageing*, **20**: 245–254.
63. Donaldson C., Gregson B. (1989)   Prolonging life at home: what is the cost? *Commun. Med.*, **11**: 200–209.
64. Dellasega C. Ling L. (1996)   The psychogeriatric nurse in home health care: use of research to develop the role. *Clin. Nurse Spec.*, **10**: 64–68.
65. Spillman B. (1992)   Long term care arrangements for elderly persons with disabilities: private and public roles. *Home Health Care Quarterly*, **13**: 5–35.
66. Bell D. (1987)   *Home Care in New York City: Providers, Payers, and Clients*, United Hospital Fund of New York, New York.
67. Nutting P. (1991)   AHCPR studies examine impact of disabilities in the elderly. *J. Family Pract.*, **32**: 131–132.
68. Hagestad G. (1986)   The aging society as a context for family life. *Daedelus*, **115**: 119–139.
69. Busschbach J., Brouwer W., Donk V.D. (1998)   An outline for a cost-effectiveness analysis of a drug for patients with Alzheimer's disease. *PharmacoEconomics*, **15**: 21–34.
70. Netten A. (1992)   Costing informal care. In *Costing Community Care* (Eds A. Netten, J. Beecham), pp. 43–57, Ashgate, Aldershot.
71. Koopmanschap M., Brouwer W. (1998)   Indirect costs and costing informal care. In *The Health Economics of Dementia* (Eds A. Wimo, G. Karlsson, B. Jönsson, B. Winblad), pp. 245–256, Wiley, Chichester.
72. Becker G. (1965)   A theory of the allocation of time. *Economic J.*, **75**: 493–517.
73. Drummond M., Stoddart G., Torrance G. (1987)   *Methods for the Economic Evaluation of Health Care Programs*, Oxford University Press, Oxford.

74. Karlsson G., Wimo A., Jönsson B., Winblad B. (1998) Methodological issues in health economic studies of dementia. In *The Health Economics of Dementia* (Eds A. Wimo, G. Karlsson, B. Jönsson, B. Winblad), pp. 161–169, Wiley, Chichester.

75. Wimo A., Winblad B., Grafström M. (1999) The social consequences for families with Alzheimer's disease: potential impact of new drug treatment. *Int. J. Geriatr. Psychiatry*, **14**: 338–347.

76. Reisberg B., Franssen E., Souren L., Kenowski S., Auer S. (1998) Severity scales. In *The Health Economics of Dementia* (Eds A. Wimo, G. Karlsson, B. Jönsson, B. Winblad), pp. 327–357, Wiley, Chichester.

77. Folstein M., Folstein S., McHugh P. (1975) Mini-Mental State: a practical method for grading the cognitive state of patients for the clinician. *J. Psychiatr. Res.*, **12**: 189–198.

78. Ernst R., Hay J., Fenn C., Tinklenberg J., Yesavage J. (1997) Cognitive function and the costs of Alzheimer's disease. *Arch. Neurol.*, **54**: 687–693.

79. Jönsson L., Lindgren P., Wimo A., Jönsson B., Winblad B. (1999) Costs of MMSE-related cognitive impairment. *PharmacoEconomics*, **16**: 409–416.

80. Fratiglioni L., Forsell Y., Torres H.A., Winblad B. (1994) Severity of dementia and institutionalization in the elderly: prevalence data from an urban area in Sweden. *Neuroepidemiology*, **13**: 79–88.

81. Winblad B., Wimo A. (1999) Pharmacoeconomics and dementia: perspectives for clinicians. *Int. Psychogeriatrics*, **11** (Suppl. 1): 85.

82. Katz S., Ford A.B., Moskowitz R.W., Jackson B.A., Joffe M.W. (1963) Studies of illness in the aged: the index of ADL, a standardized measure of biological and psychological function. *JAMA*, **185**: 914–919.

83. Hux M., O'Brien B., Iskedijan M., Goeree R., Cagnon M., Gauthier S. (1998) Relation between severity of Alzheimer's disease and costs of caring. *Can. Med. Assoc. J.*, **159**: 457–465.

84. Sonnenberg F., Beck J. (1993) Markov models in decision making: a practical guide. *Medical Decision Making*, **13**: 322–338.

85. Lubeck D., Mazonson P., Bowe T. (1994) The potential impact of tacrine on expenditures for Alzheimer's disease. *Medical Interface*, **7**: 130–138.

86. Knapp M., Knopman D., Solomon P. (1994) 30-week randomized controlled trial of high-dose tacrine in patients with Alzheimer's disease. *JAMA*, **271**: 985–991.

87. Glennie J. (1997) *The Efficacy of Tacrine and the Measurement of Outcomes in Alzheimer's Disease*, Canadian Coordinating Office for Health Technology Assessment, Ottawa.

88. Knopman D., Schneider L., Davis K., Talwalker S., Smith F., Hoover I., Gracon S. (1996) Long-term tacrine treatment: effects on nursing home placement and mortality. *Neurology*, **47**: 166–177.

89. Rogers S.L., Farlow M.R., Doody R.S., Mohs R., Friedhoff L.T. (1998) A 24-week, double-blind, placebo-controlled trial of donepezil in patients with Alzheimer's disease. Donepezil Study Group. *Neurology*, **50**: 136–145.

90. Foster R., Plosker G. (1999) Donepezil: pharmacoeconomic implications of therapy. *PharmacoEconomics*, **16**: 99–114.

91. Neumann P., Hermann R., Kuntz K. (1999) Cost-effectiveness of donepezil in the treatment of mild or moderate Alzheimer's disease. *Neurology*, **52**: 1138–1145.

92. Stewart A., Phillips R., Dempsey G. (1998) Pharmacotherapy for people with Alzheimer's disease: a Markov-cycle evaluation of five years therapy using donepezil. *Int. J. Geriatr. Psychiatry*, **13**: 445–453.

93. O'Brien B., Goeree R., Hux M. (1999)   Economic evaluation of donepezil in the treatment of Alzheimer's disease in Canada. *J. Am. Geriatr. Soc.*, **47**: 570–578.
94. Lanctôt K., Risebrough N., Oh P. (1998)   Factors affecting the economic attractiveness of cognitive enhancers in Alzheimer's disease. *J. Clin. Pharmacol.*, **38**: 870.
95. Jönsson L., Lindgren P., Wimo A., Jönsson B., Winblad B. (1999)   The cost-effectiveness of donepezil therapy in Swedish patients with Alzheimer's disease: a Markov model. *Clin. Ther.*, **21**: 1230–1240.
96. Fenn P., Gray A. (1999)   Estimating long term cost savings from treatment of Alzheimer's disease. A modelling approach. *PharmacoEconomics*, **16**: 165–174.

# Commentaries

6.1
## Dementia: the Challenges for Economic Analysis
Wendy Max[1]

Dementia is an increasingly prevalent and horrible illness that affects millions of people and their families worldwide. A body of literature has developed that looks at the economic aspects of dementia. Jönsson *et al* have done a fine job of reviewing and synthesizing this literature. A number of issues emerge that make dementia a particularly challenging area for economic analysis.

*International differences.* A comparison of studies of the costs of dementia reflects the differing ways in which people are cared for internationally [1]. In some cultures, care of the elderly is primarily the responsibility of the state or of paid professionals. In most, substantial hours of family time are involved. In some countries, home-based community care is the norm, whereas in others the typical demented person is institutionalized. There are also differences internationally in the access and financing of care. Thus, differences in costs reflect far more than resource use and may in fact include cultural differences and the characteristics of the health care system as a whole.

*Medical models, non-medical needs.* The use of medical care services, particularly hospital care, dominates the cost of treating most diseases. Dementia patients, however, particularly in the early stages of the disease, often require other types of care. For example, social services may be required to enable a patient to remain living in the community or to provide the respite care needed by a caregiver whose services permit the patient to remain at home. Many other patients are cared for in non-medical settings, such as intermediate care or residential care facilities. Few studies have analyzed costs in such settings and the impact of the disease here is little understood.

*Caregiving: treat the patient, impact the entire family.* Dementia impacts the entire family of the patient. While most studies have focused on the cost of caring for the patient him- or herself, many others also incur costs. For

[1] *Institute for Health and Aging, University of California, San Francisco, CA 94143–0646, USA*

example, a caregiver may change his or her labour market plans by retiring early or working fewer hours [2]. The caregiver may spend many hours providing care and supervision. Caregivers have been found to require more medical services themselves. Yet, few studies have addressed these economic ramifications of the disease. Furthermore, while it is often accepted as a worthwhile policy goal to permit people to remain living in their homes for as long as possible, the economic implications of shifting the burden of care to caregiving families has been largely ignored.

*Dementia as a comorbid condition.* Dementia patients often have comorbid conditions [3] that cause them to seek health care and social services. Hence, these comorbidities must be considered before attributing costs to the dementia. Similarly, dementia may be a comorbid condition that increases the cost of care for non-dementia conditions. The analysis of comorbidity poses analytic challenges that must be addressed.

*Measuring outcomes: whose, what and how?* Economic evaluations typically involve the comparison of the cost of an intervention or therapy with an outcome. For dementia, defining and measuring outcomes poses several challenges. (a) Whose outcome should we evaluate? In the light of growing evidence and documentation of the impact dementia has on the caregivers and other family members, both patient and family outcomes should be evaluated. (b) What is the outcome of interest? It is important to define the outcome that may be affected by a given intervention. However, outcomes experienced by dementia patients are often qualitative in nature (e.g. changed quality of life) rather than quantitative (reduced hospitalization costs). (c) How can outcomes be measured? Patient outcomes can be assessed by asking the patient directly or relying on a proxy measure from the caregiver or the health care provider. Dementia patients, particularly in the early stages of the disease, have been found capable of assessing their own outcomes [4].

*The context of the study: clinical vs. economic.* Another challenge for the economic analysis of dementia is the context in which most economic studies are done. Commonly, data collected from a clinical trial are subjected to economic analysis after the fact. Other times, economic measures are added on to a trial that is primarily clinical in nature. Rarely is the economic outcome data collected in a study with purely economic hypotheses as the key goal. Furthermore, due to the nature of the studies done, only care actually received is measured. However, it would be far preferable to design a study that is primarily economic in nature and that would permit a thorough consideration of the relevant issues.

Dementia is a costly illness no matter how or where it is studied. While there are a number of challenges to quantifying the burden from an economic perspective, it is clear that the burden is large and likely to grow. Therefore, it is imperative that economists and other health care researchers continue to address these issues so that we may be able to make rational policy and treatment decisions, informed by an understanding of economic implications.

## REFERENCES

1. Sokolovsky J. (Ed.) (1990)  *The Cultural Context of Aging. Worldwide Perspectives*, Bergin and Harvey, New York.
2. Max W., Webber P., Fox P. (1995)  Alzheimer's disease: the unpaid burden of caring. *J. Aging Health*, **7**: 179–199.
3. Fox P.F., Maslow K., Zhang X. (1999)  Long-term care eligibility criteria for people with Alzheimer's disease. *Health Care Financing Rev.*, **20**: 67–85.
4. Brod M., Stewart A.L., Sands L., Walton P. (1999)  Conceptualization and measurement of quality of life in dementia: the dementia quality of life instrument (DQoL). *Gerontologist*, **39**: 25–35.

6.2
### Costs of Dementia: More Questions than Answers
Caroline Selai[1]

In the past decade, the once arcane terminology of the health economist has quietly seeped into the clinician's everyday language. As pressures to control health care spending have increased, terms such as "cost-effectiveness", "cost-per-QALY" and "pharmacoeconomics" are now ubiquitous. They remain, however, poorly understood and, as a result, are often the source of much controversy and debate.

The importance of knowledge about *costs* (of health conditions, of interventions, of medical equipment) is confirmed by one sobering fact. No country in the world, not even the richest, can afford to do all the things that it is now possible to do to improve the health of its citizens. It is not enough, in the competition for resources, solely to show that a particular intervention is beneficial, although that still is (or should be) one basis for funding. To be successful in that competition, an intervention should be demonstrably more beneficial, per unit of resource used, than some mini-

[1] *Institute of Neurology, National Hospital for Neurology and Neurosurgery, Alexandra House, 17 Queen Square, London WC1N 3BG, UK*

mum cut-off level [1]. The crucial policy decisions within the health care system are thus concerned with the setting of priorities.

Prioritizing or rationing of health care raises a huge number of methodological issues. The subject is also very emotive. Debate on the subject between researchers from a large number of academic disciplines, including economics, medicine, operations research, philosophy and public health, is difficult to follow because each group brings a particular set of concepts and terminology or uses the same terms in slightly different ways. Because of the complexity of the rationing debate, all health care professionals must remain alert to the technical and ethical issues. This vigilance is particularly important in the area of dementia.

All research into dementia is complex. For example, a recent Cochrane review to determine the efficacy of tacrine for Alzheimer's disease (AD) highlighted a number of problems, including the wide variety of outcome measures used, some of which were unvalidated [2]. Few trials had any scales in common and there were high patient drop-out rates. The review produced no clear results. There are also ongoing debates in many areas of health economics. It is no surprise, therefore, that the problems at the interface of these two areas (i.e. the economics of dementia) are both large in number and complex.

The key message arising from the review by Jönsson *et al* is that, whilst a considerable amount of research has been done into the costs of dementia, there are, at present, more questions than answers.

Although a number of cost of illness (COI) studies have been published showing the costs of dementia in several countries, different methods have been used and different costs included, making it extremely difficult to compare the different studies. Other problems include the controversy over the most appropriate method for costing resources, particularly "non-medical" direct costs. A number of ways of measuring informal care have been used. It is difficult to cost the caregiver's time, particularly leisure time and the time spent by a retired spouse, since there are no market prices available. The list goes on.

The main types of economic evaluation are COI studies, cost-minimization analysis (CMA), cost–effectiveness analysis (CEA), cost–benefit analysis (CBA) and cost–utility analysis (CUA) [3]. They differ in their approaches to the measurement of costs and consequences [4]. In cost-minimization analysis, only the costs of alternative treatments are compared. The consequences are assumed to be equal and are thus disregarded. Since defining and measuring outcome in dementia is so difficult, cost–minimisation is the most frequently used economic evaluation. There are, however, a number of developments in assessing outcome in dementia.

One area of much recent research is the development of quality of life (QOL) measures. A number of techniques are available for patient self-report, carer-proxy ratings and observational techniques, although full validation is ongoing [5,6]. QOL is an important outcome for a number of reasons, including economic evaluation. CUA is a technique which uses the Quality Adjusted Life Year (QALY) as an outcome measure. For its calculation, the QALY requires well-being or QOL to be expressed as a single index score. The Quality of Well-being Scale is a utility weighted measure of health-related QOL used in CUA. This has recently been validated for use in patients with AD [7]. Other groups are also looking at ways to obtain "utilities" for stages of AD [8].

Finally, we must be aware of the ethical issues raised by economic analyses in dementia. In a recent study of the measurement of preferences for health states, respondents rated dementia and coma as worse than death [9]. In debates about the allocation of scarce health care resources, it has been argued that older people face discrimination [10,11]. In an area that often relies on carer-proxy or observational ratings, we must remain vigilant, ask ourselves what the data mean and carefully scrutinize the development of all measures.

What we learn from this review of the costs of dementia is that whilst there are a number of published studies, a variety of methods have been used, making inter-study comparisons difficult. Moreover, for the costing of some activities, no techniques are yet available. In summary, many questions remain unanswered.

## REFERENCES

1. Williams A. (1993)  The importance of quality of life in policy decisions. In *Quality of Life Assessment: Key Issues in the 1990s* (Eds S.R. Walker, R.M. Rosser), pp. 427–439, Kluwer, Dordrecht.
2. Qizilbash N., Birks J., Lopez-Arrieta J., Lewington S., Szeto S. (2000)  Tacrine for Alzheimer's disease (Cochrane Review). In *The Cochrane Library*, Update Software, Oxford.
3. Jefferson T., Demicheli V., Mugford M. (1996)  *Elementary Economic Evaluation in Health Care*, BMJ Publishing Group, London.
4. Drummond M.F., O'Brien B., Stoddart G.L., Torrance G.W. (1997)  *Methods for the Economic Evaluation of Health Care Programmes*, 2nd edn, Oxford University Press, Oxford.
5. Selai C.E., Trimble M.R. (1999)  Assessing quality of life in dementia. *Aging Ment. Health*, **3**: 101–111.
6. Albert S., Logsdon R. (1999)  Assessing quality of life in Alzheimer's disease. *J. Ment. Health Aging*, **5**: 3–6.
7. Kerner D.N., Paterson T.L., Grant I., Kaplan R.M. (1998)  Validity of the Quality of Wellbeing Scale for patients with Alzheimer's disease. *J. Aging Health*, **10**: 44–61.

8. Sano M., Albert S.M., Tractenberg R., Schittini M. (1999) Developing utilities: quantifying quality of life for stages of Alzheimer's disease as measured by the Clinical Dementia Rating. *J. Ment. Health Aging*, **5**: 59–68.
9. Patrick D.L., Starks H.E., Cain K.C., Uhlmann R.F., Pearlman R.A. (1994) Measuring preferences for health states worse than death. *Medical Decision Making*, **14**: 9–18.
10. Harris J. (1998) More and better justice. In *Philosophy and Medical Welfare* (Eds J.M. Bell, S. Mendus), pp. 75–96, Cambridge University Press, Cambridge.
11. Smith A. (1987) Qualms about QALYs. *Lancet*, **1**: 1134–1136.

# 6.3
## Toward the Economics of Dementia
### Agnes E. Rupp[1]

The German psychiatrist Alois Alzheimer first described Alzheimer's disease (AD) in 1906. At that time, the disease was rare, because most people died young enough to avoid it. But life expectancy has risen dramatically since the beginning of the century (approximately 30 years in the USA), and the economic burden of AD and other dementias have grown accordingly.

The new concepts of the economic burden of disease and the methods of assessing resource consumption and econometric analyses moved the field of health economics from the 1960s to be able to assist policy makers in setting priorities in life science research and health care service development [1].

Jönsson *et al* are involved in developing the economics of dementia for health care policy and practice decision purposes. This is reflected in their international literature review and the discussion of conceptual and methodological issues of cost of illness COI studies.

The authors have chosen to review the most common, *human capital* theory based COI studies. The human capital approach has been developed by Becker [2] and others [3–5] and it is rooted in labour economics. Its basic assumption is that an individual's value to society is his or her production potential. Mortality and morbidity associated with a specific disease reduces the production potential of an individual by causing premature death and reducing time spent in productive work. The COI studies based on the human capital approach distinguish "direct" and "indirect" costs as two key components of costs. A disease creates a loss to individuals and to society and this productivity loss is captured as indirect costs by the human capital approach. The authors note that, since

[1] *Mental Health Economics Research Program, National Institute of Mental Health, Room 7139, MSC-9631, 6001 Executive Blvd., Bethesda, MD 20878, USA*

dementia effects primarily the aging population that is no longer in the labour force, the role of indirect costs is less relevant. Whereas the indirect costs are those for which resources are lost, the direct costs are the resources used for treatment.

As expected, the literature review indicates great differences between the indirect cost estimates, depending on the data source, the scope of the study as well as the variation in the service system for patients suffering from dementia in different countries. In addition to calculating the cost/user measure from the estimates, it will be useful in future studies to publish the direct (treatment) cost/national health care expenditures as a relative burden measure in the different countries.

In a literature review one could also ask for economic burden studies based on alternative approaches. The *willingness to pay approach* proposed by two researchers [6,7] attempts to determine the objective value that individuals would place on being free of the disease. In the neuropsy-chiatric disease category, no studies have been conducted based on this approach. However, as the authors implicitly indicate in the theoretical discussion of the value of informal care, there might be a place for this approach to ask relatives of patients with dementia how much they are willing to pay for research to improve the QALYs (Quality Adjusted Life Years, as applied in the reviewed cost–effectiveness analyses) of their loved ones.

The QALYs measure positive utility in the health economics literature, while DALYs (Disability Adjusted Life Years) are based on the *utility loss approach,* and have developed into a new economic burden measure [8]. According to the weighting system of the DALYs, the relative value of a year of life at different ages varies; increasing from birth until approx-imately the mid-30s and then decreasing in later years. The comparative index of DALYs estimates the number of disability-adjusted life years that are lost as a result of premature death, measured by years of life lost (YLL), and years lived with disability (YLD). An especially important appli-cation of the DALYs is the neuropsychiatric illness area: the mortality rate is relatively low but the incorporation of the long-term disabling nature of the disease provides a more realistic burden measure [9].

The rank order of the burden of neuropsychiatric illnesses expressed in DALYs between ages 0 and 60 + in 1990 in the world [8] is the following: (1) unipolar depression; (2) alcohol use; (3) bipolar disorder; (4) schizophrenia; (5) obsessive-compulsive disorder (OCD); (6) dementia; (7) drug use; (8) epilepsy; (9) panic disorder; (10) post-traumatic stress disorder (PTSD), (11) multiple sclerosis; (12) Parkinson's disease. The economic burden of demen-tia is probably underestimated, just as in the case of the human capital approach, given that in the DALY concept the relative value of life decreases after the mid-30s.

It still seems to be a worthwhile effort from researchers in different countries (e.g. [10]) to calculate the DALYs for their own country, taking into consideration some of the unique sociocultural aspects of life in the country, as pointed out by Jönsson *et al* while analyzing how sociocultural differences may affect the treatment modalities and their cost–effectiveness for people suffering from dementia.

Dealing with a complex, progressing, incurable illness which affects an increasing number of the population in the developed countries is a challenging task for basic, clinical and economic researchers. There are variations in the data, controversial empirical findings, uncertainties in outcome measures and many other methodological issues. However, the ongoing intensive basic and clinical research activities in several countries may bring exciting new developments in cost-effective medical technology which can reduce the increasing economic costs of dementia on society.

## REFERENCES

1. Rupp A., Keith S.J. (1993) The costs of schizophrenia: assessing the burden. *Psychiatr. Clin. North Am.*, **16**: 413–423.
2. Becker G. (1964) *Human Capital*, National Bureau of Economic Research, New York.
3. Mushkin S.J. (1962) Health as an investment. *J. Political Economy*, **70**: 129–157.
4. Rice D.P. (1966) *Estimating the Cost of Illness*, Health Economics Series, No. 6, US Department of Health, Education and Welfare, Rockville.
5. Hodgson T.A., Miers M. (1982) Cost-of-illness methodology: a guide to current practices and procedures. *Milbank Memorial Fund Quarterly*, **60**: 429–462.
6. Schelling T.C. (1968) The life you save may be your own. In *Problems in Public Expenditures Analysis* (Ed. S.B. Chase), pp. 127–176, The Brookings Institution, Washington, DC.
7. Mishan E.J. (1971) Evaluation of life and limb: a theoretical approach. *J. Political Economy*, **79**: 687–705.
8. Murray C.J.L., Lopez A. (1996) *The Global Burden of Disease*, World Health Organization, Geneva.
9. Rupp A., Sorel E. (in press) Economic models. In *The Mental Health Consequences of Torture and Related Violence and Trauma* (Eds E. Gerrity, T. Keana, F. Tuma), Kluwer/Plenum, New York.
10. Kissimove-Skarbek K., Kowal A. (1999) Creation of the burden of schizophrenia study in Poland. Presented at the WPA Regional Meeting on Mental Health Economics and Psychiatric Practice in Central and Eastern Europe, Warsaw, August 3–5.

6.4
## A Cautionary Commentary on Costs of Dementia Studies
Justine Schneider[1]

Jönsson *et al* review a large volume of research. Here, I set out to clarify some of the issues which may complicate the interpretation of the review. I see these issues as *cost-related*, concerned with *research design* and with the *context* of the studies.

*Cost-related issues.* A first issue is defining types of care. There is a notional hierarchy of health care, ranging from the most technologically sophisticated to the least. The hierarchy also reflects the ranking of average costs. Thus, for example, in the UK, acute hospital care is followed by long-stay hospital care, nursing homes with skilled staff, residential homes where staff are not professionally qualified, and group living arrangements, where there are untrained staff but the accommodation is superior to average domestic housing. Within these settings, individuals may receive more or less inputs from formal or informal (paid or unpaid) carers. Formal care might include the services of a doctor, nurse, lawyer, accountant, cleaner, cook or paid companion. Informal care might include all these services if they are delivered by family or friends for no pay. Sleeping in hospital does not obviate the need for all of these services, but they are provided mainly by hospital personnel, and covered by the unit cost of hospital care. If people living in domestic settings have to purchase each of these services separately, this has a significant impact on the costs of care. In nursing homes, residential homes or group living situations, there is a danger that some of these expenses are overlooked, because they do not figure in the central accounts but come out of the residents' pockets. A careful and critical approach to making costs comparisons will need to take account of such questions.

A second issue is defining types of costs. Jönsson *et al* rightly note that different approaches to costing probably explain much of the range of results which they report. What are the cost components which make up most of the costs of caring for people with dementia? Leaving aside for the moment the cost of new pharmaceuticals, to which I will return later, we know that there is a "reduced list" of costs which can usually account for over 90% of total costs [1]. This list includes accommodation, hospital inpatient and outpatient treatment and day care. In several studies of people with severe mental health problems living in the community, these services accounted for up to 96% of total costs. In comparing studies of the costs of dementia, it may be helpful to identify these cost elements and ensure that

[1] *University of Durham, 15 Old Elvet, Durham, DH6 1EN, UK*

they are all included. If the study indicates that the costs are not comprehensive, the exclusion of any items on the "reduced list" cited above, or of informal care costs, is cause for questioning the comparability of different studies. Jönsson *et al*'s review does touch on the difficulties of costing informal care. This is a challenge, but not an impossible task. Dementia has vast repercussions for the family members, who often have to compensate for any shortfall in health and social services. Therefore, cost evaluations which omit informal care can only be regarded as partial.

*Research design questions.* In studies of dementia, samples are rarely drawn from a representative population. Most often, they are taken from clinical caseloads. This raises questions of differential access to that caseload, whether primary or secondary care. In addition, when we count the cost of dementia, we seldom include people at the onset of the illness, in terms of job loss, the disappearance of personal belongings, accidents, limitations in social activity and a drastically reduced quality of life. These high personal costs are not included in studies of people who reach secondary care. There is probably a broad-based "iceberg" of costs of early dementia that is never measured by conventional clinical studies.

Economic evaluations of interventions for dementia include cost–effectiveness analysis, which raises the question of meaningful outcomes in dementia. In a disease characterized by progressive deterioration, can staying the same be seen as a positive outcome? Is maintaining a person in his or her home a desirable outcome *at all costs*? What weight is to be given to the carer's health and mental well-being? These are some of the dilemmas presented by economic evaluations in this field. This brings me to the implications of new pharmaceutical interventions for dementia. Unless an ethical, acceptable, clinically significant outcome can be agreed upon, economic evaluations may have little relevance.

*Study context.* In conclusion, I have to express some reservations about the usefulness of making cost comparisons between countries with different cultures and health care systems. There are wide variations between "developed" countries; comparisons are even more difficult when "developing" countries are included. While it is often illuminating to compare countries, the differences that emerge are more likely to be related to national idiosyncrasies than to anything else. This is illustrated by a study of carer burden in dementia in 14 countries, where we found that 11% of the variation in carer burden (by far the largest component) was explained by the factor "country" [2]. Moreover, low costs may simply reflect a lack of services; where nothing is provided, no costs are incurred.

The impact of new technology in dementia care, both pharmaceutical and genetic, will be felt in rich nations first, and it will change dramatically the costs of dementia prevention and treatment. It is safe to predict that we have not seen the last cost study of dementia. Therefore, Jönsson *et al* have made an invaluable contribution in summarizing research to date, and I hope to have offered some sign posts for applying their research.

## REFERENCES

1. Knapp M.R.J., Beecham J.K. (1995)   Reduced-list costings. In *The Economic Evaluation of Mental Health Care* (Ed. M.R.J. Knapp), pp. 195–206, Arena/Ashgate, Aldershot.
2. Schneider J., Murray J., Banerjee S., Mann A. (1999)   Eurocare: a cross-national study of co-resident spouse carers for people with Alzheimer's disease. I— factors associated with carer burden. *Int. J. Geriatr. Psychiatry*, **14**: 651–661.

6.5
## Costs of Dementia: Valuable Information for Economic Evaluations

Christian Kronborg Andersen[1]

Jönsson *et al*'s review demonstrates that the health economic research in the area of dementia has been dominated by studies of the costs of dementia, the so-called cost of illness  (COI) studies. Such studies are useful to demonstrate how society is affected economically and who bears the economic burden of the disease. However, they cannot *per se* be used in priority setting, because the costs of dementia do not provide any information on the health benefits, e.g. quality of life, that are associated with the resource use that causes the costs [1–3]. Nonetheless, estimates of the direct costs can inform decision makers about how much money is spent for the treatment of a specific disease [4], e.g. dementia, and thus give an idea of how resources are currently being used [2]. Another limitation of COI analyses is the methodological issues in costing. Inclusion of some cost components and exclusion of others may significantly influence the result. However, carefully designed COI studies are useful for economic evaluations, because information on resource use can serve as input in modelling costs [5].

In order to collect information on resource use for economic evaluation purposes, the correlation between health care costs, i.e. medical costs,

[1] *Health Economics Research Unit, Institute of Public Health, University of Southern Denmark, Winsløwparken 19, DK-5000 Odense C, Denmark*

nursing home costs, costs of assistance in the home, and disease severity measured on the Clinical Dementia Rating (CDR) scale was analysed in a study of the costs of dementia in Denmark [6,7]. Classifying patients in four groups by their severity of dementia (very mild, mild, moderate and severe), the Danish study found that costs were higher for groups of more severely demented patients than for mildly demented patients. The annual health care costs in Denmark, estimated as the difference between a demented patient and a non-demented elderly person, was DKK 25 300 for a very mildly demented patient, DKK 57 500 for a mildly demented patient, DKK 57 500 for a moderately demented patient, and DKK 171 600 for a severely demented patient (US$1 = DKK 7) [7]. In addition, health care costs for patients who had a spouse were about half of the costs for a patient who was single or widowed.

One important limitation in most studies of the costs of dementia is the use of cross-sectional study designs [3]. In principle, such designs allow comparison across different groups at a point in time, but do not explore changes in the same patient groups over time. In order to get valid estimates of cost changes with disease progression, follow-up studies will be needed. However, the Danish study indicates that such designs are not straightforward, because diagnoses may change over time and, furthermore, many patients die or are lost to follow-up.

It is not possible to meet total needs in society, because resources are limited. Inevitably choices have to be made. Knowing how resources are currently being used, and, additionally, knowing the benefits they generate to patients, family and society, it is possible to analyse the consequences of shifting resources between various programmes, for example, shifting resources from institutional care to home care or to pharmaceutical treatment. In other words, will benefits in terms of patients' well-being increase, decrease or remain unchanged with a change in the way resources are used? Likewise, will benefits in terms of caregiver distress increase, decrease or remain unchanged? If total benefits, i.e. benefits under programme A plus benefits under programme B, increase when shifting resources from A to B, then it is suggested that resources should be shifted. Such an approach is also useful for analysing how to allocate extra resources that are made available in order to create most extra benefits, or the other way around, if expenditures are to be cut, where the cut should occur to minimize the loss of benefits [2].

Informal care is of central importance in caring for demented patients, but valuation and quantification of such care is rather troublesome. Jönsson *et al* mention three ways of including the costs of informal care in economic evaluations. They recommend including them all in the sensitivity analysis as a first step of handling this methodological problem, but further research is needed in developing methods to value informal care. As drugs that delay dementia progression become available, relatives of demented patients will be capable of providing care for a longer time than hitherto and will make it necessary to develop methods for evaluating informal care.

## REFERENCES

1. Shiell A., Gerard K., Donaldson C. (1987)   Cost of illness studies: an aid to decision making? *Health Policy*, **8**: 317–323.
2. Mooney G. (1996)   *Key Issues in Health Economics*, Harvester Wheatsheaf, Hempstead.
3. Koopmanschap M.A. (1998)   Cost-of-illness studies. Useful for health policy? *PharmacoEconomics*, **14**: 143–148.
4. Behrens C., Henke K.D. (1988)   Cost of illness studies: no aid to decision making? Reply to Shiell *et al*. *Health Policy*, **10**: 137–141.
5. Hodgson T.A. (1994)   Cost of illness in cost-effectiveness analysis. *Pharmaco-Economics*, **6**: 536–552.
6. Andersen C.K., Søgaard J., Hansen E., Kragh-Sørensen A., Hastrup L., Andersen J., Andersen K., Lolk A., Nielsen H., Kragh-Sørensen P. (1999)   The cost of dementia in Denmark. The Odense Study. *Dement. Geriatr. Cogn. Disord.*, **10**: 295–304.
7. Andersen C.K., Andersen K., Kragh-Sørensen P.   Cost function estimation. The choice of a model to apply to dementia. Submitted for publication.

**6.6**
## Cost of Illness Study in Dementia: a Comment
J.-Matthias Graf von der Schulenburg[1]

It is not surprising that ageing populations are confronted with a growing number of people suffering from dementia. Whilst only 2.4–5.1% of Germans suffer from dementia in the age group 65–69 years, the prevalence of dementia rises to 10–12% for the group 75–79 years and 20–24% for 80–90 years. We estimate about 1.24–1.68 million dementia patients in Germany.

However, the costs of treatment of dementia compared to all other health care costs are still very low. There are a number of reasons for this, which are discussed in the very informative review by Jönsson *et al*. Only a small share of the costs are found in traditional hospitals. Most care is delivered by day care, home care or by nursing homes. Those costs do not show up in national statistics on health care costs, because they are

[1] *North German Centre for Health Services Research, University of Hannover, 30617 Hannover, Germany*

not covered by health insurers or by the national health service in most countries. A great share of these costs has to be paid out of pocket by the patient or his or her family. The other part is covered by social aid, general public expenditure or special nursing insurance programmes [1]. A further reason is that medicine still has little to offer to patients suffering from dementia.

In contrast to Jönsson *et al*'s observation, our research suggests that the medical treatment costs of dementia are not much correlated with the severity of the disease. However, the costs of care and the need for care increase sharply with the severity of dementia.

In a German study [2], treatment costs and nursing insurance data were collected for 158 patients with dementia of Alzheimer's type. The patients were recruited by 10 office-based physicians, all working in collaboration with three university psychiatric departments. The severity of dementia was classified according to the Mini-Mental State Examination (MMSE). The results are given in Table 6.6.1.

**TABLE 6.6.1**  Annual costs of dementia (in DM) per patient in Germany according to severity

| MMSE score | 30–26 (very mild) | 25–21 (mild) | 20–16 (moderate) | 15–11 (severe) | 10–0 (very severe) |
|---|---|---|---|---|---|
| Total treatment costs | 1337 | 1974 | 3198 | 3405 | 1568 |
| *Outpatient physician* | 623 | 634 | 709 | 637 | 911 |
| *Hospital* | 0 | 574 | 1686 | 2197 | 120 |
| *Medication* | 620 | 526 | 517 | 434 | 460 |
| *Diagnostic* | 94 | 240 | 286 | 137 | 77 |
| Nursing costs (institutional care) | 381 | 2592 | 9383 | 18662 | 23571 |

MMSE, Mini-Mental State Examination

The total costs of treatment per year which are covered by the German social health insurers do not increase monotonically with severity. In moderate and severe cases, hospital costs are higher than in other cases. However, medication costs do decrease with severity. On the other hand, nursing costs covered by the German social nursing insurance are highly correlated with severity.

To sum up, medical costs of treating dementia are low, and in most cases lower than the sickness fund contributions or health insurance premiums paid by the patients. We should focus, therefore, more on the nursing costs and how society can help and does help patients and their families to manage the heavy burden of long-term care.

## REFERENCES

1. Campell J.C., Ikegami N. (Eds) (1999)  *Long-term Care for Frail Older People*, Springer, Tokyo.
2. Schulenburg J., Schulenburg I., Horn R. (1998)   Cost of treatment and cost of care for Alzheimer's disease in Germany. In *The Health Economics of Dementia* (Eds A. Wimo, G. Karlsson, B. Jönsson, B. Winblad), pp. 217–230, Wiley, Chichester.

6.7
## Dementia: Whose Burden is it Anyway?

Sudhir K. Khandelwal[1]

Ageing is a worldwide phenomenon and people all over the world are surviving longer, with the result that all regions of the world are having a larger population of elderly people than ever before. Increased life span has meant increased morbidity too in the elderly age group, and a major question before us is now how to bring down morbidity, cut down costs of care, and add meaningful life to the years gained. The paper by Jönsson *et al* reviews the evidence on the costs of dementia, the difficulties in computing costs of care, and how to reduce costs while caring for patients of dementia. This Swedish group is credited with commendable work in cost analysis of dementia care programmes.

Although the life expectancy at birth in the developed countries is much higher than that in the developing world, the rate of growth in the elderly population in the developing countries has exceeded that of the rich nations in the last few decades. Although more and more elderly people will live in the so-called developing countries, practically all the studies focusing on costs of dementia have come from the developed countries such as the USA, the UK, Sweden, Germany, Holland, Norway, etc. Cost analysis studies in the field of psychiatry are essential for a number of reasons. Many of the psychiatric disorders run a long and disabling course, and the consequences of the disability and the costs of care can put a severe financial burden on any society or nation. In a time of scarce resources and high economic costs for care of dementia, to search for improved methods of treatment and efficient use of resources has become increasingly important. Besides helping us to select type of care, such studies help us to determine our priorities for research funding. They also help us to examine the burden caused by a disorder on the health and social services.

[1] *Department of Psychiatry, All India Institute of Medical Sciences, New Delhi 110029, India*

Dementia is one of the most expensive disorders per sufferer, and remains a highly significant independent predictor of cost, which is associated with high use of nursing care and social services [1]. However, calculating the cost of care of a disorder like dementia is not an easy task, considering the fact that in dementia multiple aetiologies are involved and health care practices are not uniform, with the result that, as the review points out, a dementia patient can receive institutional care, home care or informal care (provided by family members and friends), depending on the resources and facilities available both to a given patient and the society. The decision to select a type of care rests on many facts other than the medical factors alone. The costs have differed not only from country to country but within the same country in different estimates. Evidence is mounting that dementia is a costly disease, but comparison of costs is difficult to make, due to the varieties of care available and the stages of illness which heavily influence the choice and cost of treatment.

A major limiting factor has been the total absence of such studies from developing countries. Treatment alternatives differ between developed and developing countries. For example, in India family still remains the main nucleus for care of the dementia sufferer. Although now under pressure due to increasing industrialization and urbanization, the joint family system still strives to provide support to its elderly members. Most dementia patients continue to stay with their families, where family members look after all their needs. Institutional care in any form is not prevalent. The spouse and the children of the dementia victim will look after him or her, considering it as part of their duty, and will not like to calculate their time and efforts so spent in terms of costs, notwithstanding the fact that dementia may have a heavy impact on caregivers in terms of psychosocial burden, quality of life and leisure time activities [2]. The same is true for other societies where informal care is provided by the family members without cost to the government or insurance companies [3]. Jönsson et al have analysed in detail the controversies related to the costing of informal care and how to measure it. They have argued that informal care as provided by the family members should be interpreted as a direct cost, since the time and energy spent by a family member could have been utilized in work on the labour market. It may be a good strategy to calculate the total burden of cost of a given disorder, or to compare different management plans of the disorder, but its cross-cultural appeal is doubtful.

Health economics or pharmacoeconomics are new research areas in psychiatry. In a time of increasing population of older people, new diseases and new therapies, it has become increasingly important to evaluate new treatments and to compare differences in treatment effects between new and older methods. A drug that preserves function or delays loss of function may help postpone the need for professional caring services or nursing home placement and thereby hold down the cost of caring in the dementia population. Lately, a few drugs (tacrine, donepezil) have been introduced for the treatment of mild or moderate Alzheimer's disease, and these also have undergone economic evaluation for considering their cost–effectiveness. Cost–effectiveness is a comparative analysis where the costs are measured in money but the effects of a treatment are measured by improvement in symptomatology, or an improved quality of life. Similar to cost–effectiveness analysis is cost–utility analysis, where the costs are measured in money and the utility in QALYs (Quality Adjusted Life Years) or DALYs (Disability Adjusted Life Years). A major initiative in the management of dementia has been the study of the effects of these drugs on various outcome measures of the illness, namely cognition (as measured by the Mini-Mental State Examination, MMSE), nursing home placement, quality of life, and mortality. Initial results have shown some promise with these drugs in cost saving, but long-term studies on larger samples will be required to study the full impact of these drugs on various parameters of cost and effect measurements in caregiving of dementia. The MMSE, although influenced by educational and cultural factors, has been shown over the years to be a highly sensitive instrument for assessing the severity of cognitive impairment and consequently the staging of a dementing illness. Only long-term studies will show if any changes in MMSE scores during the course of treatment are likely to have any cost implication for the illness. Such studies will help in allocating resources to those interventions that generate reduction in DALY loss.

Dementia is a serious illness and a major source of disability and death in elderly people. To date there is no cure and little can be done to stop its progression. Lately there have been systematic attempts to calculate the costs involved in different kinds of care available for dementia. Such studies are necessary for a variety of reasons, as already discussed. However, at this time there are a number of methodological issues that limit the application of findings of this research. Since so far we neither know the cause of most cases of dementia nor have curative treatments for them, the management largely depends on: (a) the resources available in a given society; (b) the expectations of a society from its health care system; and (c) the socio-cultural milieu of the individuals. Also, management of dementia involves more caring than curing, which may have important bearing in those societies where insurance and managed care determine health care strategies. Hence, the information gathered from this kind of work needs to be interpreted and applied very carefully. Market mechanisms may be ill-suited for the needs of the chronically medically ill. Costs should be viewed not as a basis of cutting down on services but to emphasize research that can prevent the disease, improve the quality of life and decrease the burden subsequently [1]. Development of preventive measures will certainly lower the costs of health care for the aged.

## REFERENCES

1.  Livingston G., Manela M., Katona C. (1997)  Cost of community care for older people. *Br. J. Psychiatry*, **171**: 56–59.
2.  Khandelwal S.K., Gupta S. (1996)  Caring for dementia sufferers: impact on caregivers. *J. Ment. Health Hum. Behav.*, **1**: 41–48.
3.  Topinkova E. Callahan D. (1999)  Culture, economics, and Alzheimer's disease: social determinants of resource allocation. *J. Appl. Gerontol.*, **18**: 411–422.

# Acknowledgements for the First Edition

The Editors would like to thank Drs Paola Bucci, Umberto Volpe, Andrea Dell'Acqua, Andrea Fiorillo, Francesco Perris, Massimo Lanzaro, Vincenzo Scarallo, Giuseppe Piegari, Mariangela Masella, Pasquale Saviano and Enrico Tresca, of the Department of Psychiatry of the University of Naples, for their help in the processing of manuscripts.

The publication has been supported by an unrestricted educational grant from the Lundbeck Institute, which is hereby gratefully acknowledged.

# Index

Note: Page numbers in **bold** refer to Tables; those in *italics* refer to Figures

*Index compiled by Annette Musker*

# Second Edition

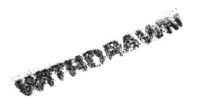

*WPA Series*
Evidence and Experience in Psychiatry

# Other Titles in the *WPA Series* Evidence and Experience in Psychiatry

Volume 1—Depressive Disorders, Second Edition
*Mario Maj and Norman Sartorius*

Volume 2—Schizophrenia, Second Edition
*Mario Maj and Norman Sartorius*

Volume 4—Obsessive-Compulsive Disorder, Second Edition
*Mario Maj, Norman Sartorius, Ahmed Okasha and Joseph Zohar*

Volume 5—Bipolar Disorder
*Mario Maj, Hagop S. Akiskal, Juan José López-Ibor and Norman Sartorius*